Dr. Naomi Breslau
Dept. of Epidemiology &
   Community Health
Case Western Reserve University
School of Medicine
2119 Abington Road
Cleveland, Ohio 44106

Motherhood and Mental Illness

Motherhood and Mental Illness

I.F. Brockington

Department of Psychiatry
University Hospital of South Manchester, England

R. Kumar

Institute of Psychiatry,
University of London, England

1982

ACADEMIC PRESS London Paris San Diego São Paulo
Sydney Tokyo Toronto

GRUNE AND STRATTON New York San Francisco

ACADEMIC PRESS INC. (LONDON) LTD.
24/28 Oval Road
London NW1

United States Edition published by
GRUNE & STRATTON INC.
111 Fifth Avenue
New York, New York 10003

British Library Cataloguing in Publication Data

Motherhood and mental illness.

I. Women—Mental health 2. Childbirth
I. Brockington, I F. II. Kumar, R.
616.89 RC451.4.W6

ISBN (Academic Press) 0-12-790666-5
ISBN (Grune & Stratton) 0-8089-1481-2

LCCN 82-82595

Printed in Great Britain by
St Edmundsbury Press, Bury St Edmunds, Suffolk

Contributors

I.F. Brockington MD FRCP *Senior Lecturer, Department of Psychiatry, University Hospital of South Manchester, West Didsbury, Manchester M20 8LR, England.*

Christine Dean BA MRC Psych *Research Worker, University Department of Psychiatry, Royal Edinburgh Hospital, Edinburgh, and Consultant Psychiatrist, Manchester Royal Infirmary, Oxford Road, Manchester, England.*

J.A. Hamilton MD *490 Post Street, San Francisco, California 94102, USA, formerly Clinical Professor of Psychiatry, Stanford University School of Medicine, Stanford, California, USA.*

R. Kumar MD PhD MRC Psych *Senior Lecturer, Department of Psychiatry, Institute of Psychiatry, De Crespigny Park, London SE5 8AF, England.*

F. Margison MSc MRC Psych *Consultant Psychiatrist, University Hospital of South Manchester, West Didsbury, Manchester M20 8LR England.*

R. Paffenbarger Jr. MD *Professor of Epidemiology, Department of Family, Community and Preventive Medicine, Stanford University School of Medicine, Stanford University Medical Center, California 94305, USA.*

Elisabeth Powell BSc *Graduate Student, Department of Psychology, University College Hospital, Gower Street, London WC1E 6BT, England.*

Kay Robson PhD *Research Psychologist, Institute of Psychiatry, De Crespigny Park, London SE5 8AF, England.*

G. Stein M Phil MRC Psych *Consultant Psychiatrist, Farnborough Hospital, Farnborough, Kent, England.*

G. Winokur MD *Paul W. Penningroth Professor and Head, Department of Psychiatry, University of Iowa, 500 Newton Road, Iowa City, Iowa 52242, USA.*

Preface

Puerperal mental disorders have been recognized for centuries but research into their nature and origins, prevention, management and consequences has not kept pace with advances in other areas of psychiatry. Severe puerperal psychoses are relatively rare, but they continue to occur at a rate of one or two per thousand deliveries. Less severe disturbances, consistent with the diagnosis of depressive neurosis, occur in 10–20% of women and "postnatal depression" has been much talked about in the past decade. Yet, in spite of increasing awareness of the risk of neurotic disturbance in childbearing women, the majority of sufferers neither seek, nor are given, any help at a critical time for themselves and their families. The ways in which childbearing may be linked with psychiatric disorder remain uncertain and controversial. The antenatal period would seem to provide an ideal opportunity for prevention, but how and in whom?

In the past few years there has been a growing body of research into the psychopathology of reproduction, but there has been little communication between workers. With the aim of drawing together the different strands of research, the University of Manchester Department of Psychiatry (with generous financial support from, in particular, Boots Pure Drug Company) held an international conference in June 1980. The meeting was attended by many of the active researchers in the field and resulted in the foundation of a society, named after L.V. Marcé, the French psychiatrist and student of Esquirol, who wrote the first treatise entirely devoted to puerperal mental illness. The conference demonstrated the vitality as well as the disorganization of this field of medicine and a publication of its proceedings might have been valuable. It seemed to us, however, that there was a need for a more general statement of art and knowledge in this area. About 20 years have elapsed since the publication of Hamilton's *Postpartum Psychiatric Problems*, which attracted many into this field of work and a new text might serve as a platform for more coherent research. For this reason we selected nine important areas discussed at the conference and invited one or more participants to review the field.

The first chapter by Hamilton urges the recognition of postpartum psychosis as a nosological entity and describes the foundation of the Marcé Society. Paffenbarger's chapter presents his own classic epidemiological investigation of puerperal psychosis, with some further analyses. Brockington, Winokur and Dean review clinical studies of puerperal psychosis, distinguishing between the florid psychoses of early onset and another condition specifically related to childbirth — depression accompanied by failure to develop and sustain maternal attachment. Robson and Powell focus upon the normal process of attachment between mothers and their babies — a field of research which has suddenly begun to grow extremely fast and Margison surveys the pathology of mother–infant bonding. A review of psychiatric mother and baby units by Margison and Brockington describes the history of this form of service and contains hitherto unpublished information about one such unit in Manchester. Kumar reviews the background and research into the neurotic disturbances occurring in pregnancy and the puerperium. Stein considers the syndrome of the postpartum blues and its possible relevance to more severe mental breakdowns. Finally, Brockington and Kumar examine the vexed question of drug use and abuse by pregnant and lactating mothers and the problems of prescribing psychotropic medication to childbearing women.

It is our hope that this volume will serve as a summary of present knowledge and as a stimulus to those interested in the psychiatric hazards of motherhood. Because of the pervasive effects of maternal mental illness on the family and on the psychological development of young children, this is a matter which deserves our best efforts.

April 1982

I.F. Brockington
R. Kumar

Contents

1

The Identity of Postpartum Psychosis

J.A. Hamilton

Status of Postpartum Psychosis

This chapter supports the position that postpartum psychosis is a disease entity. Patients with postpartum psychosis share organic etiological mechanisms and psychological stresses and responses. For these patients, therapeutic opportunities exist which will not be well utilized unless and until this disease is appreciated as an entity.

During and before the nineteenth century, psychiatric illness which began in the puerperium was regarded as a disease. Thousands of cases were studied and hundreds were described in a very extensive literature. Quite a number of distinguishing characteristics, symptoms and features which set postpartum psychosis apart from other illnesses, were discovered. Then, early in the twentieth century, as psychiatrists adopted the classification system of Kraepelin, it was found that "postpartum psychosis" did not fit into the categories which were being established. The simple solution was to expunge "postpartum psychosis" from the favored list. The distinguishing characteristics of postpartum psychosis were first minimized, then forgotten. This has done a disservice to patients and to the advance of knowledge.

This chapter reviews distinguishing characteristics of postpartum psychosis which were discovered many years ago, adds a few more, and suggests that these distinguishing characteristics may afford valuable clues to the understanding and treatment of psychiatric illness which follows childbearing.

Before the distinguishing characteristics of postpartum psychosis are presented, it may be useful to review briefly the steps which led to the exclusion of "postpartum psychosis" as a disease entity.

From the mid-eighteenth century the tools of morbid anatomy, cellular pathology and bacteriology led to giant steps toward the understanding of a great

1

many varieties of human illness. Diseases were defined and classified in terms of etiological agents and tissue pathology. Medicine moved rapidly toward becoming a science as well as an art. It seemed reasonable for psychiatrists to try to move in the same direction. Emil Kraepelin was among those who believed that psychiatric diseases would also eventually be defined precisely in terms of etiological mechanisms and tissue pathology. Adolph Meyer, a brilliant Swiss transplanted to Baltimore, tried to follow Kraepelin but found it impossible to do so. Gradually, Meyer moved toward the practical expedient of defining many psychiatric illnesses in terms of constellations of symptoms, groups of symptoms which often occurred together. The broad categories of schizophrenia and the affective psychoses were thought to be constellations of this kind, although modern investigators find it increasingly difficult to establish "natural boundaries" between them (Kendell and Gourlay, 1970).

Psychiatric illness after childbirth did not, and does not, fit nicely into one or another of the broad categories which were defined in terms of constellations of symptoms. Illness in the puerperium presents itself as depression, mania, delirium, or with delusions and aberrant thinking resembling schizophrenia. With even more intransigence, some patients may move from one constellation to another, or display symptoms from more than one constellation at the same time. Depressed or "schizophrenic" patients may display "organic" symptoms, such as confusion or delirium.

In short, a great variety of symptoms are displayed by patients who become ill after childbearing. The fact that a group of patients who appeared to have a uniform etiology straddled the boundary between major clinical categories posed a threat to the new classification system. For most twentieth-century psychiatrists, Kraepelinian classification seemed a more valid approach than the practice of classifying by etiological association, so they disregarded the distinguishing characteristics of puerperal psychosis and forced all puerperal psychosis patients into symptom-oriented categories. Among the most vigorous proponents of this proposal were Adolph Meyer's followers, E.A. Strecker and F.G. Ebaugh (1926), whose textbook of psychiatry, *Practical Clinical Psychiatry*, had a dominant influence on psychiatric education in the United States for a quarter of a century. These authors had published a paper on illness following childbirth, based on examination of 50 charts from three hospitals. Patients were divided neatly into three separate categories, dementia praecox, manic-depressive insanity and toxic-exhaustive reaction. The patients in the manic-depressive and dementia praecox categories had an unexpectedly high incidence of "organic symptoms;" i.e., delirium and confusion, but this anomaly was not addressed by the authors. They suggested that their study supported the position that the term "postpartum psychosis" should be abolished; whereas, good evidence within their own paper supported a contrary position.

By the time the American Psychiatric Association published its first Diagnostic and Statistical Manual, in 1952, the leaders of psychiatry could echo

Macbeth: "I have done the deed". Twenty-eight years later, in 1980, the index of DSM III attests to the fact that the official position is virtually unchanged: "Postpartum psychosis. See Schizophrenic disorder, Brief reactive psychosis, Major affective disorders, Organic brain syndrome". Textbooks of psychiatry and of obstetrics over the past half-century, if they mention puerperal illness at all, state that childbearing occasionally acts as a trigger to bring out latent tendencies for one kind of mental illness or another.

In this chapter, I will suggest that the act of dismembering "postpartum psychosis" was misguided. It was incompatible with many facts which were known in the nineteenth century and it is equally incompatible with facts which have emerged in the twentieth century. Psychiatric illness after childbearing has many common features and many characteristics which distinguish it from other varieties of mental illness. The distinguishing characteristics of postpartum illness could be clues to increased understanding and improved treatment of psychiatric illness after childbearing. These distinguishing characteristics will now be outlined.

Clinical Features of Postpartum Psychosis

A Symptom-free Phase

When large numbers of cases are studied and the first symptoms are tabulated by date of onset, these symptoms sometimes begin on the fourth day postpartum, sometimes on the tenth day postpartum, sometimes on the thirtieth day postpartum, or even later. There are virtually no cases in which symptoms appear on the day of delivery or on postpartum days one or two. This was first stated clearly by Fürstner in 1875, though many centuries before, Hippocrates noted that psychiatric symptoms often began when lactation began, rather than with delivery itself (Adams, 1886). Many observers have noted a relationship between the onset of symptoms and lactation, the time when lactation was expected, or the onset of problems related to lactation, the latter as recounted by Bernhard Pauleikhoff (1964). In 1937, Karnosh and Hope reviewed studies of the symptom-free phase and speculated that hormonal events paralleling or overlapping those which induce lactation must take place before psychiatric symptoms occur.

Confusion, Delirium, Hallucinations, Insomnia

Nineteenth-century medical literature was remarkable for its detailed descriptions of the signs and symptoms of various diseases. This literature contains literally hundreds of word-pictures of mental illness after childbearing, most of which stress the high incidence of postpartum cases which present one or more of the four symptoms mentioned above. Three languages were strained to find words to describe what was observed: Marcé (1858) coined *délire triste*, Fürstner spoke of *Verwirrtheit*, translated as "distressed perplexity", and Jones (1902) spoke of miserable sleeplessness.

Confusion, delirium and hallucinations are now generally recognized as symptoms which suggest that brain function is adversely affected by toxic infectous, traumatic or hormonal influences. Fürstner distinguished the delirium of postpartum psychosis from that of childbed fever, noting that the former was afebrile. "Miserable sleeplessness" remained an enigma during the nineteenth century; now it is recognized that insomnia may be a symptom due to toxic influences or hormonal changes.

Among those who prefer to minimize or disparage the unique qualities of postpartum psychosis, a favorite argument is the following: the vivid descriptions of postpartum delirium were written, for the most part, in the nineteenth century. In those days, it is likely that many cases of childbed fever were missed. The described delirium was probably a symptom of infection.

The foregoing hypothesis is belied by the 235 cases of postpartum illness described by Pauleikhoff, spanning the years 1930-60. This investigator, and the physicians with whom he worked, was thoroughly familiar with modern diagnostic techniques for infection. The mental states which he described, with hyperactivity, "busyness," evanescence of hallucinations, and apparent good physical condition, are quite different from the picture of an individual suffering from infection.

Organic/Psychological Correspondences

One of the most astute observers of psychiatric illness which follows childbearing was Louis V. Marcé. His book summarized knowledge at mid-century and presented his own meticulous observations of 44 cases. Marcé described many instances in which the development and progression of psychiatric symptoms paralleled recognizable physical changes. He noted the association between the onset of lactation and symptoms, and stated that a remarkably large proportion of his psychiatric cases had had difficulty in producing milk. He observed that prolonged psychiatric illness was associated with prolonged amenorrhoea, and that when these patients began to recover, their periods resumed. He noted that postpartum cases who had had manic symptoms and who had recovered were particularly vulnerable to premenstrual recurrences of symptoms.

When Marcé's book was published in 1858, hormones and their actions were unknown. Nevertheless, Marcé insisted that there must be a connection between the uterus and the brain. He said, *"Ce qui donne à la folie puerpérale son charactère spéciale, c'est la coexistence d'une modification organique et fonctionelle de l'utérus et de ses annexes."*

Marcé was convinced that the development and course of postpartum psychosis was determined by organic factors. Lacking the concept of hormones and lacking any anatomical explanation for the influence of the generative organs on the brain, he invented a hypothetical mechanism, "*sympathie morbide.*" It is unfortunate that early in the twentieth century this astute physician was misquoted as having said that there is no such thing as postpartum psychosis. This misquotation was repeated over and over, obviously without reference to Marcé's text. What Marcé had said was that postpartum psychosis has a number of symptoms which also occur in other diseases.

Laboratory and clinical study of hormones accelerated after the turn of the century. For example, the first description of the action of desiccated thyroid in postpartum illness was made by Stössner in 1910. In 1962 I suggested that thyroid medication might have a place in the treatment of depressive symptoms which develop or persist to six or more weeks after childbearing. A similar suggestion was made independently by A.A. Baker in 1967.

The Swiss investigator, V.S. Bürgi, directed attention in 1954 to the pituitary and associated structures by the title of his paper "*Puerperalpsychose oder Diencephalosis puerperalis?*" Bürgi noted that headache, tiredness, insomnia, excessive sleeplessness, dizziness, decrease in blood pressure, hair and skin changes, constipation, marked change in appetite which was reflected in weight (in the direction of marked loss or marked gain), and a decrease in sexual responsiveness were all found in chronic cases where onset had followed childbirth. He recalled that Marcé had noted that postpartum patients who remained ill for some time were inclined to exhibit one or more of the following symptoms: weakness, pallor, anemia, gastro-intestinal disorders, excessive sweating and menstrual disorders. Reviewing all of these symptoms, Bürgi argued that they created a strong suspicion of pituitary involvement.

An exploratory study of the adrenal chemistry of postpartum illness was made by Jacobides in 1957. He compared 17-hydroxysteroids in postpartum psychiatric patients with normal postpartum controls and found that the variability, the movement from high to low values, was greater in the psychiatric patients. When patients suffered exacerbations of symptoms, there was a tendency for the 17-hydroxysteroids to rise several days before the relapse, even while the patients appeared well.

The foregoing citations represent a sample of observations which collectively suggest that postpartum psychiatric illness could involve one or more of the following endocrine systems: the pituitary, the thyroid and the adrenals. There is additional evidence which implicates gonadotrophic hormones. Very little has been done to translate information regarding endocrine parameters into applications for prevention and treatment. The majority of psychiatrists, and certainly the vast majority of American psychiatrists, have been content to treat patients with regimes and medications which are used for non-puerperal psychiatric cases.

Changeability and Progression

Many nineteenth-century writers reported that patients with illness in the puer-perium often exhibited a remarkable degree of changeability and unpredictability. Delirium appeared and disappeared, often clearing after sleep. On occasion, the hallucinations of delirium stabilized into states which resembled paranoid schizophrenia. Clouding of the sensorium or deep depression could move to a state of apparent lucidity. The temporary clearing of depression could lead to a mistaken impression of recovery. This error could lead to premature release from a controlled hospital environment and the opportunity for a suicide attempt.

In 1875, Savage commented on the changeability of postpartum patients as follows:

> We cannot classify them with any degree of precision into mania, melancholia, and dementia. We shall note typical cases of each of these varieties, but I must premise by saying that it is common for one to pass through all of these forms.

When I had a large hospital practice with postpartum patients, I was particularly aware of the possibility that significant changes could occur during the 18 hours when I was not in the hospital. To compensate for this, the psychiatric staff were trained to look for changes and to summon me at once. Some patients remained quite stable, or improved steadily from depression to normal mood and activity. Others exhibited very marked changes, often very rapidly. We were inclined to treat episodes of marked agitation or mania with large doses of parenteral barbiturates. When patients awoke, a few hours later, they were often quite calm and the incident was forgotten. As the shift of symptoms, or the exacerbation and remission of symptoms was observed, it seemed that these changes sometimes occurred spontaneously, not necessarily in response to medication or external events.

It is quite possible that the current extensive use of long-acting drugs such as the phenothiazines may tend to obliterate or obscure the changeability which was observed in the nineteenth century and which we observed. While we had phenothiazines, we used them in small to moderate doses, fearful of an additive effect to what we regarded as an inherent propensity of these patients toward confusion.

Distinguishing Psychological Characteristic

Among the characteristics which distinguish postpartum psychiatric illness is the impact of this illness on the patient's thinking, mood and possibly even on her physiology. The quality and the enormity of this impact was captured effectively by R. Gundry in 1859:

> Surely no affliction appeals more strongly to our sympathy than this fearful disease, which, when a household rejoices at the happy issue of its matron from the "hour of Nature's need", turns its joy into mourning by the approach of a far greater evil than just vanished—where the fulfillment of the maternal function, woman's crowning joy and glory, forms the alembic in which is distilled a most bitter cup of sorrow.

Written in the prosaic language of the twentieth century, here is what appears to take place: during pregnancy, women accept increasing discomfort and limitations, and at parturition, they experience fear and pain. When it is over, relief and a sense of accomplishment and happiness ensue. The mother and the newborn child together form a center for admiration. When great discomfort and severe symptoms develop out of this situation, physical illness is the first thought. The thermometer and the careful physical examination are followed by "reassurance" that there is no physical illness. Instead of comforting the patient, this report turns her mind to other explanatory hypotheses for her symptoms. If there is no physical illness, as she has been "reassured," she fears the symptoms may represent "incompetence," failure as a mother, or "mental illness." These interpretations provide fertile soil for the growth of the great variety of psychological aberrations which are so characteristic of postpartum psychiatric illness.

Most varieties of psychiatric illness develop slowly, over periods of weeks, months or years. To some extent, the patient becomes acclimatized to symptoms and to aberrant thinking patterns. Postpartum illness, and certainly those cases which develop within the first fortnight after delivery, is characterized by sudden onset, developing in periods measured in hours or days. Almost always it is unanticipated, but its impact on mood and thinking is great.

The role of the patient's denigrating interpretation of her illness is often seen during the first 24 hours after psychiatric intervention. If hospitalization in a psychiatric facility is warranted, and if the patient is told that she has a very serious illness which requires hospitalization, the response is often favorable. Additionally, if the patient is told that several weeks of treatment may be required, but that a favorable outcome is expected, the patient is further reassured. In the hospital, a properly trained staff will concentrate on current symptoms and play down any effort of the patient to tie her illness to former problems or failures. With this approach, some improvement is often noted within hours. The concept of an acute, severe illness is acceptable, even comforting.

Thus, an acute psychiatric illness which begins in the puerperium has distinct psychological features which are different from any other psychiatric illness. First, it arises out of the special situation of happy new motherhood, and it is particularly vulnerable to notions which cast serious doubt on the capability or worthiness of the new mother, in her own mind. Second, this illness provides a special challenge and opportunity for moves which have great psychotherapeutic value. Conversely, it has psychotherapeutic hazards of great magnitude. Third, the psychological situation, itself, with a large component of fear and anxiety, may play a significant role in psychophysiological feed-back mechanisms which may perpetuate or worsen the postpartum illness.

A Possible Clue

Five lines of evidence have been assembled and presented as characteristics which distinguish postpartum psychiatric illness from other varieties of illness. For the most part, the cited distinguishing characteristics have evolved from studies and observations which date back many years and regarding which there was concurrence by many independent observers.

This final "distinguishing characteristic" is labeled a "possible clue" because it has been tested neither by experimentation nor by additional independent observers. The clue is presented here, partly because it needs confirmation and partly because, if confirmed, it could contribute to understanding physiological mechanisms in postpartum psychosis.

In 1959 I became interested in the so-called "maternity blues." In the course of consulting obstetricians about the "blues," I interviewed Dr Emory Page, who was then studying the suppression of lactation by administering various estrogens at the time of delivery. Doctor Page offered the observation that successful suppression of lactation with estrogen had one interesting side-effect: the patients seemed to be free of the "blues." Two years later I consulted another physician, S.M. Dodek (1961) who was doing research on the prevention of lactation. He confirmed Page's (1959) observation; administration of estrogen to prevent lactation appears to prevent the "blues".

The next step in this account must be viewed in the light of morbidity figures. For well over a hundred years, hospital statistics have been remarkably consistent in their assessment of the incidence of postpartum psychosis. If one defines "psychosis" as a mental illness of such severity as to need hospitalization, then about one delivery in 1000 results in a postpartum psychosis. However, if a patient has had a prior postpartum psychosis, the probability of having *another* postpartum psychosis is 1:4 to 1:6. The low-risk situation now changes to a high-risk situation.

In the early 1960s I began to see patients who had suffered a prior postpartum psychosis, who were again pregnant and who were determined to carry their pregnancies to term. As I searched for a way to counter the high-risk hazard that psychosis would be repeated, the observations of Page and Dodek came to mind. "If the 'blues' can be aborted by estrogen, perhaps the risk of a recurring psychosis can be diminished." The recommendation was made, and over a period of 18 years, 40 high-risk patients have been treated without a single recurrent postpartum psychosis.

In point of fact, most of the 40 patients received a mixture of estrogen and testosterone in oil, delivered by injection on the delivery table. Until recently, this was a favored procedure in the United States for suppression of lactation. Some obstetricians supplemented the parenteral medication with oral estrogen for a few days. My advice was simply to take the same steps as would be used to suppress lactation. (Recently, a number of physicians have moved away from the use of hormones to suppress lactation. Instead, the prolactin inhibitor bromocriptine has been used. My experience does not include the use of bromocriptine.)

The foregoing experience with lactation-inhibiting hormones is not submitted as a recommendation that high-risk patients should be treated with lactation-inhibiting hormones. Such a recommendation would depend on a controlled experiment, and this has not been carried out. The results, no recurrences in 40 trials, where the expectation was 1:4 to 1:6, are encouraging.

The foregoing observation, that estrogen administered after delivery may influence the recurrence probability in high-risk patients, is introduced as a possible clue that the postpartum fall in estrogen may be a critical component in the chain of events which initiates postpartum psychosis. If this finding is verified by others, the phenomenon could be regarded as another distinguishing feature of postpartum psychosis. No other psychosis, and indeed no other disease entity, is ignited by a 20-fold drop in serum estrogen.

A Possible Connection

Postpartum psychiatric illness has many features which distinguish it from other non-puerperal varieties of psychiatric illness. When viewed together, these characteristics convey an impression that postpartum psychosis is not only a separate entity, but that it is an entity in which organic factors play a significant role. Since the puerperium is a period of enormous changes in circulating hormones, it is tempting to look for connections between the two. One way to do this is to lay out hormonal changes on a temporal scale and then superimpose psychiatric events. It is convenient to divide the hormone changes into four phases.

The first phase extends from the last days of pregnancy through the first two or three days after delivery. During the last trimester of pregnancy the maternal blood carries a high level of many hormones. Estrogen and progesterone are found in concentrations several times as great as the highest level reached in the non-pregnant state. The source of these hormones is mainly the placenta, but in the case of progesterone, the fetus is involved. When the fetoplacental source is lost at delivery, serum estrogen levels fall to 1/20th of the pregnancy level, or lower. Progesterone levels drop a little more slowly, but at the end of 48 hours they are below the pre-pregnancy level.

During the period of time while estrogen and progesterone are falling most rapidly, patients are remarkably free of psychiatric symptoms. Provisionally, this may suggest that it is unlikely that a direct relationship exists between the drop in these hormones, especially estrogen, and the production of psychiatric symptoms. However, there are precedents in psychiatry for important agents producing effects only after delays. ECT and tricyclic antidepressants relieve depression only after a delay of some days, and in the psychological sphere, the death of a loved one may result in grief only after a period of "shock." So it is still possible that the sudden fall in hormones is the prime mover.

The second phase extends from about the third to the tenth day postpartum. At this time the production of pituitary trophic hormones and the hormones whose production they stimulate (estrogen, progesterone, cortisol) are all low. There may also be other changes which affect the action of the hormones, such as the progressive unbinding of cortisol from globulin. The adrenal cortico-steroids would be worth studying in these cases because they are known to have some association with psychotic states; for example, states of agitation and confusion have been reported in Cushing's syndrome and Addison's disease.

The third phase extends from the tenth to the thirtieth or fortieth days. During this phase, the pituitary trophic hormones remain low, as do their target organs. The turbulence of hormone changes lessens and their titres level out at below-normal values. Clinically, patients who have their first symptoms during this phase are more likely to be depressed. Florid early syndromes are likely to have moved into depressive or schizophreniform syndromes.

The fourth phase, in which hormonal events have usually reverted to the normal pattern for women of childbearing age, may still be characterized by continued psychiatric illness, or by the onset of fresh episodes. These new episodes are usually of depression, though women with other psychiatric syndromes may relapse during this time. Possibly, intermediate physical or psychological factors need to be invoked to explain psychiatric illness in this phase. On the other hand, it must be recalled that when Bürgi looked specifically for evidence of hormonal abnormalities and irregularities in these instances of late postpartum illness, he found a plethora of them. If he could observe these phenomena in 1954, it would seem that we might accomplish even more a quarter of a century later, were we to turn our enormous facilities for endocrine diagnosis and treatment in the direction of these patients.

The Cost of Lost Identity

When the classifiers of psychiatric illness expunged "postpartum psychosis" from the official list of diseases, early in this century, cases of mental illness which arose after childbirth were distributed into other categories. This action seemed rather harmless at the time, and it did conform to a system of classification which was based mainly on symptoms, rather than etiology. In retrospect, it would appear that the fragmentation of "postpartum psychosis" has led to the overlooking of many characteristics which distinguish postpartum illness from other varieties of illness. Possible disease mechanisms and possible treatment modalities may also have been overlooked.

Destruction of the identity of postpartum psychosis may have had another, more subtle effect. Many generations of medical students were taught that the term "postpartum psychosis" was archaic, and that they should think of their psychiatric patients in other categories. Textbooks of psychiatry and obstetrics reflected the same position. As a result, many physicians may be poorly qualified to cope with psychiatric problems which arise in the puerperium. This position is not amenable to laboratory or statistical analysis. Nevertheless, two cases, almost identical, contrast the medical and public sophistication of nineteenth-century England with the lack of it in twentieth-century America.

Martha Prior, a resident of a village near Waltham, gave birth to a baby boy on December 10, 1847. A few days later, neighboring ladies got word to Mr Bell, the general physican who had delivered her, that Mrs Prior was not doing well. Mr Bell made a house call on December 19 and made an immediate diagnosis of postpartum psychosis. He ordered the baby kept apart from the mother and advised round-the-clock surveillance and nursing by the neighboring ladies. Four days later there was a lapse in the availability of neighbors, and Mrs Prior's daughter, Ellen, age 13, was left in charge. Mrs Prior, exercising her maternal authority, ordered her daughter to bring in the baby. A little later she complained of a hard callous on her hand and demanded a razor to pare it. The inevitable happened.

A trial was held on March 10, 1848. Mr Bell described the case as postpartum insanity and indicated that the infant's death was the result of an unfortunate lapse in the controls he had set up. Lord Denman, the Chief Justice, pointed out that Mrs Prior may have planned the murder, since she had asked for a razor. The jury deliberated for what appears to have been only a few minutes and returned a verdict of "Not guilty by reason of insanity." Within three months from the death of the baby, the case was settled (various newspapers, 1848).

Helen Winter, who resided near Palo Alto, California, gave birth to a baby boy on August 14, 1976. About ten days later she went to her mother and insisted that something was wrong with the child, and that her "head was flying." She made the same report to the pediatrician; he assured her that the child was well. She said that the child had an animal cry.

Then, on September 20, six weeks after the baby was born, she wrenched the baby's arm, breaking it. Her pediatrician referred her to an orthopedic surgeon who set the arm and put it in a cast. He carefully explained green stick fractures and the fragility of the infant skeleton. On September 27, Mrs Winter went to her minister, described the broken arm, and said that she was afraid that she would do something more to hurt her baby. He asked her to kneel down and pray with him. A few days later she went back to the church, but the minister was not available. Throughout this period, she visited her mother daily, spending most of her time pacing and crying. On November 11, she crushed and beat her baby until it was lifeless. She shot herself in the abdomen and was hospitalized.

On December 6, she was arraigned. Bail was set at $100 000. On January 18, 1977, a plea of Not Guilty was made for her. Trial was set for March 15, but because she was still hospitalized for the gunshot wound, it was put over. On May 27, the plea of Not Guilty by reason of insanity was added. Trial was held from October 5 to 15. The result was a hung jury.

Another trial was set for November 1. While out on bail she had become pregnant again. At delivery she was given an injection of estrogen in oil, and the psychosis did not recur. Finally, she was tried from June 10 through June 28, 1978 and found "Guilty of second degree murder." Mrs Winter spent six months in prison and was released on five-years probation on January 16, 1979. Elapsed time for trials, legal actions, prison: over two years, plus five years probation (Superior Court Records, 1976-79, Santa Clara County). After the second trial her husband left her.

The 1847 case was handled with medical wisdom and sophistication. Death followed an accidental failure of a control measure. The case was completed three months after the incident.

The Helen Winter case, over a century later in 1976, was remarkable for the clear-cut symptoms which were seen and disregarded from August 24 to November 11 by her family, her pediatrician, her obstetrician, the orthopedic surgeon, the nurses and aides, and the minister. Helen Winter knew that something was terribly wrong and she made repeated and continuous efforts to get help. Nobody recognized that she had suffered a postpartum psychosis. The incarceration, trials and sentencing, carried on month after month, and year after year are an example of barbarity. Only an excellent defense saved her from conviction for first degree murder. Happily, she has survived all of this and is now productively employed in the electronics industry.

We are left with a haunting question: could the very poor performance of many physicians and others concerned with the twentieth-century case be attributable to the fact that postpartum psychosis was denied its identity and expunged from the nomenclature and the thinking of modern medicine?

Picture Puzzle Progress

Modern methods of statistical analysis were first applied to psychiatric illness which follows childbirth in 1961, by Ralph S. Paffenbarger. With 126 hospitalized patients who were compared with 252 controls, he concluded that his evidence did not support the position that postpartum illness was caused by psychological stress. "Rather," he wrote,

> the data suggest an etiology that is active during pregnancy but exerts its full effect only after loss of a hormone-producing organ, the placenta. Whatever the etiological events, their influence is first seen in subtle abnormalities of pregnancy and parturition. Then the climax of derangement bursts on the psyche in a weird accompaniment of genital evolution.

Paffenbarger added that he found postpartum problems to be a special challenge, in which factors of the perinatal period are "arranged in a tantalizing fashion, much like the pieces of a picture puzzle partly fitted together. The question remains whether all of the pieces will match, or indeed whether they are all on hand."

For two decades there was little apparent progress in finding the missing pieces of the picture puzzle, or in fitting them together. Then a conference on these matters was held at the University of Manchester on June 19–20, 1980. Over a single 48-hour period it became apparent that many new pieces of the picture puzzle were at hand, and many able workers were ready to put them together.

It is not the task of this chapter to review the findings which were reported at the Manchester meeting. It is, however, its purpose to address some of the special, overall problems which pertain to the performance of research and the communication of findings in this special field; and to outline a possible solution through the vehicle of a new international society whose goal is to advance the understanding, prevention and treatment of mental illness in mothers of young children.

The first problem begins as an exercise in terminology, but the facts have broad implication. Psychiatric nomenclature is notoriously imprecise, and physicians have often disagreed on the names which they choose to attach to various syndromes or diseases. The classic instance of institutional stupidity in this area is the policy ennunciated by the American Psychiatric Association which required that "postpartum psychosis" be expunged from the official nomenclature—but that is another story.

The terminological problem to be discussed here relates to the term "depression," or "melancholia," as it was known in former times. The classical students of postpartum illness, and many modern workers as well, were and are psychiatrists who work around psychiatric hospitals. This means that the population with which these physicians deal is a *hospitalized* population. This means, almost invariably, that at least one expert has decided that the patient cannot be cared for safely without psychiatric hospital controls. The number of such patients, as tabulated many times in the nineteenth and twentieth centuries, corresponds to about 1/1000th of the number of births in the area served by the psychiatric facility. Not all of these patients are "depressed," and diagnostic fashions have varied from decade to decade and nation to nation. A fair estimate would be that half of the hospitalized patients, overall, could be called "depressed." This is 1/2000th of all births, and this is what the classic writers meant when they talked about the incidence of depression.

At the Manchester conference, several investigators spoke about "depression" from a totally different point of view. A different population was sampled. Typically, investigators would work from the base of a maternity hospital or service. Subject patients would be recruited. Reactions would be studied, by interview, test or questionnaire, and patients would be rated or measured by degree of depression. Then those patients with high ratings would be compared with patients who did not seem to be affected at all adversely, compared with respect to all kinds of variables, physical, historical, social or other. An impressive study of this kind was described at the Manchester meeting by Dr H.R. Playfair and later reported in detail in a 1981 paper. Dr Playfair, a general practioner in Plymouth, enlisted 64 of his colleagues throughout the British Isles to participate in a joint effort to search for signs which would predict depression following childbirth. A total of 618 obstetric patients were studied intensively by interview, questionnaire and follow-up. Ten per cent had a sufficient weight of depressive symptoms three months after childbirth to be designated as "depressed," and this group was then compared with others in the search for predictive signs.

In the study by Playfair and his associates, the sampling was wide, the assessment was thorough and the statistical analysis was excellent. However, his "depressed" patients, 10% of women delivered, were not comparable to "depressed" patients in hospital studies, which represent 1/2000th of the cases delivered.

Dr Playfair is not alone is applying the term "depressed" to a very large number of patients whose symptoms date from childbearing. Katherina Dalton, a respected British gynecologist, has stated in her book, *Depression after Childbirth*, that 1/10th of all new mothers are sufficiently depressed to need medical or psychiatric help (Dalton, 1980).

The implications of the foregoing are these: (1) Different investigators may use the same psychiatric terms and mean far different things in terms of degree, and possibly diagnosis in some instances. (2) If we pay attention to the observations of Playfair, Dalton and many others, as indeed we should, then it is apparent that we are not dealing with occasional, rare, florid departures from the norm. In looking for the cause and treatment of postpartum psychiatric illness we are concerned with disabilities and afflictions which cause a great deal of distress to millions of women. It is one of the scandals of modern medicine that distress of this frequency and enormity should have been neglected for so long.

After the Manchester meeting several participants remained to discuss the events and the significance of the conference. A general impression was that the meeting presaged an imminent information explosion in the area of postpartum psychiatric problems. Optimism was expressed that the major aspects of postpartum illness might well be amenable to control within a decade. However, for this to be accomplished, it would be necessary to establish and maintain communication between the widely-dispersed investigators. The dispersion was particularly difficult, since it crossed not only national boundaries, but professional categories as well. If postpartum illness were to be conquered, a vehicle of communication had to be set up, and this vehicle had to have continuity.

The vehicle selected was the new society, mentioned above. The small group who had originally met after the conference constituted itself as a Founding Committee. It was the consensus that this society should search out the most able investigators and practitioners in the field all over the world, but that a wide range of individuals, with differing professions and contributions to make and not excluding lay people, should be encouraged to apply for membership. The Committee agreed that no steps should be taken to select officers or levy dues until the society met as a body in 1982. Thereafter, dues should be kept to a minimum.

As a name for this society, Dr Kumar had the happy thought of proposing it be named in memory of Louis Victor Marcé, the great nineteenth -century investigator of postpartum psychiatric illness. The suggestion met with immediate approval, and The Marcé Society was launched officially.

Louis Victor Marcé made enormous contributions to the understanding and treatment of postpartum psychiatric illness. His life history reveals an exemplary sense of mission. Born in 1828, he attended medical school at Nantes and had an outstanding record. After completion of his medical training, and in need of funds to support a newly-acquired wife, he accepted a salaried position in the mental hospital at Ivry-sur-Seine, near Paris. This hospital had been founded by the famous J.E.D. Esquirol and had a long tradition in the treatment of psychiatric cases associated with childbearing. Concurrently, Marcé became affiliated with the University of Paris, where he received high honors and, in 1853, a gold medal prize.

At Ivry-sur-Seine, Marcé moved rapidly to follow in the tradition of Esquirol. He quickly familiarized himself with the literature regarding postpartum cases, reviewed cases which had been studied by Esquirol and others and accumulated many of his own. Synthesizing the literature and 310 cases, he published *Traité de la folie des femmes enceintes, des nouvelles accouchées et des nourrices* in 1858. He was 30 years old at the time and was listed on the title page as *"Ancien interne, lauréat des hôspitaux et de la faculté de médecine."* Four years later, in 1862, he published his 672-page *Traité pratique des maladies mentales.* At that time he was listed as *"Professeur agrégé à la faculté de médecine de Paris."* He died in 1864 at the age of 36.

As indicated earlier, Marcé's position on postpartum illness was that it displayed many and varied symptoms, and that these symptoms are similar to those in non-puerperal cases. Further, he noted that the syndromes of postpartum illness, the combinations of symptoms, the way one syndrome moves to another, and the consistent association between the changes in psychiatric syndromes and changes in the generative organs were unique to postpartum illness.

Marcé's writings are the key to his mind. Through them, we know that he approached every subject, even in the broad scope of his general textbook, with scholarly knowledge of the research and opinions of his colleagues and predecessors. He studied their clinical approaches and results and analyzed their opinions. He studied what was known about anatomy and physiology and tried to relate his knowledge of physical states to what he observed in behavior. He tested treatment methods on his own patients, developing and modifying his thinking through meticulous, continuous observation. Every step was thought through and documented. When information was insufficient, he looked further. When this failed, he used reason and came to what he considered the best conclusion.

Marcé's career was terminated prematurely by his death at the age of 36. During his short professional life he made many contributions which revealed great scope and vision. A case in point: Marcé was struck repeatedly by the simultaneous march of psychiatric symptoms and the physical changes which follow childbearing. He believed that a very definite connection must exist between the organs of reproduction and the brain. He found nothing in the structure of the body to account for the relationship which he saw. He knew, however, that "something" was connecting perturbed or abnormal physiology to abnormal behavior and he gave it a name, *sympathie morbide*. His conclusions foresaw endocrinology.

The Marcé Society was launched, hopefully, with the vision and sense of mission which so characterized Marcé. At the time of writing it has a Bulletin, and a growing membership of over 200 persons. Officially, it is a public service scientific body, approved by the US Federal Government for tax-exempt status.

The Marcé Society has several purposes. In general, and for the immediate future, the Society will continue to act as a medium of communication, analogous to the central processor in a computer system. To carry the computer analogy further, the Society proposes to act as a bridge between quite a few languages, linguistic and technical.

Related to communication is the function of stimulating new activity. Quite a few scientists, once they realize the enormous opportunities which exist, seem to be ready to turn their minds and facilities to postpartum problems. The Society encourages meetings concerned with postpartum matters, and at least two have been stimulated in addition to the Society meeting and Conference scheduled at the University of London in 1982.

Additional activities are under consideration. The information explosion has resulted in the scattering of papers into many journals, some of which are inaccessible. In time, the Bulletin may become a journal. The Society hopes to attract the attention of medical leaders, teachers and writers of medical and obstetrical textbooks, so that the results of research can be extended into practice. The Society should develop a public relations and a public information capacity, so that an informed public can insist on optimal care for postpartum patients.

Conceivably, most of the goals of the Society could be accomplished within a decade. A wealth of relevant knowledge, not only in psychiatry but in endocrinology, obstetrics and pharmacology as well, awaits synthesis and application. Innovative treatment methods, such as mother and baby hospitalization, are being explored. A timetable of ten years is ambitious, but not irrational.

References

Adams, F. (1886). *The Genuine Works of Hippocrates*. Wood, New York.
Baker, A.A. (1967). *Psychiatric Disorders in Obstetrics*. Blackwell, Oxford.
Bürgi, V.S. (1954). Puerperalpsychose oder Diencephalosis puerperalis? *Schweizerische Medizinische Wochenschrift* **84**, 1222-1225.

Dalton, K. (1980). *Depression after childbirth: how to recognize and treat postnatal depression.* Oxford University Press, London.

Dodek, S.M. (1961). Personal communication.

Fürstner, C. (1875). Ueber Schwangerschafts- und Puerperalpsychosen. *Archiv für Psychiatrie und Nervenkranken* 5, 505-543.

Gundry, R. (1859). Observations upon puerperal insanity. *Am. J. Insan.* 16, 294-320.

Hamilton, J.A. (1962). *Postpartum psychiatric problems.* L.V. Mosby, St. Louis.

Jacobides, G.M. (1961). Adrenocortical function in puerperal psychoses. MD thesis, University of Athens.

Jones, R. (1902). Puerperal insanity. *Br. med. J.* 1, 579-585.

Karnosh, L.J. and Hope, J.M. (1937). Puerperal psychoses and their sequelae. *Am. J. Psychiat.* 94, 537-550.

Kendell, R.E. and Gourlay, J. (1970). The clinical distinction between the affective psychoses and schizophrenia. *Br. J. Psychiat.* 117, 261-266.

Marcé, L.V. (1958). *Traité de la Folie des Femmes Enceintes, des Nouvelles Accouchées et des Nourrices.* Baillière, Paris.

Paffenbarger, R.S. Jr. (1961). The picture puzzle of the postpartum psychoses. *J. chron. Dis.* 13, 161-173.

Page, E. (1959). Personal Communication.

Pauleikhoff, B. (1964). *Seelische Störungen in der Schwangerschaft und nach der Geburt.* Ferdinand Enke Verlag, Stuttgart.

Playfair, H.R. and Gowers, J.I. (1981). Depression following childbirth—a search for predictive signs. *J. R. Coll. Gen. Pract.* 31, 201-208.

Savage, G. (1875). Observations on insanity in pregnancy and childbirth. *Guy's Hospital Reports* 20, 83-117.

Stössner, K. (1910). Ein Fall von Myxödem im Anschluss an Gravidität. *München Medizinische Wochenschrift* 57, 2531-2534.

Strecker, E.A. and Ebaugh, F.C. (1926). Psychoses occurring during the puerperium. *Arch. Neurol. Psychiat.* 15, 239-252.

2

Epidemiological Aspects of Mental Illness Associated with Childbearing

R.S. Paffenbarger, Jr.

Mental illness associated with childbirth has probably been recognized for thousands of years. During the reproductive age span, mental illnesses display a higher incidence in women than in men (Jaco, 1960; Pugh and MacMahon, 1962), and when associated with pregnancy these mental illnesses in women tend to have onset shortly after delivery rather than at other stages in the childbearing process (Thomas and Gordon, 1959). The incidence and tragic nature of this disease are ample reason to ask whether modern research can lead to better understanding and control of its causes.

Despite much interest, the epidemiological literature on the subject is not conclusive. Marcé claimed to have distinguished postpartum mental illness as a syndrome different from prepartum disturbances and from various psychoses and neuroses unassociated with pregnancy or motherhood (Marcé, 1858). More than a century ago an attempt was made to differentiate the clinical features of prepartum and postpartum mental illnesses. Disorders occurring during pregnancy were considered clincially indistinguishable from those unrelated to childbirth, but disorders following delivery were considered quite distinct. Abrupt or slow in onset, varied and fluctuating in course, the postpartum disturbances most often included elements of confusion or delirium together with depression or excitement.

The early concept of a distinct clinical entity gradually fell into disrepute (Strecker and Ebaugh, 1926; Boyd, 1942), and its convenient terms such as "postpartum psychosis" were removed from standard nomenclature. Now, however, the more recent publication of new clinical material (Hamilton, 1962; Jansson, 1964; Brockington *et al.*, 1981) has revived the concept of a separate disease entity, and recommendations for treatment have been advanced (Dalton, 1980), although hypotheses of causation have remained uncertain (Kendell *et al.*,

19

1976; Kumar chapter 4; Kendell *et al.*, 1981). Meanwhile, further distinctions between prepartum and postpartum mental illnesses have been found in obstetric and perinatal variables (Paffenbarger, 1961, 1963, 1964; Paffenbarger and McCabe, 1966).

These last-mentioned findings were the results of epidemiological studies concerned with frequency distributions of obstetric variables as possible determinants of parapartum mental illnesses. The epidemiological techniques were employed in a search for clues to a practical understanding of the disease by assessing the relative risks of developing a first mental illness in the presence and absence of certain obstetric variables and other circumstances of childbearing. Whereas clinical studies tend to focus on individuals and a case-history approach, epidemiological studies look at larger numbers and calculate the risk of disease in the presence of a characteristic versus its risk in the absence of the characteristic. This relativity of risk can suggest what relationship may exist between the characteristic and the disease. Analysis is not quite that simple, as there may be confounding influences, but relative risk estimates can be helpful, especially in conjunction with other data on the same or other variables. In epidemiology it is not unusual to analyze characteristics and risks in terms of person-years of experience instead of simply per capita, as this technique again tends to focus on the trait being studied rather than on the individuals who possess that trait. In the present instance, for example, one woman or several women may contribute to a single woman-year of experience with a particular trait, and except for that trait their individualities have no part in the analysis. By the same token, it is possible to calculate rates of disease per person-years of experience with a characteristic, thus providing an expression of the degree of risk of disease that is attached to that characteristic. Such an observation, of course, reveals only part of the risk that a particular individual may have of contracting a given illness, since other traits or experience may also be contributing to risk of the same illness. By considering a number of variables, however, an epidemiological study can assemble a quite suggestive set of data applicable to some or a number of individuals, and the findings may be very persuasive even though the study cannot identify specifically which individuals with the high-risk trait will contract the probable disease. Epidemiological information of this kind can be very helpful to clinical activities. This is the general approach by which the present report will now undertake to review and extend the earlier findings on parapartum mental illness and perhaps to assist in updating impressions as newer information is brought up for study. It examines relative risks of mental illness during pregnancy, delivery, and new motherhood. The data are analyzed as prepartum, first month postpartum, and two to six months postpartum.

Methods

Medical records were surveyed for all women aged 15 through 44 who were inpatients on any public or private psychiatric service in Hamilton County, Ohio, in the years 1940 through 1958. The county includes Cincinnati, which was then the second largest metropolitan area in the state. All patients experiencing a psychotic or psychoneurotic attack were included for study, while those with a behavior disorder or mental deficiency were excluded. Patients were identified who were pregnant at the onset (diagnosis) of a mental illness or in the prior six months. Only those who produced a viable infant, i.e. who were pregnant for 20 or more weeks, were included. Those patients with a record of multiple parapartum mental illness attacks were considered only as of their first attack, except in the computation of incidence and of recurrence rates. The rationale of the described procedure for selection of study subjects was, obviously, to identify those women whose mental illness was most likely to have been associated with their childbearing circumstances if any such association did in fact exist. The search for association would then be pursued by studying obstetric and other variables of these patients in comparison with the same variables in control subjects free of mental illness.

Data on commonly recorded obstetric variables were compiled for parapartum mental illness patients from their maternity hospital records. Comparison data were obtained from the records of control subjects arbitrarily chosen as the two maternity patients of the same race who delivered just before and after each mental illness patient in the same obstetric unit. This method of choosing controls would preserve a randomness necessary to avoid bias, while also simplifying access to records and promoting uniformity of record-keeping and diagnostic procedures regarding the childbearing experiences of both mental illness patients and control subjects. Obstetric variables were reported as group averages or proportional distributions wherever significant disparity existed between mental illness patients and controls. As frequencies of these variables differed little among the control subjects, whether chosen for prepartum or postpartum mental illness patients, all the control subjects were combined into one group for reference. A review of county and state vital statistics showed that race-specific values in the general population for maternal age and parity; for perinatal mortality and infant birth weight; for birthplace, residence, and occupation of father; and for legitimacy or marital status were closely approximated in the control group. In other words, the control subjects could be regarded as representative of the general or normal experience of childbearing women in the study area, and any significant differences noted for the mental illness patients could be considered as departures from that criterion for motherhood.

The epidemiological analyses reported here assess relative risks (odds ratios) of mental illness in relation to specific obstetric variables, using a summary chi-square procedure with adjustment as necessary for differences between mental illness patients and control subjects in age and parity (Mantel and Haenszel, 1959). Multivariate estimates of mental illness risk were based on a logistic model, using maximum likelihood estimates (Cornfield, 1962) related to specific variables adjusted for other variables found to alter risk.

Although definitions and diagnostic criteria of the psychoses and psychoneuroses varied during the 18-year period surveyed, the patients hospitalized for these variously described mental illnesses showed no corresponding differences in obstetric variables or by black or white race: therefore they could be combined in the analysis as a total group of childbearing mental illness patients. On the other hand, several obstetric variables differentiated prepartum from postpartum mental illness patients, and these two categories are reported separately in all analyses. Also, because of the remarkable clustering of onsets in the first month after delivery, postpartum mental illnesses are distinguished wherever possible as having had onset in the first month after childbirth or during the next five months. Examination of data for patients who had onset in the first week postpartum showed no significant differences from findings for those with onset in the second through fourth weeks, so the results were combined for all with onset in the first month postpartum. Incidentally, the postpartum patients afforded obstetric data recorded before overt mental illness appeared, and hence seemingly unbiased by psychiatric symptoms, while this was not so for gestational and obstetric data on prepartum mental illness patients.

Computation of incidence (attack rates) of mental illness was limited to the two most recent years of study, 1957 and 1958, so as to set aside variations in hospital policies, standards, and facilities. Attack rates per 10 000 woman-years were computed for new episodes (i.e. initial, recurrent, or reactivated attacks of mental illness) in the two-year sample. Incidence was equated both to the number of women of childbearing age and to the number of infants born alive in the county during that period. Because selection of parapartum mental illness patients was based on childbirth during 1957–8, the incidence data include some illnesses developing outside that time but exclude some that had onset within it.

Birth certificates of infants and marriage license applications of subjects married within the country furnished additional social data.

Recurrence rates of parapartum mental illness during the 18 years included for study were equated to the number of women at risk and to the number of their pregnancies subsequent to the first episode.

Findings

A total of 247 first mental illnesses among parapartum women was identified in the 18-year period available for study, 57 with onset during pregnancy and 190

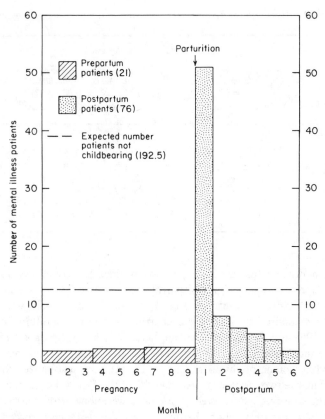

Fig. 1. Onset of mental illness in parous ever-married women aged 15–44 years, Hamilton County, Ohio, 1957–8.

Table 1. Attack rates[a] of mental illness by childbearing status, Hamilton County, Ohio, 1957-8.

Age	Prepartum No. of Patients	Rate	1-6 months Postpartum No. of Patients	Rate	Non-childbearing No. of Patients	Rate
15-24	5	3.4	24	24.2	175	20.0
25-34	15	10.2	46	46.9	401	44.4
35-44	2	5.9	13	57.9	461	40.5
Total	22	6.7	83	37.8	1037	35.5
Age-adjusted		7.1[b]		40.3		35.1

[a]Per 10 000 woman-years at risk.   [b]$P < 0.01$.

Table 2. Relative risks *(RR)* of first mental illness, by childbearing status, age, and parity.

	Prepartum (N=57)		1 month Postpartum (N=123)		2-6 month Postpartum (N=67)		Control subjects (N=494)
	%	RR	%	RR	%	RR	%
Age							
25-44	64.9	1.36	63.4	1.28	70.1	1.73	57.6
15-24	35.1	1	36.6	1	29.9	1	42.4
Parity[a]							
1	15.8	0.53	38.2	2.04	19.4	0.76	27.7
2+	84.2	1	63.8	1	80.6	1	72.3

Mental Illness Patients

[a]Age-adjusted

in the six months postpartum. The prepartum illnesses were evenly distributed by trimester of pregnancy, but postpartum onsets were clustered shortly after delivery. This pattern is seen in Fig. 1, which presents incidence data for parapartum mental illness among ever-married women in Hamilton County for the period 1957 and 1958. Since only mothers are at risk of a parapartum mental illness, the incidence figures expressed on this basis may be more realistic.

In all, 1142 women of childbearing age (15–44) were hospitalized for mental illness during the two years, or fewer than 1% of the 173 000 women in that age range in the county. Age-adjusted attack rates were lowest for married women (54 per 10 000), progressively higher for single, widowed, and divorced women, and highest for separated women (196 per 10 000).

As Table 1 shows, mental illness attack rates are substantially lower during pregnancy (7.1 per 10 000 woman-years) than among women not in childbearing status (35.1 per 10 000 woman-years). Rates during the six months postpartum

Table 3. Interval [a]since prior childbirth for multiparae.

	Prepartum (N=53)	1-6 month Postpartum (N=148)	Control subjects (N=393)
	Mental Illness Patients		
Years	3.2[c]	3.0[b]	2.5
±1SD	±2.0	±2.4	±2.4

[a]Age-and parity-adjusted mean ± 1SD
[b]$P<0.05$ [c]$P<0.01$

(40.3 per 10 000 woman-years) trend slightly higher as a group than for non-childbearing women, but markedly higher in the first month following delivery. Although not shown here, the same unique pattern that Fig. 1 gives for parous ever-married women is found if the analysis is extended to include all women of childbearing age. Thus, the sharp temporal differences observed in the parapartum occurrence of mental illness appear to be specific to childbearing.

Normal childbearing women aged 25 through 44 were at 36% higher risk (relative risk $RR = 1.36$) of a first mental illness during pregnancy than pregnant women under age 25 (Table 2). The corresponding risk of first postpartum mental illness was 28% higher for the older women than for younger mothers during the first month after delivery, and 73% higher in the next five months after parturition. With data adjusted for age differences, women bearing their first child were at 47% lower risk ($RR = 0.53$) of first mental illness during pregnancy than women bearing a second or later child (Table 2). In contrast, however, primiparae were at doubled risk ($RR = 2.04$) of first mental illness during the first month postpartum as compared with multiparous women, but at 24% lower risk ($RR = 0.76$) during the next five months.

Comparisons of mental illness patients with control subjects showed them to have equivalent onsets of maturity, i.e. to have been of the same ages at menarche, at marriage, and at each parity—until the particular pregnancy associated with onset of first parapartum mental illness. At that point the women who developed mental illness during pregnancy averaged two years older than

Table 4. Relative risks $(RR)^a$ of first mental illness, by childbearing status, gestation, and infant weight.

| | Mental Illness Patients | | | | | | Control subjects (N=494) |
| | Prepartum (N=57) | | 1 month Postpartum (N=123) | | 2-6 month Postpartum (N=67) | | |
	%	RR	%	RR	%	RR	%
Gestation							
<40 wks	28.3	1.00	35.2	1.35	43.3	1.92^b	28.5
40+	71.7	1	64.8	1	56.7	1	71.5
Infant weight							
<3350 g	57.4	1.67	67.8	2.43^d	59.7	1.65	48.2
3350+	42.6	1	32.2	1	40.3	1	51.8
<2500 g	5.6	0.63	17.4	2.43^c	11.9	1.55	8.2
2500+	94.4	1	82.6	1	88.1	1	91.8

^{a}Age- and parity-adjusted $^bP<0.05$ $^cP<0.01$ $^dP<0.001$

control subjects, and those who became mentally ill postpartum were 1.3 years older than controls. Table 3 shows that paraparatum mental illness patients had significantly longer intervals since their last previous pregnancy than the control subjects had.

Table 4 shows that relative risk of postpartum mental illness was higher among women whose gestation period was less than 40 weeks. The hazard was significant for postpartum mental illness in the second through sixth month. The risk in the first month after delivery was 35% greater after short gestation, and in the next five months 92% greater, than for women whose pregnancies lasted 40 or more weeks. As might be expected, postpartum risk of mental illness in the first month was significantly higher (more than doubled) for women whose infants weighed less than 3350 g (7.4 lb) at birth, although nearly half the birth weights for infants of normal women were in this category. The first-month relative risk of postpartum mental illness for women delivered of premature infants (birthweight less than 2500 g, or 5.5 lb) likewise was more than twice the risk for women who bore heavier infants. Similarly, risks during months two through six after delivery with low birthweight were up respectively 65 and 55% for mothers of lightweight and premature infants, though more likely due to chance.

Dystocia was experienced by 6% of the control women, and 2% lost infants to perinatal death. Table 5 shows that risk of mental illness developing within the first month postpartum was nearly tripled among women who experienced dystocia and still greater for those who lost an infant. These relationships were not significant for prepartum or later postpartum mental illness, perhaps because

Table 5. Relative risks $(RR)^a$ of first mental illness, by childbearing status and perinatal variables.

| | Mental Illness Patients | | | | | | Control |
| | Prepartum (N=57) | | 1 month Postpartum (N=123) | | 2-6 month Postpartum (N=67) | | subjects (N=494) |
	%	RR	%	RR	%	RR	%
Dystocia							
Yes	3.5	0.64	15.4	2.62^b	9.0	2.13	5.8
No	96.5	1	84.6	1	91.0	1	94.2
Perinatal death							
Yes	0	0.0	10.3	4.77^c	3.0	1.30	2.3
No	100	1	89.7	1	97.0	1	97.7

^{a}Age- and parity-adjusted $^bP<0.01$ $^cP<0.001$

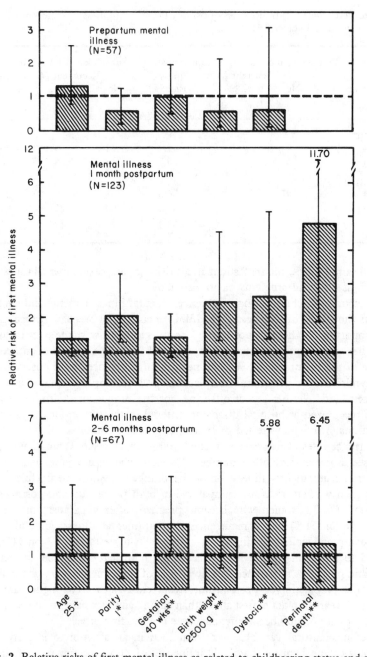

Fig. 2. Relative risks of first mental illness as related to childbearing status and selected obstetric variables

*Adjusted for age   **Adjusted for age and parity | 95% confidence limits

Table 6. Percentage recurrence rates of parapartum mental illness by childbearing status and age at first attack.

Status and Age	Women with Subsequent Childbirths			Subsequent Childbirths		
		Recurrent Mental Illness			Recurrent Mental illness	
	No.	No.	Rate(%)	No.	No.	Rate(%)
Prepartum						
15-24	7	3	42.9	12	3	25.0
25-44	6	4	66.7	11	4	36.4
Postpartum						
15-24	19	7	36.8	38	9	23.7
25-44	40	23	57.5	64	26	40.6
Total	72	37	51.4	125	42	33.6

of small sample sizes. Figure 2 summarizes risks of parapartum mental illness by the various obstetric problems mentioned above.

In the surveyed childbearing experiences, mental illness patients and control subjects showed no differences in scheduling or amount of prenatal medical care. The proportions of these groups whose labor was induced were the same (4%), as were the proportions hospitalized in false labor (4%) or with spontaneous rupture of the membranes (8%). No meaningful differences were observed for such syndromes as pre-eclampsia, placenta praevia, abruptio placentae, and prolapsed cord. Neither sex of offspring nor the proportions with congenital defects recognized at hospital discharge differed in the two groups, and equal proportions of infants were fed by breast, bottle, or a combination.

Recurrence rates of parapartum mental illness are given in Table 6. Whether expressed as percentages of the number of women who became pregnant after a first parapartum mental illness, or of the number of subsequent childbirths among such women, risks are comparable in both prepartum and postpartum categories. Of 72 women who became pregnant after a parapartum mental illness, 37 (or 51%) had a recurrence of their mental illness; and, of their successive pregnancies reaching 20 or more weeks of gestation, 42 (or 34%) of 125 led to recurrent mental illness. Although it may represent an artifact of diagnostic practices, recurrence was invariably of the same category as the first attack, i.e. prepartum or postpartum. Recurrence rates were higher among patients 25 years or older at first attack than among younger patients, but did not differ by parity or number of pregnancies since the first attack.

Some sociocultural variables were examined in an attempt to identify any psychological mechanisms that might influence risk of parapartum mental illness (Paffenbarger, 1961). Geographic mobility was rated in terms of birthplace versus residence at successive deliveries. Parapartum mental illness patients and control subjects were similar in distribution by birthplace and urban/rural residence. They did not differ in mean number of residential addresses reported or in occupational distributions listed for their husbands. Similar proportions (6 to 8%) of patients and controls bore children out of wedlock.

Discussion

Some concomitants that differ for prepartum and postpartum mental illness patients may imply relationships to a common set of circumstances. For example, women who developed a first mental illness prepartum were more parous and less often primiparous than the controls, while women who first became mentally ill postpartum were less parous and more apt to be primiparae. Moreover, there were no reports of women developing both prepartum and postpartum mental illness or shifting from one category to the other in connection with any subsequent pregnancy. These data could result if the experience of a postpartum mental illness after first childbirth tended to dissuade or deter women so affected from undergoing another pregnancy and parturition: there would be a surplus of primiparae among the postpartum mental illness patients. On the other hand, multiparous women would *ipso facto* be increasing their opportunities of developing mental illness during pregnancy, and the onset of such an illness would in these data rule out their opportunity of becoming a postpartum mental illness patient. Since pregnancy precedes parturition, the multiparous woman would have a further likelihood of becoming a prepartum rather than a postpartum mental illness patient. In view of these potential tendencies, it is striking that postpartum mental illness was almost four times as frequent as prepartum mental illness. This sharp reversal of what might be the expected pattern is not readily explained away as due to diagnostic variations or availability, since in either category, prepartum or postpartum, the mental illness had to be sufficiently evident to require the woman to become an inpatient of a psychiatric service. There is no good reason to suppose that this level of mental illness would be more likely to be overlooked in a pregnant woman than in a recently delivered mother, if it was present.

There are other contrasts to consider. The attack rate of prepartum mental illness in age-comparable women was substantially lower than that of mental illness among women not in childbearing status. The prepartum mental illness patients did not differ from normal women in most events of pregnancy, labor, delivery, and puerperium, but fewer were primiparae and they were older, more parous, and had had a longer interval since their last previous viable pregnancy. Although their risk of a first attack of mental illness was lower, their risk of recurrence of it was high, therefore pregnant women with a history of prepartum mental illness should be carefully observed and could serve as valuable subjects for etiological studies of such illness.

The attack rate of mental illness in the six months following delivery was only minimally higher than that of mental illness in age-comparable women not in childbearing status, but it was noted for its peak in the first month after delivery. This skewed temporal distribution is one of the distinctive features of mental illness associated with childbirth. It leads us to ask whether the low attack rate during pregnancy is the result of some protective physiological, psychological or social process, and whether the sudden increase immediately following delivery is due to a release of that defense. Or, is the postpartum peak of onset a result of some physiological surge or aberration associated with parturition or involution. In fact both of these prepartum and postpartum influences could be acting to produce the pattern of experience observed.

If there is no evident clinical difference between mental illness in pregnancy and that without any association with childbirth, some explanation (endocrine or metabolic?) may be sought for the decline in mental illness during pregnancy. However, if mental illness in the first month postpartum is somehow quite different clinically from others, we may ask what distinctive circumstances develop at parturition to produce this startling result. In contrast to prepartum mental illness patients, women with a first mental illness in the first month postpartum differed in many ways from control subjects. They were older than the controls and had had a longer interval since their last preceding childbirth. They were less parous than controls and more were primiparae. If this significant difference in age, which developed in a relatively short interval within the childbearing age span, is causally associated with increased risk of parapartum mental illness, or if we interpret it as a clue to a condition that was sufficient to delay the pregnancy involved (Table 3 shows intervals since prior childbirth), perhaps we can conclude that the influence responsible for the mental illness was of relatively recent origin before the disease became manifest.

The epidemiological data as to timing cannot explain what happened, but they can at least give us a hint as to how far back in time we should look for causes of a parapartum mental illness. Perhaps the physiological or psychological hardship responsible for the overt mental illness was not simply the ordeal of gestation or parturition itself, but some precursive experience that added a new danger to the childbearing process. In multiparae, the pregnancy associated with the mental illness was delayed as compared with the experience of control women. The postpartum mental illness patients had shorter gestational periods than controls; their pregnancies were complicated by more dystocia and attended by higher perinatal death rates; and they delivered infants of lighter weight than those produced by normal women. The association of these differences with mental illness was more pronounced in the first month postpartum than in the next five months. Most of these observations could support a hypothesis of an extraneous influence as well as the possibility of an intrinsic circumstance of parturition.

Specificity versus Generality

The categories of prepartum psychoses and reactivated postpartum psychoses involved groups too small to offer profitable analysis. Therefore, to test the specificity of findings associated with first attacks of postpartum psychoses, additional control groups were studied. One group included mothers developing late postpartum uterine hemorrhage, and the other consisted of mothers whose infants developed hypertropic pyloric stenosis. Each group was compared independently with the postpartum psychotic patients, and adjustments were made for age, race, and parity (Paffenbarger, 1964).

Of 87 women discharged from the hospital following parturition and readmitted because of hemorrhage, fewer had experienced the complications associated with postpartum psychoses than had the psychotic group. (Patients with late postpartum hemorrhage had experienced significantly more uterine bleeding during pregnancy, as might occur with low implantation or premature separation of the placenta. The obstetrician is thus offered a basis for special watchfulness after delivery of patients with a history of such prior bleeding.)

Hemorrhage and psychosis groups showed complete parallelism in their frequency distributions for length of gestation. Infant weights in the two groups were also similar. Hence, like the psychotic patients, women with hemorrhage had shorter gestational periods and lighter infants than average mothers not so afflicted. These common factors may be of importance in the etiology of both late postpartum uterine hemorrhage and postpartum psychosis.

A total of 76 mothers whose infants developed pyloric stenosis was studied. They too experienced fewer complications than shown to be associated with postpartum psychoses. Their gestational periods averaged 40 weeks, and infants with pyloric stenosis weighed more at birth than infants born to psychotic patients, as did newborn offspring of the original control group.

The mothers in the pyloric stenosis group included more primiparae than the other groups of control subjects or the patients with postpartum psychosis. Also they produced a larger proportion of male infants, but the excess of males did not affect weight comparisons.

This review of two additional comparison or control groups was sufficient to show that the patients with postpartum psychosis were not the only ones who displayed many of the characteristic somatic phenomena that appeared to differentiate them from normal mothers. Hence, postpartum psychoses may be linked in etiology with other postpartum abnormalities.

Postpartum mental disturbances are distinctive for their timing, early in the puerperium, coincident with uterine involution and marked alteration of endogenous hormones, and may be characterized clinically by a delirium or confusion with depression or excitement. Their time of onset and high level of

recurrence with subsequent pregnancies point to appropriate candidates for
more specific endocrinological studies during and after any of their pregnancies
following a first episode of mental illness associated with childbearing.

Summary

Attack rates of mental illness (psychoses and neuroses) among women of
childbearing age in Hamilton County, Ohio, in 1957 through 1958 were
compared by various stages of womanhood. Age-adjusted rates for pregnant
women were substantially lower than for women not in childbearing status.
Rates for the first six months postpartum were slightly higher than those for non-
childbearing, parous, ever-married women, but were marked by an explosive
peak in the first month following delivery.

Obstetric, perinatal, and certain social characteristics were studied in women
with a first mental illness during pregnancy or the six months postpartum, and
in normal childbearing women, for the period 1940 through 1958. Mental illness
patients and control subjects were similar in sociocultural indices such as place
of residence, mobility pattern, occupation of spouse, and legitimacy of offspring.
Marked differences were noted in several obstetric and perinatal variables, which
distinguished prepartum from postpartum mental illness patients and both from
normal childbearing women.

Contrasted to normal mothers, prepartum mental illness patients were older,
more parous, and fewer were primiparae. Multiparous patients with a first
mental illness had had a longer interval since their last viable pregnancy,
suggesting a shift toward controlled or otherwise lowered fertility. The lower
attack rate of mental illness among pregnant women implies a salutary or
protective influence in pregnancy.

Women with a first mental illness postpartum also tended to be older, and
multiparous patients had had a delayed latest pregnancy as compared with
normal women, but differed further in being more likely to be primiparae and in
having fewer children, shorter gestation, more dystocia, lighter infants, and
higher perinatal mortality of offspring. These differences were more pronounced
for, and in some instances confined to, women diagnosed with onset of mental
illness in the first month postpartum as opposed to the next five months. The
characteristic sudden development of mental illness in the month after
parturition coincides with violent endocrine readjustments. Delayed latest
pregnancy and lower parity alike suggest either lowered fertility or a deliberate
reduction in risk of pregnancy.

One-half of the parapartum mental illness patients who became pregnant again
suffered recurrence of mental illness in one-third of their subsequent
pregnancies, each mental illness repeating in the same stage as the original
attack, prepartum or postpartum. This consistent replication suggests that the

two categories of mental illness differ in their causes.

Because they relate parapartum mental illness to age and to temporal, obstetric and perinatal variables, and show high recurrence rates with subsequent pregnancies, the present findings should be extended further with specific endocrinological studies of parapartum mental illness patients during and after any pregnancies following a first episode, especially if that illness occurred in the month immediately following parturition.

Acknowledgements

The assistance of Dexter L. Jung, Robert T. Hyde, and Elinor Kamath is gratefully acknowledged.

Editor's Comment

It is interesting to compare Paffenbarger's findings with the more recent epidemiological investigations of Kendell and his colleagues in Camberwell and Edinburgh (Kendell *et al.*, 1976; Kendell *et al.*, 1981).

In the Camberwell study they located all women giving birth during 1970 and used the Camberwell Case Register to search for those making psychiatric contact in the two years before and after the birth. 2257 women gave birth and 99 had contact with the psychiatric services during the four-year period. Only 24 were admitted to hospital, the rest being out-patient appointments. The four-year period was divided into 16 trimesters. The number of new episodes, and the number with a psychotic diagnosis are shown in Table 7.

In the Edinburgh study they used a computer link between obstetric and psychiatric record systems to locate 71 240 women giving birth during the seven-year period 1971–7. 704 of these women were admitted to the Royal Edinburgh (psychiatric) Hospital during this time. In order to study the same four-year period used in the Camberwell study, they used only those 195 mentally ill women who delivered between 1972–5. The distribution of these admissions by trimester and number with psychotic diagnoses is also shown in Table 7.

Kendell's results confirm the prominent peak of new episodes or admissions during the first trimester after childbirth. The increase is even more dramatic for functional psychoses. Nine of the 28 Camberwell psychotic episodes and 28 of the 63 Edinburgh psychoses occurred in that trimester. Over half the Edinburgh psychotic patients, who were admitted in the first trimester, were admitted in the first month after delivery.

In the Camberwell study there was a drop in new referrals in the second and third trimesters after delivery, followed by a second surge 9–18 months after. This was not confirmed in the Edinburgh study, but instead the admission rate

Table 7. Camberwell and Edinburgh epidemiological surveys

Trimester	Camberwell New Episodes (psychoses)	Edinburgh Admissions (psychoses)
−8	5 (nil)	16 (2)
−7	10 (nil)	9 (nil)
−6	11 (nil)	13 (nil)
−5	5 (2)	3 (1)
−4	9 (1)	9 (3)
−3	10 (1)	7 (2)
−2	3 (2)	9 (3)
−1	9 (1)	8 (3)
Birth		
+1	22 (9)	43 (28)
+2	7 (nil)	10 (3)
+3	6 (nil)	14 (6)
+4	14 (5)	15 (3)
+5	12 (2)	13 (4)
+6	10 (1)	15 (2)
+7	9 (nil)	10 (2)
+8	6 (4)	11 (1)

remained high after delivery compared with the rate during the year before delivery. The British studies give only slight support to Paffenbarger's low rates of mental illness during pregnancy itself. In the Camberwell study the mean of the three pregnancy trimesters was 7.3 new episodes, compared with 9.3 for the whole four-year period (though the second trimester had the lowest rate of all with only three new episodes). In the Edinburgh study the mean was eight per trimester for pregnancy and 12.2 for the whole four years.

In both studies comparisons were made between women falling ill in the puerperal trimester and other women. In the Camberwell study they were compared with those developing psychiatric episodes at other times, and the only significant difference was the higher proportion of puerperal breakdowns occurring in foreign born women. Puerperal breakdown was not associated with childbirth out of wedlock. In the Edinburgh study they were compared with all other women, and there were three statistically significant associations. Women with puerperal mental illness were less often married (79% compared with 91%), though this was not significant for psychotic women, 82% of whom were married. Secondly, they were more often delivered by Caesarian section (17% compared with 8%), and this was even more true of those with a psychotic diagnosis, 22% of whom had a Caesarian section. Thirdly, puerperal mental illness was commoner in those with no living children (i.e. primiparous women). Sixty-two percent of them were primiparous compared with the general frequency of 47%, and an even higher proportion of the psychotic women had no living children (65%). The risk for first confinements was thus 2.6/1000, and for later confinements only 1.4/1000. This confirms Paffenbarger's findings, and the conclusions of Thomas and Gordon (1959), based on a review of thirteen British and American reports, that puerperal mental illness is particularly associated with the first pregnancy.

The Edinburgh study did not confirm Paffenbarger's findings that women with puerperal mental illness were older and had shorter gestation periods, lighter babies and more obstetric complications, which must call in doubt Paffenbarger's conclusion that these illnesses are primarily somatic in origin. On the other hand they did not reveal any increased risk after twin deliveries or after stillbirths or other neonatal deaths, as might have been expected if the role of childbirth was primarily as a psychological stress or "life event".

References

Boyd, D.A. Jr (1942). Mental disorders associated with childbearing. *Am. J. Obstet. Gynec.* **43**, 148-163 & 335-349.

Brockington, I.F., Cernik, K.F., Schofield, E.M., Downing, A.R., Francis, A.F. and Keelan, C. (1981). Puerperal psychosis phenomena and diagnosis. *Arch.J. Psychiatry* **38**, 829-833.

Cornfield, J. (1962). Joint dependence of risk of coronary heart disease on serum cholesterol and systolic blood pressure: a discriminant function analysis. *Fed. Proc.* **21**, 58-61.

Dalton, K. (1980). *Depression after childbirth: how to recognize and treat postnatal depression.* Oxford University Press, London.

Hamilton, J.A. (1962). *Postpartum Psychiatric Problems.* Mosby, St. Louis.

Jaco, E.G. (1960). *The Social Epidemiology of Mental Disorders—A Psychiatric Survey of Texas.* Russell Sage Foundation, New York.

Jansson, B. (1964). *Psychic Insufficiencies Associated with Childbearing.* Munksgaard, Copenhagen.

Kendell, R.E., Wainwright, S., Hailey, A. and Shannon, B. (1976). The influence of childbirth on psychiatric morbidity. *Psychol. Med.* **6**, 297-302.

Kendell, R.E., Rennie, D., Clarke, J.A. and Dean, C. (1981). The social and obstetric correlates of psychiatric admission in the puerperium. *Psychol Med.* **11**, 341-350.

Marcé, L.V. (1858). *Traité de la Folie des Femmes Enceintes, des Nouvelles Accouchées et des Nourrices.* Baillière, Paris.

Mantel, N. and Haenszel, W. (1959). Statistical aspects of the analysis of data from retrospective studies of disease. *J. Nat. Canc. Inst.* **22**, 719-748.

Paffenbarger, R.S. Jr. (1961). The picture puzzle of the postpartum psychoses. *J. Chron. Dis.* **13**, 161-173.

Paffenbarger, R.S., Jr. (1963). Susceptibility to late postpartum hemorrhage. *Am. J. Obstet. Gynocol.* **87**, 263-267.

Paffenbarger, R.S. Jr. (1964). Epidemiological aspects of postpartum mental illness. *Br. J. Prev. Soc. Med.* **18**, 189-195.

Paffenbarger, R.S. Jr. and McCabe, L.J. Jr. (1966). The effect of obstetric and perinatal events on risk of mental illness in women of childbearing age. *Am. J. Publ. Health* **56**, 400-407.

Pugh, T.F. and MacMahon, B. (1962). *Epidemiological Findings in United States Mental Hospital Data*. Little Brown, Boston.

Strecker, E.A. and Ebaugh, F.C. (1926). Psychoses occurring during the puerperium. *Arch. Neurol. Psychiat.* **15**, 239-252.

Thomas, C.L. and Gordon, J.E. (1959). Psychosis after childbirth: ecological aspects of a single impact stress. *Am. J. Med. Sci.* **238**, 363-388.

3

Puerperal Psychosis

I.F. Brockington, G. Winokur and Christine Dean

Definition

Psychiatric research is beset by problems of definition. Diseases can be defined at various levels: initially they are often defined in terms of their clinical picture and course, or their pathology, but as the pathogenesis is unravelled they come to be defined eventually by their aetiology. Puerperal psychosis, however, is one of the few psychiatric diseases defined from the start by an aetiological association. Although the connection between parturition and psychosis is not understood at all, the association is so obvious that it was among the first wave of observations to be made when the Greeks turned their attention to medicine. It became epidemiological fact when Paffenbarger (1961, 1964; Paffenbarger *et al.*, 1966) showed that 18 times as many women were admitted to mental hospital in the first month postpartum (164) as in each month of pregnancy (9). This sudden influx of acutely psychotic women is the only reason for having a concept of puerperal psychosis. It follows that the work of reaching an accurate and agreed definition must begin by establishing the limits of the time interval after childbirth to which this increased incidence applies.

Paffenbarger's figures suggest that only women becoming ill in the first month should be considered to be suffering from this disease, because there is no excess of patients admitted during the second month. As an index of illness he used admission to hospital which is an exact measure, liable to clerical errors only. However, this time interval has two components—the time between delivery and the onset of symptoms or behavioural changes (which is due to the march of the disease), and that between onset and hospitalization, which may also be related to the severity of the illness, but is heavily influenced by social and nosocomial factors. It seems preferable to define the illness by the onset, if this can be satisfactorily determined. Unfortunately there is some loss of precision when we

37

try to define the disease by its onset, because the data are usually retrospective and come from a mentally ill patient and her relatives; they are often of poor quality, and Cernik and Brockington, independently rating the onset of 103 patients at Manchester, achieved an inter-rater reliability of only 0.61 (Cohen's kappa) when selecting those patients whose illness began within two weeks of parturition.

Accepting these limitations, one can still search for the optimum interval between delivery and onset with which to define the disease. As Thomas and Gordon (1959) point out in their thoughtful review, a great variety of intervals have been used, ranging from 18 days to six months or even a year. A glance at some clinical data, however, suggests that even the shortest of these may be too long. Figure 1 shows some data collected from the Mothers and Babies Unit at Manchester by Kate Cernik: of 239 women admitted during a five-year period, 51 had an illness starting in pregnancy, 80 had an onset in the first week after delivery, 46 in the second, 13 in the third, 8 in the fourth and the remaining 41 spread out over the rest of the first year. A similar analysis of 56 patients at Edinburgh (Dean and Kendell, 1981) showed that 15 began in pregnancy, 21 in the first week, four in the second, five in the third and the remaining 11 during the remaining eight weeks of the first trimester. All the manic patients became ill

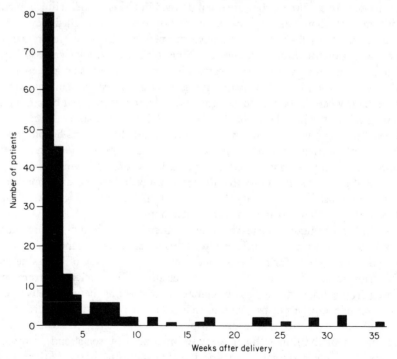

Fig. 1. Onset of illness in patients admitted to the Manchester Mothers and Babies Unit.

within the first 19 days. Marcé (1858) found the same 120 years ago, 33 of his 44 episodes beginning within 10 days of delivery, while Karnosh and Hope (1937) found that almost all postpartum illnesses which had a component of delirium began within two weeks. These figures suggest that the fuse lit by the birth of a baby is a short one, exploding into psychosis within the space of two to three weeks at the most. It is not possible at the moment to make a rational decision between 12, or 14, or 18 or 21 days as the optimum interval, but it already seems fairly certain that six weeks is too long a time, because there is no evidence of an increased risk of mental illness in weeks five and six after childbirth. It follows that we must treat with reservation those studies which have used a longer time interval to define the puerperium. This includes Esquirol's observations (1845) which were based on 92 women, only a minority of whom (37) became insane before the 15th day. His finding, for example, that mental alienation is common among unmarried mothers (29 of his 92 patients) may apply to those admitted during lactation, not immediately after delivery.

A definition expressed purely in terms of timing can never be wholly satisfactory, not only because of difficulties in establishing the onset, but also because completely different illnesses may start within that interval, either by chance or because they have their own independent causal link with childbirth. The fortuitous onset of illnesses like schizophrenia and manic depression, which have a lifetime risk of only 1 or 2%, is not very likely, because the risk for any two week period is less than 1/100 000. It is more likely that there will be contamination by other psychiatric disorders which are also precipitated or aggravated by childbirth. An analogy from general medicine may help to make this clear. Heart failure is a well recognized complication of childbearing, and at least three different cardiopathies seem to be connected with it, namely bacterial endocarditis, thromboembolic pulmonary hypertension and "cardiomyopathy" in negro women. Thus childbirth triggers at least three different causal chains leading to congestive heart failure. In the field of mental illness we can at present tentatively identify two forms of severe mental disturbance which have a specific connection with parturition, and which are probably completely different in clinical picture and cause. They are puerperal psychosis and mother–baby bonding failure (discussed in Chapter 5). If this hypothesis is correct, the two conditions will tend to contaminate each other in research studies. Attempts to isolate and study "bonding failure" will encounter patients with the depressive form of puerperal psychosis, and this will lead to dilemmas of definition and diagnosis. Although in our experience "bonding failure" presents somewhat later than puerperal psychosis on the whole, some patients present early and these will contaminate any series of puerperal psychosis defined purely by onset. The solution to these difficulties is to work out the discriminating clinical features of these different entities, so that future definitions will rest partly on timing and partly on a compatible clinical picture. Until these studies have been done, we shall have to struggle on with a temporal definition. Keeping this to within two to three weeks of childbirth, however, should keep contamination to a minimum and lead to more clear-cut findings in future research.

Early Descriptive Accounts

The systematic study of puerperal psychosis began with Esquirol's (1845) chapter on "mental alienation of those recently confined, and of nursing women" in his *Treatise on Insanity*. It was based on his work at the *Salpetrière* in Paris during the Napoleonic wars. He recognized four distinct forms—dementia (eight cases), mania (49 cases), lypemania (melancholia) and monomania (35 cases between them), but it is not clear how these were distributed between the smaller group of 37 beginning within the first 15 days, and the remaining 55 patients.

Conolly (1846), physician at Hanwell Lunatic Asylum in Middlesex, England, distinguished two varieties In his "Clinical Lectures on the Principal Forms of Insanity"—the maniacal and the melancholic:

The maniacal attack is most frequently of a lively character. The patient sings, talks incoherently, and laughs much; is sleepless and restless, and very active; dancing, undressing herself, running about, overturning chairs, breaking windows, kneeling down and praying loudly, and sometimes manifesting sexual excitement.

In the melancholic form there is general apathy and listlessness, mingled with anxiety about domestic affairs, and self-reproach for neglecting them; the patient is indifferent to food, very silent, and exhibits no affection towards her infant or her husband. The countenance is anxious, the brow wrinkled; fretfulness, vague suspicions, various delusions and a disposition to self-destruction ensue.

The Parisian alienist Louis Marcé gave a detailed account in his *Treatise on Insanity in Pregnant, Puerperal and Lactating Women* in 1858. He devoted 133 pages of his monograph to puerperal psychosis, of which he gives 31 case vignettes. His diagnostic breakdown was 29 cases of mania, 10 of melancholia, five of partial insanity and two of transitory intellectual enfeeblement. This appears to add up to 46, but he claims only 44 cases, 33 with onset in the first 10 days and the other 11 becoming ill towards the sixth week after delivery. He does not say how many of his manic patients began within the first 10 days, but nine of his quoted examples did so, the remaining three beginning on the 11th day (two cases) and towards the end of six weeks. The majority of the manic episodes developed progressively with talkativeness, labile mood, almost complete insomnia, violent agitation dangerous to the patient and the whole family, exaltation of all intellectual and nervous functions, delusions and hallucinations, erotic excitement, excessive sensitivity to sound and light, headache, incoherence and albuminuria. Three of the patients, however, had a very brief attack of excitement, e.g. his thirty-fourth case:

A 30 year old woman delivered 6 days ago of her 4th infant was suddenly seized by a "délire furieux". The first sign was that she wanted to put her baby (whom she was suckling) in a stove to cook him. The family managed to stop her, but only against her vociferous and violent resistence. When the doctor arrived it required 4 men to restrain her. She didn't recognize anyone and repeated the same words in a strident voice. She was treated with ether and immediately fell asleep for 2 hours. When she awoke she was in a rational frame of mind, though tired, and remembered nothing of the incident. She resumed her normal life 2 days later. Some years later (unrelated to childbirth) she had a similar attack.

We have seen similar cases at Manchester, for example the following:

A patient who was delivered 7 days earlier of her second infant suddenly became over-active, babbling away 19 to the dozen and writing pages and pages of absolute rubbish. She was convinced she had appendicitis and that some of the patients had been planted to spy on her. She lost her normal shyness and was swearing her head off. At times she showed great fear, trembling so much that she could not hold a cup. She seemed confused about time and place but realized that she was having a recurrence of the illness she had had after her first baby. Her motility varied between extremes. One morning she stood for 15 minutes without moving, but a few hours later she was intensely active and takative. By the 6th day she had completely recovered and forgotten most of what happened.

Marcé's cases of melancholia suffered from depression often accompanied by delusions (including delusions of persecution) and various hallucinations; six of them had a melancholic disposition or had suffered severe stresses such as stillbirth, bereavement or unwanted pregnancy. His group of patients with "partial insanity" were a mixture of different states including hypnogogic hallucinations, religious preoccupations, and unexplained suicidal or infanticidal attempts.

"Transitory intellectual enfeeblement" is an interesting condition of which he gives one example which can be compared with a similar case seen at Manchester:

A 29 year old unmarried mother, whose uncle died in an asylum from prolonged depression, had lost her memory and wandered about the streets during the early stages of her 9th pregnancy. [This was an earlier attack of psychosis in pregnancy] After the birth of her 10th baby she lost a good deal of blood. She immediately became completely incoherent, wandered here and there, made purchases for which she could not pay, chewed coal, ate candles, and made soup from kippers. On admission to hospital she was very weak, could do no work, would occasionally become agitated without reason, leave her bed and wander here and there like a dement, but she answered all questions and showed no delusions or hallucinations. She recovered completely within 2 months, worked all day in the workshop and remembered all that had happened".

Compare this with the following:

A young woman of sound premorbid personality, a Jehovah's Witness married to a Spaniard, became ill 3 days after the birth of her first baby. Her illness was dominated by one striking symptom—a marked inability to think clearly. At her first interview she said, "I'm walking around in a dream. I seem to be stuck on one thing. Thoughts don't come. I keep forgetting things. I am very slow and have to be organized by others. I'll be doing something and my mind will wander on to something else. I spent all my time on the maternity unity just trying to organize myself and my locker. I found myself wandering around and my legs got awfully tired just like when I'm tense and worrying. I am fed up with being a cabbage and having to be led around." Retrospectively she said, "I really did not know whether I was coming or going. I was very confused and did not quite understand things". The nurses described her as vague and woolly, showing little interest in the baby and strikingly incompetent. "She was very disorganized and vacant and unable to attend to the baby properly, so that she had to be removed completely from its care". There was no other marked or consistent symptom, no prominent disorder of affect, no consistent biological symptoms, no delusions or hallucinations. She had some insight—"I'm just accepting the fact that I'm a hopeless case at the moment". She spoke little and after long delays, and would stop in the middle of a sentence. She was fully orientated but made 2 errors out of the 5 subtractions she was able to do on the serial 7s test. She took her own discharge on the 4th day, and made a gradual recovery over the next 2 months without treatment, returning to her normal life.

These three early accounts of Esquirol, Conolly and Marcé recognized that contrasting forms of manic and melancholic illness accounted for most of the cases. Yet Marcé described clinical pictures which are not commonly seen in episodes of non-puerperal affective disorder.

The Debate about the Unique Features of Puerperal Psychosis

From the time of Esquirol, psychiatrists have debated whether or not this psychosis is a distinct disease entity. It appears that orthodox opinion has always held that there are no pathognomonic symptoms, while defensively aware of the heretics who believed otherwise. Marcé wrote (1858, p.204) that "puerperal mania has neither in its psychotic manifestations nor its physical symptoms anything specific to itself", and the only way to distinguish it from other cases of mania was to search for the signs of recent delivery.

Gundry (1860) who collected a large series of cases at Ohio Lunatic Asylum, stated even more categorically that "no man who passes into the company of insane women unacquainted with their history can pick out those labouring under puerperal insanity in any of its forms".

Towards the end of the century we find Sir James Crichton Brown belabouring Dr Savage (who had just expressed the view that there was no special definite form of insanity deserving the name "puerperal mania") for being "rather too apt to seize upon the puerperium and connect it with the insanity. They did not refer to measles occurring during the puerperium as 'puerperal measles' ". Dr Jacobs of Edinburgh (1943) considered the matter finally settled, concluding "It has been proved that 'puerperal insanity' does not exist and that every reaction type defined in clinical psychiatry may occur in the puerperium". By that time at least 10 diagnostic analyses had appeared (Table 1). They all recognized that affective and schizophrenic psychoses occurred in the puerperium and most showed quite a high proportion of toxic psychoses too. Further diagnostic studies have appeared (Table 1) and in 1957 Foundeur et al. published a comparison between a large series of "postpartum mental illness" and 100 controls, carried out at the New York Hospital, Westchester Division, in the 1950s. They found the same high proportion of schizophrenic cases in both groups (50%). They defined postpartum mental illness very loosely as "any mental illness in a female patient in which childbirth is a major precipitating factor independent of the time of onset", including illnesses which began during pregnancy. Another odd feature of their patient selection was that the mean duration of illness before admission was 13.9 months in the postpartum group and 19 months in the controls. It seems almost certain that their series was heavily contaminated with episodes not closely related to the puerperium. As for the diagnoses of schizophrenia, we now know that they were made at a time when Americans had an extremely broad concept of schizophrenia almost equivalent to psychosis (Cooper *et al.*, 1972). Foundeur's study was probably influential in consolidating opinion against the recognition of puerperal psychosis as a specific entity, so that it has been steadily eliminated from official nosologies. A vestigial remnant appeared in the eighth Revision of the International Classification of Diseases, under heading 294.4 "Psychosis associated with Childbirth", where "unspecified psychosis" occurring within six weeks of delivery could be coded if not classifiable under headings 295–298

Table 1. Hospital diagnoses made in patients with puerperal psychosis.

	First author	Country	Number of patients	Schizo-phrenia	Affective psychosis	Toxic psychosis	Other
					Percentage of patients		
1911	Runge	Germany	—	37	20	25	—
1924	Gregory	USA	114	16	46	27	11
1926	Kilpatrick	USA	72	14	50	32	4
1926	Strecker	USA	50	26	36	34	4
1927	Ellery	Australia	89	24	30	44	2
1928	Stone	USA	85	45	35	19	1
1929	Saunders	USA	75	60	40	—	—
1933	Anderson	UK	50	18	70	8	4
1940	Smalldon	USA	220	29	49	4	18
1942	Boyd	USA	150	18	31	29	22
1950	Brew	USA	83	51	41	5	3
1952	Hemphill	UK	140	22	58	—	20
1955	Polonio	Portugal	244	28	3	48	21
1957	Foundeur	USA	100	50	25	—	25
1958	Martin	Ireland	75	58	37	2	1
1958	Madden	USA	116	65	15	—	20
1968	Melges	USA	100	51	31	—	18
1969	Protheroe	UK	134	28	67	5	—
1971	Shah	India	102	35	28	12	25
1978	Hyde	UK	50	26	42	—	32

(schizophrenia, affective psychosis, paranoid and other psychoses). In the ninth Revision it is necessary to turn to the section on obstetrics to find any mention of it. In the third edition of the American Psychiatric Association Diagnostic and Statistical Manual (DSM III), it is mentioned under 298.9 "atypical psychosis", with the proviso that disorders thus classified "do not meet the criteria for an organic mental disorder, schizophreniform disorder, paranoid disorder or affective disorder".

There have, however, always been mavericks ready to assert the contrary opinion. Esquirol (1845) was the first to mention the matter:

> Mental alienation which makes its appearance during or after lactation presents little difference in character from insanity which breaks forth under any other circumstances. Notwithstanding there is something peculiar in its aspect which causes it to be recognized by one who is accustomed to the care of the insane.

In 1847 James McDonald, who collected 49 cases from the Bloomingdale Asylum, wrote

> Is there anything in the character of puerperal insanity to distinguish it from other forms of madness? In the acute form of the mania which succeeds parturition we observe an intensity of mental excitement, an excessive incoherence, a degree of fever and, above all, a disposition to mingle obscene words with the broken sentences, things which are rarely noted in other circumstances.

Robert Jones, Medical Superintendent of the Claybury Asylum, made a clear statement in favour of its specificity in 1902. He had an extensive experience of 120 cases (65 manic, 52 melancholic) occurring within six months of confinement. He wrote

> My experience leads me to conclude that there is no type associated with pregnancy or lactation, but with parturition and the period immediately succeeding it the case is different ... The gibberish nonsense, erotic immodest conduct and bad language, the evolutions of shameless indecency, accompanied by noisy delirium and marked religious exaltation, with purposeless restlessness, characterize—sum up if I may say so—the insanity of the puerperal period ... it presents with such a marked delirium, with wildness and delusions of a hallucinatory character in which religious and erotic features become so prominent ("wild delirious excitement") that I recognize an almost distinct nosological entity, a view I am bound to confess is not supported by high authorities.

In 1937 Karnosh and Hope stated that delirium was the special attribute of the puerperal psychoses. They wrote

> By far the most common denominator in these acute puerperal psychoses is delirium; the more abrupt the onset the more profound is the clouding of the sensorium.

The delirium is described in these terms:

> panic, confusion, sudden aversion to and distrust of relatives, misidentification, hallucinosis, sing-song jargon and disintegration of normal affect together with a rapid pulse, tremor, quick dehydration and a fever ranging from 99° to 102° were the most common features.

They seem to be claiming that a large proportion of their patients (51/78 of those starting within two weeks, according to their Figure 2) were suffering from an acute organic syndrome.

In modern times the champion of the view that postpartum psychoses are a specific disease entity has been Dr James Hamilton of San Francisco, especially in his monograph *Postpartum Psychiatric Problems* (1962). In Chapter 1 of this volume he has set out his reasons for holding this opinion, and he also participated in one of the diagnostic studies which will now be described.

Recent Clinical Investigations

The problem of the specificity of puerperal psychosis deserves to be tackled with the more precise tools of clinical investigation introduced in the last 20 years, including the structured inventory of symptoms and operationally defined definitions (Wing *et al.*, 1974; Spitzer *et al.*, 1975). In this section some modern studies carried out in Iowa (USA), Manchester (England) and Edinburgh (Scotland) will be reviewed.

The Manchester studies began with a pilot study of the records of patients admitted to the Mothers and Babies unit during its first five years. There were 135 patients admitted, including 50 whose illnesses began within two weeks of delivery, the remainder beginning during pregnancy or later in the first puerperal year. (These are a different set of patients from those whose onset was analysed by Kate Cernik, see p.38.) Dr Hyde made transcripts of the mental state of these patients, and of 50 non-puerperal psychotic controls, eliminating all clues to the presence of recent childbirth. The transcripts were then studied by two doctors (Dr Hamilton and Dr Brockington) and two social workers (Mrs Baynes and Mrs Monkhouse). The psychiatric social workers were thoroughly familiar with psychopathological concepts but had little experience of puerperal mental illness, and they were not able to pick out the postpartum patients any better than by chance, thus demonstrating that Dr Hyde had successfully eliminated all non-clinical clues. The psychiatrists, however, were able to identify patients with onset within two weeks of delivery. This was especially true of Dr Hamilton who diagnosed 53 cases as puerperal and was correct in 27 instances ($P < 0.01$), thus vindicating his claim that there was something different about these psychoses.

Following this pilot study, a prospective clinical investigation was begun, and has now been in progress for over five years. The phenomena of the illness were documented by a broad clinical approach, using multiple information sources, multiple raters and extensive narrative descriptions (a method outlined by Brockington and Meltzer, in press). The observations included structured interviews held with the patient and the next-of-kin, a brief videotaped interview with the patient, systematic nursing observations (Downing *et al.*, 1980) and a self-rating procedure. At the end of the admission, these research data (excluding the self-ratings) were reviewed together with the hospital case notes by three raters, who made their own ratings independently and then compared their findings. Computer averaging was used to derive a set of "master ratings" for each patient. So far the results have been analysed for 58 patients with puerperal psychosis (admitted up until May 1979) and 52 non-puerperal episodes of psychosis in women of the same age range (17–37 years).

The results support the views of Esquirol, McDonald, Jones, Karnosh and Hope and Hamilton—that puerperal psychoses can be distinguished from others by their psychopathology. Out of 214 variables studied, 52 showed statistically significant differences. Sixteen items, scales or factors derived from observation and two scales derived from self-rating (which had the advantage of being free from observer bias) showed differences at the 0.01 level of significance (Table 2). The largest differences were concerned with incompetence and confusion (two items and two scales), which were much more severe in the puerperal group. Most of the other differences were concerned with the relative lack of schizophrenic phenomena in the puerperal patients (eight items and scales and the two self-rating scales). A wide range of schizophrenic phenomena appeared to be less frequent or less severe in the puerperal patients, including persecution, delusional systematization, auditory hallucinations and affective flattening. In addition to the phenomena shown in Table 2, a number of manic symptoms also showed differences, but at a lower level of significance. Elation, lability of mood, rambling speech or flight of ideas, distractibility, euphoria, excessive

Table 2. Differences between puerperal and other psychoses (Manchester study).

Variable	Frequency or mean score Puerperal psychosis	Controls	P
Systematized delusions (item)	4	15	0.005
Systematization of delusions (scale)	21	35	0.004
Persecution (scale)	13	24	0.003
Persecution (self-rating)	2.8	4.4	0.002
Paranoid symptoms (factor)	78	116	0.007
Auditory hallucinations, quality (scale)	17	31	0.006
Auditory hallucinations, frequency (scale)	15	31	0.004
Auditory hallucinations (factor)	27	52	0.004
Odd affect (scale)	14	24	0.003
Psychosis (self-rating)	1.7	2.7	0.006
Social withdrawal (scale)	19	31	0.0007
Needs supervision for tasks (item)	40	14	0.0001
Cannot help with ward chores (item)	20	5	0.004
Incompetence (scale)	44	32	0.009
Confusion (scale)	19	11	0.0008
Unrealistic in expressing feelings (item)	6	20	0.001
Asks for reassurance (item)	28	10	0.002
Alcohol abuse (item)	0	8	0.006

activity and a manic factor score were all more frequent or more severe in the puerperal group ($P < 0.05$).

These results do not establish that puerperal psychosis is a specific entity. They support this position, but there are other explanations for the findings. It may be, as Clarke suggested in 1913, that "some forms of insanity are far more frequently associated" with the puerperal state than others. The frequency of various diagnoses was examined in the Manchester patients, using the Research Diagnostic Criteria (RDC, Spitzer *et al.*, 1975). This showed a marked difference in the diagnostic profile of puerperal and non-puerperal psychoses ($P < 0.001$). Twenty-five of the puerperal group qualified for a manic diagnosis (17 mania and eight schizo-affective mania) compared with only 11 controls (10 mania and one schizo-affective mania). The number of depressions was equal (26 puerperals and 25 controls), but there was a large difference in the number who met criteria for schizo-affective depression (four puerperals and 12 controls). The largest difference was in the number of schizophrenic patients (five puerperals and 16 controls). Even these five puerperal patients seemed atypical of schizophrenia, since three had manic self-ratings, and two had manic or schizo-affective manic episodes after another pregnancy. Thus it appears that Clarke was right, and that a segment of the psychotic spectrum, roughly equivalent to the paranoid psychoses, is missing from the puerperal group. This is not to deny that typical schizophrenic symptoms are to be found in these patients (including catatonic symptoms, auditory hallucinations and delusions of possession), but generally speaking they only occur in the context of a manic mood disorder.

A similar diagnostic analysis was done at Edinburgh (Dean and Kendell, 1981). Using the Edinburgh Case Register, all women admitted to mental hospital within 90 days of childbirth from 1971 to 1977 were identified, and RDC diagnoses made from the case records. It was found that 49 (69%) were suffering from depression, nine (13%) from mania or hypomania, four from schizo-affective disorder, eight from other conditions and only one from schizophrenia. The number of manic admissions was much higher than was found among all female hospital admissions during the same period (3%, $P < 0.0001$). If puerperal psychosis was strictly defined as beginning within two weeks, there were 24 cases of whom nine (38%) were suffering from mania or schizo-affective mania. Both British studies, therefore, agree that using RDC very few puerperal patients are schizophrenic and nearly 40% are manic. About 90% of the patients in both series were suffering from affective disorders. When looking for a parsimonious solution to the nosological problem of the puerperal psychoses, the first hypothesis to be considered is that they are manic depressive psychoses. This is an attractive hypothesis because it has already been demonstrated that manic patients have a high puerperal breakdown rate (Reich and Winokur, 1969).

One way to test this hypothesis is to compare the symptomatology of puerperal psychosis with non-puerperal affective disorders. The first attempt to do this was by Kadrmas *et al.* (1980) using the records of women admitted to the University of Iowa Psychiatric Hospital between 1920 and 1950. During that time the case records were all typewritten, making it possible to carry out extensive chart studies. In that 30-year period, 157 patients with an RDC of mania were admitted, of which 21 began in the postpartum period. A study of their psychopathology showed that 13 of the 21 (62%) had "first rank symptoms of Schneider", compared with only 38 of the 136 controls (28%), the difference being highly significant ($P < 0.005$). Schneider's first rank symptoms include third person auditory hallucinations, passivity experiences and some other phenomena thought by some to be diagnostic of schizophrenia, and the implication is that the puerperal mania is more severe in certain parameters of psychopathology.

Attempts to compare puerperal with non-puerperal mania have also been made in Edinburgh and Manchester. At Edinburgh, puerperal manics were compared with control manics, and puerperal schizo-affective manics with schizo-affective controls; no differences were found, though the numbers were small. At Manchester, 21 puerperal manics and schizo-affective manics (taken together, excluding four of the original 25 who also had depressive phenomena) were compared with the eleven patients from the comparison series who had either of these diagnoses. In spite of the small numbers, there were many differences. There were 11 significant differences among 180 items and scales, including 4 at the 1% level of significance or better (Table 3). The largest were concerned with the two scales "confusion" and "disorganized speech", recalling the "excessive incoherence" of McDonald (1847) and the "wild delirious excitement" and "gibberish nonsense" of Jones (1902). Although a statistically significant excess of first rank symptoms was not found, the excess of schizo-affective mania ($P < 0.10$, Fisher's exact test) was in line with the Iowa findings. Both studies show striking differences between puerperal and non-puerperal mania.

The corresponding study in the realm of depression would be the comparison of puerperal depressive illness with the depressed form of manic depressive

Table 3. Differences between puerperal and non-puerperal mania (Manchester study).

Variable	Frequency or mean score		*P*
	Puerperal mania	Non-puerperal mania	
Number of patients	21	11	
Needs supervision in tasks (item)	11	1	0.001
Incompetence (scale)	52.9	27.9	0.006
Confusion (scale)	23.8	8.5	0.0005
Disorganized communication (scale)	32.2	17.8	0.0009

Table 4. Differences between puerperal and other depressions (Manchester study).

Variable	Frequency or mean score Puerperal depression	Non-puerperal depression	P
Sadness (self-rating)	2.7	3.9	0.004
Anger (self-rating)	1.6	2.8	0.008
Hostility (scale)	29.7	43.7	0.005
Increased tempo (item)	9	1	0.003
Confusion (scale)	13.0	5.8	0.005
Obsessional checking and repeating (item)	2	16	0.007

illness. In practice this is a difficult study to undertake because it is hard to recognize bipolar depression except by the occurrence of mania at other times in the patient's life, and it takes years to assemble a sufficient group of patients carefully studied during the depressed phase. Attempts have been made to approach this problem, both at Manchester and Edinburgh, by different routes. At Manchester, 40 puerperal depressions (26 admitted up to the time of the first analysis, and 14 admitted since then) were compared with 54 other cases of depression admitted to the Mothers and Babies unit, starting during pregnancy or more than two weeks after delivery. The findings are preliminary because the rating of the dossiers is not yet complete, so there are no "master ratings", and only the separate sets of mental state ratings, nurse ratings and self-ratings (which are likely to be less sensitive) are available for the comparison. Even so, numerous differences have been found between the strictly defined puerperal depressions and other depressive illnesses. There were 22 significant differences among 218 variables studied, including six at the 1% level (Table 4). Puerperal depressives showed less anger, sadness and neurotic symptoms, higher confusion scores and (unexpectedly) more complaints of "increased tempo", i.e. they experienced the outside world as moving too fast for them. The scores on a discriminant function, using the 10 items and scales showing the largest differences, showed a bimodal distribution, suggesting that it might (with further work) be possible to distinguish sharply between puerperal and non-puerperal depression.

At Edinburgh, 33 of the 71 patients admitted within 90 days of childbirth who had research diagnoses of "major depressive disorder" were compared with 33 non-puerperal women of the same age admitted with this diagnosis. The results are shown in Table 5. Forty-two items were examined (the 38 syndromes of the Present State Examination and four others—lability of mood, disorientation, perplexity and "psychosis", i.e. the presence of delusions or hallucinations.) Seven showed differences at the 5% level. When the comparison was made

Table 5. Differences between puerperal and non-puerperal depression (Edinburgh study).

Item	Non-puerperal	Puerperal All	Puerperal Starting within 14 days
Number of patients	33	33	14
Delusions or hallucinations	5	15^a	8^b
"Non-specific psychosis" (PSE)	11	18^a	10^c
Depressive delusions (PSE)	4	13^a	7^a
Slowness (PSE)	9	19^a	8
Agitation (PSE)	7	16^a	7
Lability of mood	1	9^a	5^b
Perplexity	6	13	8^a
Disorientation	none	6^a	3^a
Organic impairment (PSE)	none	4	3^a

PSE = syndrome defined by Present State Examination (Wing et al., 1974).
$^aP = <0.05$, $^bP = <0.01$, $^cP = <0.001$, comparing puerperal groups with controls.

between the 14 patients with onset in the first two weeks, and the controls, the differences were more striking. A high proportion of the puerperal group showed the PSE syndrome "non-specific psychosis", delusions or hallucinations, perplexity and retardation. Three of the 14 patients were disorientated.

These results suggest that there is a difference in the quality of depression starting in the immediate puerperium and that which leads to hospital admission at other times. The points at issue are whether the clinical picture is compatible with that of bipolar depression, or whether it has special features of its own. Unfortunately not much is known about the clinical picture of bipolar depression. The most successful attempt to demonstrate differences between it and other depressions was that of Beigel and Murphy (1971) who showed that these patients exhibit less pacing, anger, somatic complaints and anxiety. Brockington et al. (1980) have also found evidence that bipolar depression less often presents in schizoaffective form. The Manchester findings suggest that the clinical picture is compatible with bipolar depression, in that the patients showed relatively little hostility, and were seldom given a diagnosis of schizo-affective depression. Both studies, however, found that "confusion" was often present and this has not, to our knowledge, been reported as characteristic of manic depressive illness.

Another study which suggests that there is a difference between puerperal psychosis and manic depression is that of Hays (1978). He carried out a cluster analysis on 147 "schizophrenic" patients collected in Edmonton, Canada and obtained three stable clusters—Kretchmer's sensitive psychosis, puerperal psychosis and atypical manic depressive disease. A canonical variate analysis of these groups indicated that the main differences between the last two were that puerperal psychosis was more often depressive in its mode of onset, and was more often associated with catatonic symptoms, auditory perceptual distortions and delusions of reference, while atypical manic depression had a relatively high frequency of visual hallucinations and primary delusions. It would be interesting to see whether puerperal psychosis emerged as a distinct cluster if the item "physical stress: childbirth" was not included in the analysis, because the symptomatic differences between the two groups seemed relatively weak.

The only symptom which has so far consistently emerged as "specific" of puerperal psychosis is "confusion". This element keeps cropping up in descriptive accounts of the disease (e.g. Clarke, 1913; Kilpatrick and Tiebout, 1926; Skottowe, 1942; Vislie, 1956; Protheroe, 1969; Thuwe, 1974). It is embarrassing that the nature of this "confusion" is so unclear. At the moment it is simply a clinical observation that the patient is unable to function at an elementary level and appears bewildered, perplexed or dreamy. Highly "confused" patients were consistent in their self-rating responses and performed normally on memory testing, so it seems unlikely that it is due to widespread cerebral dysfunction as in delirium. "Confusion" is one of the pathognomonic signs of the cycloid psychoses (Perris, 1974). Some of the patients seen at Manchester seem typical of this disease picture. Some believe that the cycloid and manic depressive psychoses are closely related (Brockington *et al.*, 1982). If the concept of manic depression were extended to include the cycloid patients, there would be no problem in recognizing puerperal psychosis as typical manic depressive insanity.

The Course of the Illness

Onset

Puerperal psychoses have a reputation for having an acute onset. This, however, is not so invariable or obvious as to be universally acknowledged. Marcé wrote:

> Its onset is sometimes sudden. A woman described by Dr. Reid went to sleep in good health, woke suddenly crying that her child was dead and from that moment was insane. But in the great majority of cases events proceed progressively and after a prodromal period that all authors have noted and which varies from some hours to 5–6 days, the women are sad, morose and more often excited.

(Onset over the course of five to six days is acute compared with most psychoses.) Gundry (1860) emphasized the insidious onset:

> The period of incubation in puerperal insanity varies. It is in a majority of cases gradual and progressive. It may be sudden and decisive. In the second epoque (the puerperium) the latter is more frequently the case than at either of the other periods

(pregnancy and lactation), yet it cannot be said to characterize a large proportion of these cases. Often it happens that long before any attack is apprehended the patient is exceedingly influenced by overwrought emotions.

He admits, however, that "except in a few cases it has not been my fortune to observe the actual inception of the disease", which is true of modern studies as well.

It was Clouston (1896) who particularly emphasized the acuteness of onset:

Of the 60 cases no less than 43 were very acute in character and symptoms while 17 only were mild and without acute symptoms. 29 of the 43 acute cases were generally maniacal in character and 14 generally melancholic with motor excitement, some of each of these classes changing from one state to the other at times. I know of no clinical form of insanity that would yield so large a proportion of very acute cases. Puerperal insanity may therefore be regarded as the most acute of all forms.

It is not quite clear what Clouston means by "acute". He appears to be contrasting "acute" (with "absolute delirium" as its extreme form) with "mild", so that the quality of "acuteness" is conferred by the florid and severe symptomatology especially if this contrasts with the patient's calmness and sanity at the time of delivery. "Acuteness" should really mean a rapid change from normality to the fully developed syndrome. The rate of development of a psychosis is often hard to gauge. The time interval between onset and admission may be a measure of it, though this is also influenced by the amount of social disturbance and the risk to mother or child. Some data obliquely relevant to this matter were obtained at Manchester. It was found that puerperal psychosis had a more clearly localized onset than other illnesses, in the sense that the raters were more certain about the timing. Of those episodes beginning within two weeks of delivery, 56 out of 86 (65%) had a "certain" onset, while the remainder were hard to pinpoint. Only 27 of the 68 (40%) patients whose illness began outside that time interval had a "certain" onset.

Recovery

There is a general consensus that puerperal psychoses have an excellent prognosis. This was clearly recognized by Esquirol (1845):

Mental alienation following confinement is generally cured if the predisposition is not too energetic. More than half are restored. Among our 92 women, 55 were cured, constituting one seventh of the total number of cures at the Salpetrière during the 4 year period [Puerperal and lactational psychoses accounted for one twelfth of the women admitted].

Connolly (1846) states that "cases of puerperal insanity appear to afford a better prospect of recovery than any other". Seventeen of his 26 patients who survived recovered and nine remained in an incurable state. McDonald's (1847) figures were 53 recoveries out of 61 survivors. Marcé (1858) states that cure is the most frequent end result, 16 out of 20 surviving manic patients and eight out of 10 melancholics recovering. Gundry (1860) quotes three other authorities with 60% recovery rates, and gives his own experience as 31 recovered and four improved out of 50 survivors (70%). Clouston (1895) emphasized the "great curability" and Herman (1896) said that "there *was* such a thing as 'puerperal insanity' which is characterized by its curability". All these studies were made at a time when there was no effective treatment. It is still true, however, that this psychosis has a relatively good prognosis. Dr Hyde's record study at Manchester showed that 35 out of 50 patients had completely recovered at the time of discharge and 15 were improved. In a comparison group of non-puerperal psychoses there were 17 full recoveries, 28 partial recoveries and five treatment failures.

The Duration of the Illness

It is interesting to note the duration of the illness before modern treatments were introduced. Esquirol (1845) stated that 38 of his 55 cures took place in the first six months; the median duration in his study, and that of McDonald (1847) (who gave a detailed breakdown of the timing of recovery), was five months. It was the same 50 years later when Menzies (1893) described a series of 64 cases seen at Rainhill hospital near Liverpool, with an average duration of 5.8 months. Connolly (1846) gives a harrowing description of the difficulties of nursing manic patients for such a long period of time without potent tranquillizers:

> For 8 long months this patient was almost constantly excited by night and by day: talking incessantly; often swearing; untiringly active, running about the wards or the airing-court, and riding the rocking horses like one possessed. She used to fasten a quantity of coir to her hair, which gave her a kind of unearthly appearence; and she would stamp until one might almost have fancied that our solid stone floors would give way. [There follows an account of his treatment with leeches, blisters, warm baths and cold showers, antimony, digitalis, camphor, ammonia, ether, henbane and morphia, in spite of which] the head continued to be generally hot, and sometimes her appearence became changed and haggard. She was in a very excited state, often mistaking persons and becoming very violent. She unfortunately began to mistake Mrs Bowden for someone of whom she was jealous, and made some rather desperate attacks on her ... Then by slow degrees she became more tranquil, and at that time the matron found that the patient had become impressed with the idea that if emplóyed in her service she should recover, as others had done. The opportunity was afforded to her, and some days afterward, while waiting on the matron, she suddenly threw her arms around her neck, and asked her if she could ever forgive the attacks she had made upon her. She then told the matron that after being a few days in her kitchen, it seemed as if at thick veil was all at once removed from her, and she felt well.

Connolly, McDonald and Clouston mention some very late cures, e.g. two years, or 40 months after the onset. Clouston writes, "To prevent anything like loss of hope I mention that one of the melancholic cases with stupor recovered after the disease had existed for 4 years".

It is interesting that the prolonged duration continued right up until the second world war, according to Protheroe (1969) who followed up 134 patients admitted to St Nicholas's hospital, Newcastle-upon-Tyne between 1927 and 1961. The average stay in hospital between the years 1927 and 1936 was eight months, but by 1952–61, it had fallen to 2.4 months. It is doubtful whether we could improve on that figure at the present time.

Mortality Rate

Until quite recently a number of patients in each series died of puerperal psychosis. Summating seven nineteenth century studies (those of Esquirol, Connolly, McDonald, Marcé, Gundry, Clouston and Menzies), 36 out of 397 patients died (9%). An appreciable mortality rate continued into this century. Arentsen (1968) who followed up 168 Danish cases dating back to the 1930s gives a mortality rate of 10% in the acute stage, and Protheroe (1969) states that the mortality rate was 25% before 1950 and nil since then, attributing the deaths to "the inability to control the spread of hospital infections and the poor nutrition of patients who remained withdrawn or excited" for long periods. An exception to these findings is the study of Vislie (1956) in Oslo, who reported that only three out of 81 patients admitted between 1926 and 1950 died, only one of them in the acute stage.

It is impossible to know what were the causes of death in these women who died so long ago, but the early authorities (Marcé, Gundry and Clouston) and also Arentsen all claimed that some of their patients died from "maniacal exhaustion". Marcé lost four patients in this way, 7–26 days after delivery.

> The agitation mounts from day to day, the tongue becomes dry, abdominal function is affected; the pulse accelerates and soon reaches 120/minute, the face is flushed, the head hot, the eye haggard, the skin covered by sticky sweat; responding to incessant hallucinations the patients are consumed by a violent agitation and an unstoppable loquacity, and are no longer aware of anything around them; under the influence of their delusions or hydrophobia they refuse food and above all drink.

After a few days of continuous insomnia, they become doubly incontinent and die during a syncopal attack. Nothing is found at postmortem.

One thing that stands out in these accounts is the rarity of *suicide*. Although suicide attempts are quite common (Gundry, 1856; Vislie, 1956), it is hard to find a single report of a death by suicide during an attack of puerperal psychosis.

Infanticide

Infanticide has always been recognized as one of the hazards of this disease. A famous English case, reported in 1848, has been mentioned by Dr Hamilton in Chapter 1. Marcé emphasizes the risk to the newborn and the importance of removing him from the mother. He mentions the strange case of a "modest and virtuous woman" who disappeared shortly after childbirth and was found in a well with a tiny entrance, unable to explain how she got there. All went well for some days. Nineteen days after delivery she went to bed after dinner; while she was asleep the baby disappeared and was discovered drowned in the well. These cases, however, appear to be very uncommon. Hopwood (1927), who studied

166 women admitted to Broadmoor between 1900 and 1925 for child murder, stated that infanticide was uncommon in puerperal insanity occurring soon after confinement, and especially in mania. It was more common when the insanity took the form of melancholia with delusions of unworthiness, but most of the cases occurred during "lactational insanity". Provided that puerperal psychosis is distinguished from "bonding failure" (by its symptomatology and timing), only 3/93 mothers admitted to the Manchester Unit with the psychosis made any form of attack on the baby (see Chapter 7).

Response to Treatment

According to Protheroe (1969) there was a dramatic change in the outcome of puerperal psychosis about 1950, with a precipitous drop in the mortality rate and duration of hospitalization. This he attributes mainly to electroconvulsive therapy. The first reports of the use of ECT in these patients were published within three to four years of its introduction (Cruickshank, 1940; Kraines, 1941). Kraines reported very favourably on the new treatment: "The results of such therapy are often amazingly rapid. In many instances two or three convulsive doses result in a permanent cure". He treated nine patients, seven of whom made a complete recovery after 4–10 treatments and two improved sufficiently to return home. It appears that these recoveries occurred within one to four weeks of the beginning of treatment.

According to Impastato and Gabriel (1959), ECT was used to treat thousands of women in the postpartum period during the next 15 years, but they could find not a single article describing or analysing its use. They collected 57 cases reported in the literature and added their own experience of 14 cases. They were chiefly concerned with its safety at a time when venous thrombosis was common. They state that 69 of the 71 patients had no complications from the therapy, but two died. In both cases there was a possibility that death was due to pulmonary embolism, but in neither case was this established beyond doubt, and even if this was the cause of death, there was no certainty that ECT had contributed to its occurrence. They make no attempt to analyse the effectiveness of ECT, and to our knowledge the only study reporting a therapeutic trial is that of Baker *et al.* (1961) at Banstead hospital near London. They compared a course of 20 ECT to chlorpromazine 300–1200mg daily in 20 women, randomly assigned:

> The results from the first 20 patients showed that a good remission was not obtained by chlorpromazine alone. Many patients retained flattening of affect, lack of initiative and retardation. Only one patient of those treated with chlorpromazine recovered sufficiently to be discharged forthwith, all the others needing ECT as well. Our follow-up clinic, however, showed that though patients treated with a course of 20 ECT made a good social recovery, they often needed a small dose of chlorpromazine after discharge to maintain their remission.

This is a helpful report, but no-one has provided data to prove that the duration of this benign illness is reduced by ECT. Although many psychiatrists practising in this area believe that it is an effective treatment, there are no data to show whether it is effective in all varieties (manic and schizo-affective manic as well as depressed), and it is anyone's guess whether it is more effective than the powerful newer antipsychotic agents like haloperidol, or lithium.

There are two small treatment trials comparing neuroleptics with other drugs. Steiner *et al.* (1973) compared propranolol (600–3200mg daily) with chlorpromazine (up to 800mg daily) in 10 patients with "psychosis associated with childbearing", five patients being treated with each drug. Propranolol appeared to have some advantage, but it seems doubtful if more than a few of these patients were suffering from the early-onset psychosis, because the mean interval between delivery and onset was 14.4 days in the propranolol group and 35.2 days in the chlorpromazine group. The other study was reported by Silbermann *et al.* (1975) who report favourably on a combination of perfenazine and lithium in the treatment of "postpartum delirium". Although they do not define this condition by its onset, their description of "constantly varying degrees of consciousness", perplexity and "great motoric unrest and considerable motoric and verbal abandon" is typical of puerperal psychosis. They first mention two patients responding rapidly or completely to lithium after the failure of other treatments to control the condition; one of these patients had been given 15 drugs or combinations in 97 days and improved notably within two days of receiving lithium. Encouraged by this experience they used a combination of perfenazine and lithium in 13 patients, comparing them with six patients studied before this powerful regime was introduced. They found that the recovery time fell from a mean of 19.5 weeks to 11.6 weeks.

Scarcely anything has been written on the effectiveness of tricyclic antidepressants in puerperal depression. In the Edinburgh study it was found that puerperal depressives tended not to respond to this treatment (with an 18% response rate compared with 40% in the controls, $P < 0.10$), and that more of them were treated with phenothiazines (42% compared with 24%). This may not be true, however, of the milder cases treated at home by their general practitioners.

Some bold spirits have based their therapeutic efforts on the belief that gynaecological dysfunction or hormone deficiency lay at the root of the trouble. Delay and his colleagues (1953), believing that no patient recovered before her menses were restored, employed curettage of the womb and claimed successes. Several reports describe the use of progesterone, with or without oestrogens. Sometimes it was used in combination with ECT (Billig and Bradley 1946; Tucker, 1962). Kane and Keeler (1965) prescribed progesterone alone to two patients, who recovered. Several have reported that progesterone or the oral contraceptive "enovid" prevented relapses (Schmidt, 1943; Bower & Altschule, 1956; Keeler *et al.* 1964); the most impressive of these is the study of Bower and Altschule who found that progesterone reduced the relapse rate from 44% (17 out of 39 patients) to 6% (one out of 16 patients). Dalton (1980) uses progesterone to treat postnatal depression. At Manchester we carried out a double-blind randomized controlled trial of "duphaston" (dydrogesterone) 20mg daily, given in addition to the psychiatrist's own treatment, and found no beneficial effect in a total series of 22 patients. Other hormones have been used. Kraines (1941) used testosterone to stop paramenstrual relapses in one patient. Hamilton, in Chapter 1, has described his experience of the prophylactic effects of an intramuscular injection of oestrogen and testosterone at the time of delivery. Finally Railton (1961), who believed that postpartum depression resembled "the corticoid withdrawal syndrome", treated 16 of these patients with 10–20mg prednisolone, and compared them with 16 others not so treated. Those receiving prednisolone fared better: five with a history of previous attacks did not become depressed; eight improved after 3–4 weeks treatment and the remaining three did not, but their depressions lasted only 2–5 months compared with eight months in the comparison group. These patients treated by Railton had a mild disorder not requiring hospital admission.

There is an almost complete lack of properly conducted treatment trials in this disease, no doubt partly due to its rarity, but also perhaps to the belief that it is but a miscellaneous group of completely different psychiatric states. Although it is a benign condition, and lasts only 2–3 months in most patients, this is still a very long time for these hard-pressed families and it seems probable that careful investigations of the effect of ECT, tricyclic agents, neuroleptics (e.g. haloperidol) and lithium, in the manic and depressed subgroups separately, would cut down the duration of morbidity. These studies would probably require collaboration between Mother and Baby units in order to obtain adequate numbers.

At the present time we recommend that a patient with a severe puerperal psychosis, starting within two weeks of delivery, be admitted to hospital with or without her baby. The advantages of joint admission are discussed in Chapter 8. Within the first week a diagnosis is made, excluding the main alternative diagnosis of mother–baby bonding disorder. A patient with the clinical picture of mania, schizo-affective mania or schizophrenia should be treated with neuroleptics, lithium or both, and, if there is no response within a month, with ECT. If the clinical picture is one of depression, particularly delusional depression, we favour the use of ECT at an early stage. Expert nursing (including attention to nutrition and fluid balance in severely excited patients) and social casework to support the families are particularly important in these patients.

Recurrences after Further Pregnancies

It is well-known that these women tend to relapse after subsequent pregnancies. Esquirol's (1845) second patient had 13 successive episodes; she recovered from each and "enjoyed the perfect use of her reason". Table 6 summarizes six studies

Table 6. Recurrences after further pregnancies.

Authors	Proportion of patients	Proportion of pregnancies
Vislie (1956)	3 of 15	—
Foundeur *et al.* (1957)	3 of 22	3 of 27
Paffenbarger (1961)	21 of 41	26 of 74
Arentsen (1968)	11 of 72	16 of 114
Protheroe (1969)	25 of 61	30 of 149
Wilson *et al.* (1972)	2 of 8	4 of 13
Total	65 of 219 (31%)	79 of 377 (21%)

reporting the recurrence rate. Adding them together, 65 out of 219 women (31%) suffered a further puerperal episode, and psychosis complicated 79 out of 377 pregnancies (21%). The risk is therefore about 1 in 5 for each succeeding pregnancy. There may be a higher risk in women with more severe psychoses. Protheroe found that patients with a hospital diagnosis of schizophrenia had a 47% relapse rate overall, with 24% risk after each pregnancy. At Manchester, two of the three relapses so far seen in 56 women have occurred in the small group of five who met RDC criteria for schizophrenia. Protheroe (1969) made the interesting observation that these women who suffer from puerperal mental breakdown do not appear to be discouraged by this event from having more children, their reproductive rate being about the same as the general population.

Non-puerperal Episodes

Esquirol and Marcé knew that these women were prone to attacks of mental illness throughout their lives, not only in the puerperium. Paffenbarger states that 20 of his 83 patients from Hamilton County, Ohio, had already been admitted to hospital before the first postpartum episode, and Cruickshank (1940) with 13%, Hemphill (1952) with 13%, Vislie (1956) with 19%, and Martin (1958) with 23% give similar figures. In the great majority, however, the first episode is puerperal. This is perhaps not surprising because of the age of the patients at that time. As for subsequent episodes, the best evidence comes from two magnificent long term follow-up studies, carried out in Oslo and Newcastle-upon-Tyne. Arentsen (1968), who interviewed 92% of the survivors of a group of women admitted 6–30 years earlier, found that 46 of the 131 (35%) with adequate data had recurrences, of which the majority (96 out of 107 episodes) were not related to childbirth. Protheroe (1969) found that 45 of his 104 patients (43%) had non-puerperal recurrences. It would be interesting to know whether the symptomatology of these episodes had the characteristic features (especially the "confusion") found in the puerperal attacks, and whether the same proportion were manic and depressive. Another interesting question is whether the risk of recurrence falls as childbirth fades into the distant past; one patient at Manchester suffered from a relapsing psychosis for at least two years after each pregnancy, and then remained well for a long period. The third question which future research may answer is whether there are any clinical or epidemiological differences between the majority who succumb only in the puerperium, and the minority who have a diathesis erupting at other times. It seems obvious that some patients have a particular tendency to mental illness after a baby has been born and at no other time. The evidence for this comes from a few spectacular cases, for example Cruickshank's patient who had attacks after each of eight pregnancies. It is supported by the Iowa study of mania, in which 21 non-puerperal manic patients were followed for 5.9 years and had six recurrences all unrelated to childbirth, while 21 puerperal manics (followed for 3.4 years) had only one recurrence which followed another pregnancy. The concept of a specific disease entity might apply to these patients who become psychotic only in the puerperium, especially if it is established that their symptomatology is different from the other patients.

Aetiology

The Epidemiological Evidence

Epidemiology was the subject of Chapter 2 of this volume, so will be reviewed only briefly. Puerperal psychosis is a very uncommon disorder, at least at the threshold of hospital admission. Thomas and Gordon (1959) reviewed seven studies with rates ranging from 0.8 to 2.5 cases per thousand deliveries, and Paffenbarger (1964) computed an incidence of 1.9 per thousand. What kind of women have an increased risk?

The fact that stands out most clearly from the epidemiological studies is that primiparous women have a higher risk. Thomas and Gordon reviewed 13 studies involving a total of 1100 cases, and found that 54% were primiparous, while at that time only 31% of American women giving birth were primiparous. In Kendell's Edinburgh study (Kendell *et al.*, 1981), 62% were primiparous, compared with 47% in the general population, and the risk for first confinements (2.6/1000) was almost double that for later confinements (1.4/1000). Paffenbarger (Chapter 2) has calculated that the relative risk for primiparae was 2.04. This association with first pregnancies could be construed as favouring a psychological cause, because the first baby causes a revolution in a woman's way of life. However, there is at least one somatic illness which has a predilection for the first pregnancy, namely pre-eclamptic toxaemia.

One would expect that epidemiological studies would show whether the disease is commoner in women living in difficult circumstances. Esquirol (1845) knew that it was common among the wealthy, and Gundry (1859) observes that "All classes seem equally liable. Neither riches, with the luxury that attends, nor poverty with its supposed exemption from enervation can claim any exemption". Esquirol and Gundry did not have the benefit of the relative risk index. Paffenbarger found in his first study in Cincinnati that negro women had nearly double the rate of white women (1.9 per 1000 compared with 1.0). Kendell *et al.* (1976) in their Camberwell study found that foreign-born women had relatively more puerperal breakdowns than psychiatric illnesses at other times. Even if confirmed, these differences could have a biological basis. One sure marker of social and psychological stress is the birth of a child out of wedlock; other things being equal, this is bound to be accompanied by shame, worry and hardship when compared with childbirth within legal marriage. Unfortunately the epidemiological evidence is ambiguous. Paffenbarger and Kendell (in his Camberwell study) found no association with single motherhood, but Tetlow (1955) and Kendell (in his Edinburgh study) found a rate of 14% which was double that of controls. Esquirol also reported a high proportion of unmarried mothers (31%) but his group consisted of lactational as well as puerperal psychoses, and the high rates found by Tetlow and Kendell might also be explained by the inclusion of late onset cases, because they included patients admitted within six weeks and 90 days of delivery respectively.

The third focus of epidemiological investigation has been the link with obstetric pathology. Paffenbarger found clear evidence of dystocia and prematurity in the babies of mothers who later developed the psychosis. However, this has not been confirmed by Kendell's surveys, except that one (the Edinburgh survey) showed that a high proportion of the psychotic patients had a Caesarian section (22% compared with 8% controls). There seems to be no added risk after twin pregnancies (Hemphill, 1952; Kendell *et al.*, 1981).

The Genetic Evidence

Esquirol (1845) knew that "the causes which especially predispose the recently confined and nurses to this malady include hereditary predisposition". This fact has been confirmed many times, and was firmly established even in the last century (Marcé, 1858; Gundry, 1860). In this century, 10 studies carried out between 1911 and 1973 were collated by Thuwe (1974), showing a "positive heredity" of 22–65%. His own careful study concerned the children of 47 women admitted to Göteborg Mental Hospital between 1872 and 1926; he traced them and found that 12 out of 120 of them developed psychoses, compared with two of a comparison group taken from the population register ($P=0.014$, Fisher's exact test).

Protheroe (1969) studied the first degree relatives of 98 patients and, besides confirming that a rather higher-than-expected number had psychotic illness (though only 5% in this study), made two other observations. He found that affective psychoses and schizophrenia tended to breed true in these families; for example when he studied the relatives of his small subgroup of 19 patients who had hospital diagnoses of schizophrenia, he found that eight out of nine of them also had schizophrenia. He did not use the two-week criterion for diagnosing puerperal psychosis, and it is not clear how many of his "schizophrenic" patients met this strict definition, nor whether they would be schizophrenic by modern criteria. His other finding is quite unexpected. He reports that only two of the female relatives had puerperal psychosis! Since they had a total of 386 pregnancies, their risk of breaking down in the puerperium was hardly any higher than in the general population. Whalley reported rather similar observations at the Manchester conference in 1980 (not yet published). He compared the family histories of 17 puerperal psychotics and 20 manic depressive patients; he found that their relatives had the same risk of affective disorder (mania, depression and suicide) and the same risk of puerperal psychosis. These results are to some extent in conflict, but they both suggest that a predisposition to *puerperal* breakdown is not inherited. Obviously there is an inherited tendency to psychotic illness, but the precipitating factor linked with childbirth seems to be unrelated to this, and to be environmental (i.e. social, psychological, hormonal or somatic).

Genetic studies carried out at St Louis and Iowa have contributed several items of information. At Iowa the presence of mental illness in the families has been used to subclassify unipolar depressive illness into three classes—"depressive spectrum disease" (in which there is a family history of alcoholism or antisocial personality), "familial pure depressive disease" (with a family history of depression only) and "sporadic depressive disease" (with no family history) (Winokur *et al.*, 1978). When this classification was applied to 125 depressed patients, of whom 14 were admitted during the postpartum period, it was found that 11 of the 14 had the family history of "depressive spectrum disease" and three of "familial pure depressive disease", while none had a negative family history. A second study at Iowa looked at the family history of 21 patients with postpartum mania, comparing them with 136 other manic women. The postpartum patients had lower rates of affective illness or alcoholism in their families (24% compared with 39% in the controls). Finally there is the study of Reich and Winokur (1969) from St. Louis who investigated the families of manic patients and found that a very high proportion of these relatives suffered puerperal breakdowns: of the 29 relatives who had themselves suffered from affective illness and who had born children, 12 (41%) had an episode within six months of parturition. Expressed as a proportion of the number of pregnancies, 15 of their 75 pregnancies (20%) were followed by psychotic episodes. Again, however, there was "no significant family loading for postpartum illness . . . and in only 3 families did more than one patient with postpartum illness occur", thus confirming Protheroe and Whalley's strange discovery.

The Clinical Evidence

As we have seen, the conclusion of the most recent clinical studies is that puerperal psychoses almost always meet modern criteria for affective, or schizo-affective, disorders and not paranoid schizophrenia. If it is accepted that schizo-affective mania is closely related to mania (for which there is some evidence, eg. Clayton et al., 1968; Brockington et al., 1980; Pope et al., 1980), a high proportion are manic.

Other evidence linking puerperal psychosis to manic depression comes from the study of manic depressive disease itself. Bratfos and Haug (1966) focused on this disease in Norwegian women. They collected 218 patients attending a clinic in Oslo. Only 11 of them had mania, because manic patients were not, as a rule, admitted to the clinic. Examining the relationship of episodes to childbirth, they found that 82 women had borne children, and that 52 of their 251 pregnancies had been followed by psychosis. These 52 episodes represent about one third of the 155 episodes of affective illness suffered by these 82 women during the period of the study. Thus they showed that "manic depressive" women had a very high rate of puerperal breakdown (21%). Bratfos and Haug were probably using the term "manic depressive" to mean any affective psychosis, in accordance with the custom of the time; nowadays only a proportion would be regarded as suffering from bipolar affective disorder. They also had a low threshold for diagnosing puerperal mental illness, since only 13 of the 52 episodes led to hospital admission. All 13 episodes were depressive, which is different from the Manchester and Edinburgh experience. The authors noted that all the puerperal episodes occurred in a subset of 31 women; thus 51 women had 74 episodes unrelated to childbirth and 158 births without psychosis, while the other 31 women had 29 non-puerperal episodes and 91 births of which 52 (56%) were followed by a breakdown (which was usually treated at the out-patient clinic). This suggests a possible dichotomy between two groups of affective psychoses, one with and the other without a tendency to puerperal attacks. It would be interesting to know whether this dichotomy corresponded to that between unipolar depression and manic depressive disease.

Similar studies have been carried out in St. Louis. In 1966, Winokur and Ruangtrakool examined 71 patients with primary affective disorder. All these patients had at least one episode outside the puerperium, and the great majority were unipolar. No evidence was found that postpartum episodes were more frequent than would be expected at any other time in their lives. A second study (Baker et al., 1961) dealt with 65 women with unipolar affective disorder, who were systematically interviewed about pregnancies, depression and the coincidence of depression with the postpartum period. A postpartum depression followed 6% of all pregnancies in these patients. There was no familial tendency to develop postpartum depressions. In those patients who had suffered a non-puerperal depression, the morbidity risk for the development of a postpartum episode was no higher than the risk at any other time during the childbearing years (4%). The third study in the series dealt with bipolar affective disorder, and started with 35 women who had had at least one attack of mania. This time the postpartum attack rate was much higher. Twenty of these women had borne children (46 children in all). Eight of them had postpartum episodes (40%), occurring after 14 pregnancies (30% of all deliveries). They were able to find six women who had suffered *both* a previous attack of mania, *and* an attack of puerperal psychosis. All six developed a recurrence within six months of their next baby's delivery. Again they were not able to demonstrate an increase in the morbidity risk during the postpartum period when compared with other semesters during the childbearing years, but this may have been because they used a six month time base. Had they defined the puerperium as six weeks or two weeks, it is entirely likely that both unipolar and bipolar groups would have shown an increased morbidity risk in the puerperium.

The clinical evidence favours a relationship to manic depressive disease, but it is tempting also to postulate a relationship to another form of affective disorder—the postpartum "blues" syndrome. This has been reviewed by Stein in Chapter 6 of this volume. It is a very mild, brief and common disorder. Although evidence on its timing is conflicting, one careful study (Yalom *et al.*, 1968) showed that it occurred at any time in the first 10 days. There is no evidence at present, therefore, to show that its timing differs from that of puerperal psychosis which begins at any time in the first 14 days, or possibly between days two and 19. There is much uncertainty about the exact time limits of both phenomena. The symptoms of the "blues" are those of an affective disorder with a prominent lability of mood and, according to some, a mild impairment of consciousness, though this has never been substantiated by cognitive testing (Robin, 1962; Kane *et al.*, 1966). In general one would expect that a very common mild disorder would occasionally be so severe that it required hospital admission, and it is quite possible that some episodes of puerperal psychosis are severe cases of the "blues". If so, the most likely candidates are the brief affective episodes described by Marcé, though their symptoms were mainly manic. It is also possible that there is an interaction between the cerebral disturbance underlying the "blues" and that responsible for manic depressive disease, so that the "blues" triggers an attack of depression or mania. It is hard, at present, to investigate the relationship of the two conditions because the "blues" is such a mild and non-specific disorder. Without pathognomonic clinical signs or biological markers it appears impossible to separate symptoms of the blues from those of psychosis.

The Biological Evidence

Almost everyone suspects that puerperal psychosis is in some way related to the rapid changes in hormone levels which follow delivery, but the evidence is lacking. In the immediate puerperium at least three hormones are rapidly cleared from the body (chorionic gonadotrophic hormone, oestrogen and progesterone). Prolactin is high during the last week of pregnancy and rises further if the mother breast-feeds (Rolland *et al.*, 1975). During the second week, the pituitary resumes its normal gonadotrophic function and the normal cycle is re-established in 6–8 weeks. It used to be believed that no woman recovered from her psychosis until her menses returned, and supporting evidence for this was obtained by a courageous investigation of Delay *et al.* (1948) who took uterine biopsies 2–4 times per month from 20 psychotic women and claimed that the return of normal activity was always followed by prompt recovery. Vislie (1956), however, stated that 25 out of 67 patients resumed menstruation while still mentally ill. When it became possible to measure urinary metabolites of gonadal hormones, Rey *et al.* (1957) found that psychotic women had low levels of follicle stimulating hormone (FSH), while at the same time vaginal smears showed that they had low oestrogenic activity. Recently the discovery of radio-immune assay has made it possible to measure blood hormone levels. Stein has elsewhere reviewed the hormone measurements which have been done in patients with the "blues" (e.g. by Nott *et al.*, 1976). We hope that many centres are now studying hormone levels in puerperal psychosis, but the only results so far available are from a preliminary investigation at Manchester where 45 puerperal psychotic women were compared with a similar number of normal puerperal women. The two groups were comparable in age, type of delivery, cultural background and interval after delivery, but the psychotic patients tended to have lower parity and to breast-feed less often. Thirty of the psychotic patients were already taking phenothiazines. Thyroxin measurements done by Dr Gowland showed that the psychotic patients had higher levels ($P=0.006$). Measurements of prolactin and gonadotrophins by Dr Laing showed that prolactin was raised (even in those not taking phenothiazines, and especially when lactation was taken into account), and that luteinizing hormone was low ($P<0.02$). There were also large differences in oestrogen and progesterone levels (oestrogen high, progesterone low), but there were uncertainties about the reliability of these results. These results require confirmation, and, even if substantiated, are just as likely to be a complication of the psychosis, as to be related in any way to the cause. The definitive investigations in this field will have to take women at high risk of developing puerperal psychosis, and follow them through from the ninth month of pregnancy.

Conclusion

Marcé (1858) devoted a chapter to the causes of puerperal psychosis, and his conclusions were:

Hereditary disposition, exhaustion from numerous pregnancies, advanced age at the time of delivery, previous attacks of madness (especially of puerperal psychosis), the psychological state of the woman during pregnancy, anaemia complicating prolonged lactation, the sex of the infant — these are the principal causes we can allow. Among the occasional causes, dytocia, postpartum haemorrhage, eclampsia and breast abscess seem to have a certain influence.

In the last 120 years only the hereditary element and the lifetime tendency to mental illness have been amply confirmed. In spite of the publication of hundreds of papers, and the introduction of powerful investigatory tools including the disciplines of epidemiology and genetics, statistical methods, and hormone measurements, embarrassingly little has been added. All we now know is that primiparous patients are more at risk and that there is a link with manic depressive psychosis. This is slow progress indeed, and one of the reasons must be the vagueness of clinical concepts in this field. Puerperal psychosis has been defined in too many different ways, and in general too broadly. In this volume it is argued that the term should be limited to psychoses beginning within two weeks of delivery (or three at the most), and that it should be distinguished from depression complicating the birth of a baby in psychologically painful circum-stances (e.g. when there is a failure of mother–baby "bonding"). This is only a start. The clinical characteristics of these two groups require much clearer definition, and it may later be possible to subdivide puerperal psychosis. However, it is hoped that this modest clarification will lead to the investigation of more homogeneous patient populations, and to more consistent findings.

References

Adams, F. (1886). *The Genuine Works of Hippocrates.* Wood, New York.

Anderson, E.W. (1933). A study of the sexual life in psychoses associated with childbirth. *Journal of Mental Science* **79**, 137-149.

Arentsen, K. (1968). Postpartum psychoses. *Danish Medical Bulletin,* **15**, 97-100.

Baker, A.A., Morison, M., Game, J.A., Thorpe, J.G. (1961). Admitting schizophrenic mothers with their babies. *Lancet* **2**, 237-239.

Baker, A.A. (1967), *Psychiatric Disorders in Obstetrics.* Blackwell, Oxford.

Beigel, A. and Murphy, D.L. (1971). Unipolar and bipolar affective illness. *Archives of General Psychiatry* **24**, 215-220.

Billig, O. and Bradley, J.D. (1946). Combined shock and corpus luteum hormone therapy. *American Journal of Psychiatry* **102**, 783-787.

Bower, W.H. and Altschule, M.D. (1956). The use of progesterone in the treatment of postpartum psychosis. *New England Journal of Medicine* **254**, 157-160.

Boyd, D.A. (1942). Mental disorders associated with childbearing. *American Journal of Obstetrics and Gynecology* **43**, 148-163 & 335-349.

Bratfos, O. and Haug, J.O. (1966) Puerperal mental disorders in manic depressive females. *Acta Psychiatrica Scandinavica* **42**, 285-294.

Brew, M.F. and Seidenberg, R. (1950). Psychotic reactions associated with pregnancy and childbirth. *Journal of Nervous and Mental Disease* **3**, 408-423.

Brockington, I.F., Wainwright, S. and Kendell R.E. (1980a). Manic patients with schizo-phrenic or paranoid symptoms. *Psychological Medicine* **10**, 73-83.

Brockington, I.F., Kendell, R.E. and Wainwright, S. (1980b). Depressed patients with schizophrenic or paranoid symptoms. *Psychological Medicine* **10**, 665-675.

Brockington, I.F., Perris, C., Kendell, R.E., Hillier, V.E. and Wainwright, S. (1981). The course and outcome of cycloid psychosis. *Psychological Medicine* **12**, 97-102.

Brockington, I.F. and Meltzer, H.Y. (in press). Documenting an episode of psychiatric illness: the need for multiple information sources, multiple raters and narrative. *Schizophrenia Bulletin.*

Bürgi V.S. (1954). Puerperalpsychose oder Diencephalosis puerperalis? *Schweizerlische Medizinische Wochenshrift* **84**, 1222-1225.

Cernik, K. and Brockington, I.F., Unpublished observations.

Clarke, G. (1913). The forms of mental disorder occurring in connection with child-bearing. *Journal of Mental Science* **59**, 67-74

Clayton, P.J., Rodin, L. and Winokur, G. (1968). Family history studies: 111 Schizoaffective disorder, clinical and genetic factors including a one to 2 year follow-up. *Comprehensive Psychiatry* **9**, 31-49.

Clouston, T.S., (1896). *Clinical Lectures on Mental Diseases,* 4th Edition. Churchill, London.

Connolly, J. (1846). Description and treatment of puerperal insanity. *Lancet* **1**, 349-354.

Cooper, J.E., Kendell, R.E., Gurland, B.J., Sharpe, L., Copeland and J.R.M., Simon, R. (1972). *Psychiatric Diagnosis in New York and London.* Oxford University Press, London.

Cornfield, J. (1962). Joint dependence of risk of coronary heart disease on serum cholesterol and systolic blood pressure: a discriminant function analysis. *Federation Proceedings* **21**, 58-61.

Crichton Browne, J. (1896). Prevention and treatment of insanity of pregnancy and the puerperal period. *Lancet* **1**, 164-165.

Cruickshank, W.H., (1940), Psychoses associated with pregnancy and the puerperium. *Canadian Medical Association Journal* **43**, 571-576.

Dalton, K. (1980). *Depression after childbirth: how to recognize and treat postnatal depression.* Oxford University Press, London.

Dean, C. and Kendell, R.E. (1981). The symptomatology of puerperal illnesses. *British Journal of Psychiatry* **139**, 128-133.

Delay, J., Boittelle, G. and Corteel, A. (1948). Explorations cyto-hormonales au cours des psychoses du post-partum. *Annales Médico-psychologiques* **106**, 62-69.

Delay, J., Corteel, A. and Laine, B. (1953). Traitement des psychoses du post partum. *Annales d'Endocrinologie* **14**, 428-431.

Downing. A.R., Francis, A.F. and Brockington, I.F. (1980). A comparison of information sources in the study of psychotic illness. *British Journal of Psychiatry* **137**, 38-44.

Ellery, R.S., (1927). Psychoses of puerperium. *Medical Journal of Australia* **1**, 287-292.

Esquirol, E. (1845). *Mental Maladies: A Treatise on Insanity* (translated by E.K., Hunt). Lea & Blanchard, Philadelphia.

Foundeur, M., Fixsen, C., Triebel, W.A. and White, M.A. (1957). Postpartum mental illness. *Archives of Neurology and Psychiatry* **77**, 503-512.

Fürstner, C., (1875). Ueber Schwangerschafts- und Puerperalpsychosen. *Archiv für Psychiatrie und Nervenkranken* **5**, 505-543.

Gregory, M.S. (1924). Mental diseases associated with childbearing *American Journal of Obstetrics and Gynecology* **8**, 420-430.

Gundry, R. (1859). Observations upon puerperal insanity. *American Journal of Insanity* **16**, 294-320.

Hamilton, J.A. (1962). *Postpartum Psychiatric Problems.* Mosby, St Louis.

Hays, P. (1978). Taxonomic map of the schizophrenias, with special reference to puerperal psychosis. *British Medical Journal* **2**, 755-757.

Hemphill, R.E. (1952). Incidence and nature of puerperal psychiatric illness. *British Medical Journal* **2**, 1232-1235.

Herman, (1896). See Crichton Browne above.

Hopwood, B.S. (1927). Child murder and insanity. *Journal of Mental Science* **73**, 95-108.

Hyde, C., Brockington, I.F., Hamilton, J.A., Baines, M. and Monkhouse, M. Unpublished observations.

Impastato, D.J. and Gabriel, A.R., (1957). Electroshock therapy during the puerperium. *Journal of the American Medical Association* **163**, 1017-1022.

Jaco, E.G. (1960). *The Social Epidemiology of Mental Disorders — A Psychiatric Survey of Texas*. Russell Sage Foundation, New York.

Jacobides, G.M. (1961). Adrenocortical function in puerperal psychoses. M.D. thesis, University of Athens.

Jacobs, B. (1943). Aetiological factors and reaction types in psychoses following childbirth. *Journal of Mental Science* **89**, 242-256.

Jansson, B. (1964). Psychic insufficiences associated with childbearing. *Acta Psychiatrica Scandinavica* **39**, supplement 172.

Jones, R. (1902). Puerperal insanity. *British Medical Journal* **1**, 579-585.

Kadrmas, A., Winokur, G. and Crowe, R. (1980). Postpartum mania. *British Journal of Psychiatry* **135**, 551-554.

Kane, F.J., Harman, W.J., Jr. and Keeler, M.H. (1968). Emotional and cognitive disturbance in the early puerperium. *British Journal of Psychiatry* **114**, 99-102.

Kane, F.J. and Keeler, M.H. (1965). The use of enovid in postpartum mental disorders. *Southern Medical Journal* **58**, 1089-1092.

Karnosh, L.J. and Hope, J.M. (1937). Puerperal psychoses and their sequelae. *American Journal of Psychiatry* **94**, 537-550.

Keeler, M.H., Kane, F.J. and Daly, R. (1964). An acute schizophrenic episode following abrupt withdrawal of enovid in a patient with previous postpartum psychiatric disorder. *American Journal of Psychiatry* **120**, 1123-1124.

Kendell, R.E. and Gourlay, J. (1970). The clinical distinction between the affective psychoses and schizophrenia. British *Journal of Psychiatry* **117**, 261-6.

Kendell, R.E., Wainwright, S., Hailey, A. and Shannon, B. (1976). The influence of childbirth on psychiatric morbidity. *Psychological Medicine* **6**, 297-302.

Kendell, R.E., Rennie, D., Clarke, J.A. and Dean, C. (1981). The social and obstetric correlates of psychiatric admission in the puerperium. *Psychological Medicine* **11**, 341-350.

Kilpatrick, E. and Tiebout, H.M. (1926). A study of psychoses occurring in relation to childbirth. *American Journal of Psychiatry* **6**, 145-159.

Kraines, S.H. (1941). The treatment of psychiatric states following pregnancy. *Illinois Medical Journal* **80**, 200-204.

Kumar R. and Robson K. (1978). Neurotic disturbance in pregnancy and the puerperium. In *Mental Illness in Pregnancy and the Puerperium* (Ed. M. Sandler), pp 40-51.

McDonald, J. (1847). Puerperal insanity. *American Journal of Insanity* **4**, 113-163.

Madden, J.J., Luhan, J.A., Tuteux, W. and Bimmerle, J.F. (1958). Characteristics of postpartum mental illness. *American Journal of Psychiatry* **115**, 18-24.

Mantel, N., Haenszel, W. (1959). Statistical aspects of the analysis of data from retrospective studies of disease. *Journal of the National Cancer Institute* **22**, 719-748.

Marcé, L.V. (1858). *Traité de la Folie des Femmes Enceintes, des Nouvelles Accouchées et des Nourrices*. Baillière, Paris.

Martin, M.E. (1958). Puerperal mental illness. A follow-up study of 75 cases. *British Medical Journal* **2**, 773-777.

Melges, F.T. (1968). Postpartum psychiatric syndromes. *Psychosomatic Medicine* **30**, 95-108.

Menzies, W.F. (1893), Puerperal insanity. An analysis of 140 consecutive cases. *American Journal of Insanity* **50**, 148-185.

Nott, P.H., Franklin, M., Armitage, C. and Gelder, M.G. (1976). Hormonal changes and mood in the puerperium. *British Journal of Psychiatry* **128**, 379-383.

Paffenbarger, R.S., Jr. (1961). The picture puzzle of the postpartum psychoses. *Journal of Chronic Diseases* **13**, 161-173.

Paffenbarger, R.S., Jr. (1964). Epidemiological aspects of postpartum mental illness. *British Journal of Preventive and Social Medicine* **18**, 189-195.

Paffenbarger, R.S., Jr. and McCabe, L.J., Jr. (1966). The effect of obstetric and perinatal events on risk of mental illness in women of childbearing age. *American Journal of Public Health* **56**, 400-407.

Pauleikhoff, B. (1964). *Seelische Störungen in der Schwangerschaft und nach der Geburt.* Ferdinand Enke Veriag, Stuttgart.

Perris, C. (1974). A study of cycloid psychosis. *Acta Psychiatrica Scandinavica* supplement 253.

Playfair, H.R. and Gowers J.I. (1981). Depression following childbirth — a search for predictive signs. *Journal of the Royal College of General Practitioners* **31**, 201-208.

Polonio, P. and Figueiredo, M. (1955). On the structure of mental disorders associated childbearing. *Monatschrift für Psychiatrie und Neurologie* **130**, 304-318.

Pope, H.G., Lipinski, J.F., Cohen, B.M. and Axelrod, D.T. (1980). 'Schizoaffective disorder': an invalid diagnosis? A comparison of schizoaffective disorder, schizophrenia and affective disorder. *American Journal of Psychiatry* **137**, 921-927.

Protheroe, C. (1969). Puerperal psychoses: a long term study 1927-1961. *British Journal of Psychiatry* **115**, 9-30.

Railton, I.E. (1961). The use of corticoids in postpartum depression. *Journal of the American Medical Women's Association* **16**, 450-452.

Reich, T. and Winokur, G. (1970). Postpartum psychoses in patients with manic depressive disease. *Journal of Nervous and Mental Disease* **151**, 60-68.

Rey, J.H., Nicholson-Bailey, U. and Trappl, A. (1957). Endocrine activity in psychiatric patients with menstrual disorders. *British Medical Journal* **2**, 843-850.

Robin, A.A. (1962). The psychological changes of normal parturition. *Psychiatric Quarterly* **36**, 129-150.

Rolland, R., Lequin, R.M., Schellekens, L.A. and De Jong, F.H. (1975). The role of prolactin in the restoration of ovarian function during the early postpartum period in the human female. 1 A study during physiological lactation. *Clinical Endocrinology* **4**, 15-25.

Runge, W. (1911). Die Generationpsychose des Weibes. *Archiv für Psychiatrie* **48**, 545-690.

Savage, G. (1875). Observations on insanity in pregnancy and childbirth. *Guy's Hospital Reports* **20**, 83-117.

Savage, G.H. (1896). See Crichton Browne above.

Saunders, E.B. (1929). Association of psychosis with the puerperium. *American Journal of Psychiatry* **8**, 669-680.

Schmidt, H.J. (1943), The use of progesterone in the treatment of postpartum psychosis. *Journal of the American Medical Association* **121**, 190-192.

Shah, D.K., Wig, N.N. and Akhtar, S. (1971). Status of postpartum mental illness in psychiatric nosology. *Indian Journal of Psychiatry* **13**, 14-20.

Silbermann, R.M., Beenen, F. and De Jong, H. (1975). Clinical treatment of postpartum delirium with perfenazine and lithium carbonate. *Psychiatria Clinica* **8**, 314-326.

Skottowe, I. (1942). Mental disorders in pregnancy and the puerperium. *The Practitioner* **148**, 157-163.

Smalldon, J.L. (1940). A survey of mental illness associated with pregnancy and childbirth. *American Journal of Psychiatry* **97**, 80-101.

Spitzer, R., Endicott, J. and Robins, E. (1975). *Research Diagnostic Criteria.* Instrument no. 58, New York State Psychiatric Institute, New York.

Steiner, M., Latz, A., Blum, I Atsmon, A. and Wijsenbeek, H. (1973). Propranolol versus chlorpromazine in the treatment of psychoses associated with childbearing. *Psychiatria Neurologia Neurochirugia* **76**, 421-426.

Stone, C.W. and Karnosh, L.J. (1928). Mental disturbances associated with pregnancy. *Ohio State Medical Journal* **24**, 29-32.

Stössner, K. (1910). Ein Fall von Myxödem im Anschluss an Gravidität. *München Medizinishce Wochenschrift* **57**, 2531-2534.

Strecker, E.A. and Ebaugh, F.C. (1926). Psychoses occurring during the puerperium. *Archives of Neurology and Psychiatry* **15**, 239-252.

Tetlow, C. (1955). Psychoses of childbearing. *Journal of Mental Science* **101**, 629-639.

Thomas, C.L. and Gordon, J.E. (1959). Psychosis after childbirth: ecological aspects of a single impact stress. *American Journal of the Medical Sciences* **238**, 363-388.

Thuwe, I. (1974). Genetic factors in puerperal psychosis. *British Journal of Psychiatry* **125**, 378-385.

Tucker, W.I. (1962). Progesterone treatment in postpartum schizo-affective reactions. *Journal of Neuropsychiatry* **3**, 150-153.

Various newspapers (1848). These were the Essex Standard, March 10th; the Morning Post, March 11th and the Times, March 11th.

Vislie, H. (1956). Puerperal mental disorders. *Acta Psychiatrica et Neurologica Scandinavica*, supplement 111.

Wing, J.K., Cooper, J.E. and Sartorius, N. (1974). *The Measurement and Classification of Psychiatric Symptoms.* Cambridge University Press, London.

Winokur, G., Behar, D., Vanvalkenburg, C. and Lowry, M. (1978). Is a familial definition of depression both feasible and valid? *Journal of Nervous and Mental Disease* **166**, 764-768.

Winokur, G. and Ruangtrakool, S. (1966). Postpartum impact on patients with independently diagnosed affective disorder. *Journal of the American Medical Association* **197**, 84-88.

Yalom, I.D., Lunde, D.T., Moos R.H. and Hamburg, D.A. (1968). Postpartum blues syndrome. *Archives of General Psychiatry* **18**, 16-27.

4

Neurotic Disorders in Childbearing Women

R. Kumar

Introduction

Psychiatric disturbances that arise during pregnancy and in the puerperium can have a major, and sometimes lasting, impact on the health of the mother, they may cause serious repercussions in her immediate family and, most importantly, they may exert undesirable effects upon the psychological development of the newborn child. Other contributors to this book all examine the significance of maternal psychiatric disorders from a variety of vantage points. Paffenbarger (Chapter 2) surveys the evidence on the incidence of severe puerperal mental breakdowns and Brockington, Winokur and Dean (Chapter 3) and Hamilton (Chapter 1) describe the clinical picture of the puerperal psychoses and their outcome. Margison (Chapter 7) reviews disturbances of the mother/child relationship. These authors are, however, dealing with a relatively small and selected population of severely ill women, most of whom are mental hospital in-patients. There is a much larger group of mothers who are also adversely affected by the process of childbearing, but less drastically so; these are the women who experience neurotic disturbances such as anxiety states and depression, and whose disorders were, until relatively recently, not formally acknowledged as conditions meriting study and attention in their own right. As societies develop and increase their resources and skills, it is natural that some of the interest and effort devoted to the more catastrophic mental illnesses is diverted to the neuroses. There may, however, be factors which are specific to the area of motherhood and to its medical management which have, in some way, impeded the growth of knowledge and the sharing of information about the occurrence and consequences of neurotic disturbances in pregnant and parturient women (see p.73). If, as will be described in more detail in a later section, significantly distressing and handicapping emotional problems arise afresh in between 10 and

71

15% of recently delivered mothers, then it seems worthwhile exploring all avenues which may lead to better treatment and prevention.

This review will examine neurotic disorders which may arise either in pregnancy or post-natally and the literature will be surveyed with the following main questions in mind:

(1) What is the incidence and timing of neurotic disorders in relation to childbearing?

(2) What are the clinical features of such disorders—do they differ in any significant way from neuroses in women not having babies at the time?

(3) How, if at all, does the process of becoming a mother induce such psychological disturbances?

(4) What is known of the consequences of maternal neurosis?

(5) How may these conditions be prevented or treated?

It is not possible to address these questions properly without surveying "normal" maternal mental reactions to pregnancy and childbirth. This review therefore contains a brief survey of psychosomatic reactions in normal pregnancy and of the ways in which maternity services are deployed. A mother's reactions may be critically influenced by the quality and amount of contact with professional staff. The next section consists, therefore, of a short account of patterns of care in childbearing in Britain and this is followed (p.80) by a review of psychosomatic changes in pregnancy.

The substantive part of this review (pp.90–113) covers the incidence, clinical picture and implications of maternal neurotic disorders; the survey of the literature focuses on problems of methodology and definition, with the particular aim of trying to clarify the distinctions between the various sorts of clinically important disturbances that are seen. The review ends by listing some priorities for future research into the psychology of motherhood and the care of mentally disturbed mothers.

Patterns of Care

Social Perspective

Although societies and cultures acknowledge pregnancy and childbirth in different ways, the process of reproduction is typically assigned central importance as is shown by the customs and rituals which surround it. Mead and Newton (1967) have described a variety of social reactions to the occurrence of pregnancy; it typically elicits solicitude in others and feelings of responsibility and accountability in the parents. For some cultures, pregnancy is the outward signal of sexual adequacy, but it may also evoke patterns of reactions in the mother and in those around her, which imply that it is a time of debilitation and increased vulnerability. Rules of behaviour and superstitions abound; Ford

(1945) surveyed 64 different cultures and found that dietary restrictions were imposed upon the pregnant woman in 38 of these cultures, and in only four was it mentioned that there were no such restrictions. The traditional (male) view of the pregnant woman who blooms with good health is occasionally upheld, but for most women pregnancy is a time of unpleasant subjective and bodily disturbances.

Oakley (1980) has published a trenchant critique of the ways in which important aspects of the emotional life and social behaviour of British mothers seem to be influenced by a male dominated, medical hierarchy. Maternity care is part of the wider social response to pregnancy and there is at present an important and often acrimonious debate about comparative benefits and hazards of the "medicalization" of childbirth (see also MacIntyre, 1977). By concentrating the facilities in hospital and clinic settings where the emphasis is on treating illness, the tendency is encouraged to regard healthy women as potentially malfunctioning machines. The technological invasion of ante-natal clinics and delivery suites can prevent pain, dramatically reduce the risks of harm to the mother or her child, or even death, but it also confirms her status as an object with little opportunity to have any meaningful dialogue with the person in whom control is vested. The commonest complaint by expectant mothers is that they are not acknowledged as persons who may have many questions and worries about their own and their babies' health.

Unexpressed fears and anxieties feed on uncertainty and on a lack of knowledge. Some medical and nursing staff are, however, keenly aware of the present inadequacies and are trying to redress shortcomings. Consumer guides of hospital obstetric services (Kitzinger, 1979) are as biased as any other source of highly selected information, but the very fact that they exist points to the need to treat expectant mothers as persons. Changes in the system along the lines suggested by the Short Committee (see p.78) may go some of the way, but it may also be worth undertaking a deeper enquiry into why the situation has arisen. The long-standing conflict between obstetricians and midwives (Donnison, 1977) over who has primary responsibility for bringing new life into the world may be partly responsible for the relegation of the mother to the role of a sort of anaesthetized vehicle for the baby; the presence of spouses in clinics and in delivery suites has been encouraged only relatively recently and only in a few places.

Births and Deaths

The birth rate in England and Wales reached a post-war peak in 1964 and thereafter the number of babies being born each year has declined steadily until 1975 (see Table 1; DHSS, 1977). Although there has been a slight increase in the birth rate during 1978 and 1979, nearly a quarter of a million fewer babies were born in Great Britain in 1979 in comparison with 1964 (Central Statistical

Office, 1981). Table 1 also shows the dramatic decline in the rates of maternal, neonatal and perinatal mortality as well as of stillbirths. Adelstein *et al.* (1980) have characterized a "j" shaped relationship between rates of stillbirth and perinatal mortality on the one hand, and maternal age and parity on the other—i.e. a first child is more "at risk" than the second and third, but fourth and subsequent children have the poorest relative chances of survival. Social class is another major influence on infant life expectancy; for example, mothers belonging to Social Class V had twice the expectancy of stillbirth or of their infant dying in the first month in comparison with mothers of Class I. A similar relationship with social class can be found in almost all measures of maternal and infant morbidity and mortality.

Regional variations in perinatal mortality rates have also been reported but MacFarlane *et al.* (1980) have criticized the tendency to publish "league tables" as crude indicators of the quality of service that is available in a given region. Factors other than the health services, in particular the background socio-

Table 1. Statistics for births and deaths in England and Wales during 1949–75 are shown. Figures for teminations of pregnancy carried out to women resident in England during some of these years are also shown. The corresponding numbers of legal abortions (thousands) in 1976, 1977, 1978 and 1979 are 102, 103, 112 and 119 respectively. Sources: and C.S.O. (1981) DHSS (1977)

	England and Wales				England			
Year	1949	1959	1969	1971	1972	1973	1974	1975
Thousands of subjects Number of live births (Rate per 1000 population)	731 (16.7)	749 (16.5)	798 (16.4)	740 (16.0)	685 (14.8)	638 (13.7)	603 (13.0)	569 (12.2)
Number of still births	17	16	11	9	8	7	7	6
Neonatal mortality (<4 weeks of age)	14	12	10	9	8	7	7	6
Perinatal mortality (still births and deaths of infants < 1 week of age)	28	26	19	17	15	14	12	11
Maternal mortality	0.73	0.29	0.16	0.13	0.10	0.08	0.07	0.07
Termination of pregnancy (women resident in England and Wales)	—	—	50	95	—	111	—	106

economic conditions, can markedly influence such statistics. The mother's country of origin may also be an important variable—for example, the rate of stillbirth for mothers born in the Indian sub-continent was 50% higher than in mothers born in the United Kingdom (Adelstein *et al.*, 1980).

Antenatal Care

Figures for stillbirth and perinatal mortality may seem far removed from the main subject of this review but, in fact, they are of considerable relevance. There has been much research into the adverse effects on the foetus of stress in the mother and the most well-known example of such work was the erroneous hypothesis propounded by Stott (1957, 1961) linking maternal emotional difficulties with severe mental retardation. Nevertheless, there are many possible ways, direct and indirect, in which maternal psychological problems may influence foetal well-being. Indirect effects may be mediated by the use of drugs such as nicotine and ethanol or via the teratogenic actions of psychotropic drugs that are obtained on prescription (see Chapter 9).

The relevance of socio-economic factors to perinatal mortality statistics has already been underlined and the same arguments apply to rates of maternal mortality where the overall reductions (see Table 1) can be ascribed to a complex interaction between constitutional and environmentally determined elements, e.g. social, economic, nutritional, educational, as well as to the quality of the health services. It would be patently wrong to infer that the recent decline in maternal and perinatal mortality is simply a consequence of the increasing trend towards delivering babies in hospitals and homes run by the NHS rather than at home (see Fig. 1). It is difficult, therefore, to evaluate the precise contributions of improved medical and nursing practice and recent controversies, e.g. about home v. hospital delivery tend to be characterized by arguments based more upon opinion than upon fact.

Interpretations of international league tables of mortality statistics are further complicated by variations in the way that figures are gathered and notified. Nevertheless, alarm over the fact that neonatal and perinatal mortality rates seemed to be falling more slowly in England and Wales than in many other developed countries and also the evidence for indigenous differences between regions and between socio-economic groups, led in 1978, to the setting up of a House of Commons Committee of enquiry (Social Services Committee, Chairman Mrs Short—report 1980). The aim of the enquiry was to pay special attention to ways and means of identifying and then helping "high risk" mothers. Although the enquiry was concerned with the life and death of newborn babies, social and sociomedical issues were never far from the centre of attention. Given that the vast majority of babies in this country are born in NHS hospitals or in maternity homes (see Fig. 1) the committee was forced to acknowledge that whilst antenatal care provided a potentially perfect

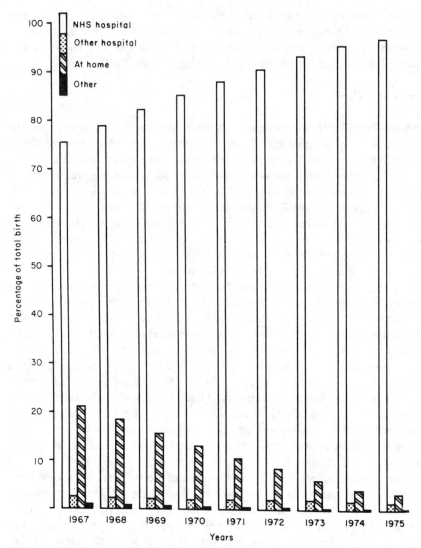

Fig. 1. The proportion of births in England and Wales by place of confinement in the years 1967–75 are shown. Source: DHSS (1979)

opportunity for preventive medicine, there was no concensus about what constituted "ideal antenatal care." Facilities and levels of staffing varied widely from place to place, the conditions in many antenatal clinics were, in the words of the Secretary of State, redolent with a "cattle-truck" atmosphere where there was little privacy and even less dignity. Other evidence indicated that mothers who attended late for antenatal care had a substantially higher rate of infant mortality. Women who were socially disadvantaged, unmarried mothers, women from working-class backgrounds, those who were faced with practical difficulties, e.g. long distances to travel, with young children at home, those with fears of hospitals, often linked with previous experiences such as stillbirth, miscarriages, terminations of pregnancy, neonatal deaths, were described as being the most likely to default on antenatal clinic attendance. Systematic investigations of the contributions of psychiatric disorder to late attendance do not seem to have been reported, but many of the features described above, e.g. lack of partner, low socio-economic status, other young children at home, were the very factors which were associated with high rates of depression in a community survey of women that was carried out by Brown and Harris (1978).

The members of the Short Committee (1980) were fully aware that simply increasing attendance at antenatal clinics would not by itself reduce perinatal mortality and they expressed their concern at "the relative lack of knowledge about the benefit to the pregnant mother and her baby of various practices and procedures which are part of established antenatal care." They went on to recommend strongly "that the DHSS and MRC should fund, as a priority, research that will determine how antenatal care can most effectively reduce perinatal and neonatal mortality and morbidity." There are several reasons why such research, if it is ever funded by the two main government grant giving bodies, should not be permitted to place psychosocial factors anywhere but at the top of its priorities. The socio-economic correlates of infant mortality have already been mentioned and there are strong grounds for suspecting that psychiatric disorders, including problems of drug abuse, are associated with erratic or late antenatal attendance. Some possible links have been drawn between maternal mental disorder and perinatal morbidity and mortality; furthermore, the impact of mental illness arising in relation to childbearing may continue to reverberate well into the child's first year of life and beyond.

The reversal in some units of "a degree of inhumanity and a lack of understanding of women's needs" and "the removal of anxiety and dread from the minds of expectant, parturient and puerperal patients" were cited by the Short Committee as being among the primary objectives for those caring for childbearing women. Ultimately, the surest way of improving a service is to base recommendations upon sound information, but sadly little is known about the wider general medical and social implications of maternal psychological illhealth in the pregnancy and in the puerperium.

Labour, Delivery and Place of Birth

Figure 1 shows that almost all babies now being born in Britain are delivered in NHS hospitals and clinics. Jokes about women "voting with their wombs" and having their babies at home ring hollow in the light of these published statistics on place of birth and they merely underline the helplessness felt by some mothers when what is, for them, a profoundly important personal experience, becomes part of an impersonal, technologically sophisticated, illness-oriented procedure. Cogent arguments against the *unnecessary* medicalization of labour and delivery have been summarized elsewhere (Cartwright, 1979; Chard & Richards, 1977; Kitzinger and Davis, 1978), and while it may be unrealistic to return to some form of home-delivery system as in Holland, there is much that could be done to improve the existing system in this country. The social services committee (Short Report, 1980) devoted a chapter of their report to recommendations for humanizing the obstetric services. Their very first point was, "it is not enough . . . . to concentrate solely on the physical well-being of the mother and her baby," and their recommendations seem simple, sensible and obvious—reduce overcrowding in clinics, facilitate attendance, choose welcoming staff (particularly receptionists and the clinic sister), explain procedures to mothers, allow a mother to have one or two people of her choice with her during labour, provide continuity of care, make delivery rooms look less clinical, avoid separating mothers from their babies, encourage breast-feeding, especially when this may be upset by the "blues" by appointing a midwife with "warmth" to listen to mothers' problems, provide practical, psychiatric and social support for parents whose babies are in special or intensive care units, appoint more staff—especially midwives. The most remarkable feature of this list of proposals is not its modesty nor its lack of novelty, but that it is the distillate of over 20 days of interviews of a galaxy of expert witnesses, who were interrogated by a distinguished committee of parliamentarians between December 1978 and March 1980. It is a sad commentary on the present state of affairs that such a list was ever needed in the first place.

Much the most potent way of altering staff attitudes and behaviour is to demonstrate that it is worth establishing relationships with antenatal clinic attenders or with mothers in postnatal wards. Quite aside from mutual benefits in the quality of life, it has to be shown that changes in procedure, e.g. allowing and encouraging every mother at least a specified amount of time to talk to a member of staff if she so wishes, has some impact on subsequent morbidity. It is, of course, quite pointless to arrange warm chats (midwives and obstetricians having been screened for this quality) unless there is some way of recording and acting upon the information that is obtained.

The other way of improving the service is to scrutinise the relevance of all aspects of it, however trivial they may seem to staff. It is now no longer normal practice to separate mothers from their babies and Robson and Powell (Chapter 6) review evidence to suggest that the actions of staff in the delivery suite can have major implications for the attachment process between mother and child. The author's own experience of a survey of recently delivered women (Robson and Kumar, 1980) revealed an unexpected and highly significant association between a lack of maternal affection immediately after delivery and the almost routine use of the procedure of fore-water amniotomy to induce or accelerate labour. This surprising association was present in mothers whose labours were felt by them as being very painful or if they received extra pethidine. It is tempting to speculate about possible physiological mechanisms, perhaps reflecting endogenous processes of analgesia (e.g. Gintzler, 1980) which may interact with mechanisms underlying the mother's psychological response to her newborn (see Robson and Powell, Chapter 6). There is a tendency to reject such findings out of hand rather than to evaluate them first. There is much that passes in medicine for science and not all potentially undesirable practices have been eliminated. Not many years have elapsed since the time when premature babies were maintained on 100% oxygen, or when mothers were kept well away from their babies who were in Intensive Care Units.

Postnatal Care

Patterns of care vary considerably between countries and this account summarizes relevant aspects of the British system. District midwives are required to pay daily home visits up to and including the tenth day after delivery and they may continue to visit until the twenty-eight day if there are any clinical complications. In such cases, the family doctor is usually informed and may also attend the mother and her baby. Typically, however, the health visitor takes on the statutory responsibility for visiting the mother and baby from the tenth day onwards:

> At the first visit the health visitor will observe the physical, mental and social condition of the family while giving advice on the physical and emotional needs of the baby and control of its environment. She may also explain the relevant services available in the vicinity, drawing attention to the value of attendance at child health clinics and to the importance of immunization and, if appropriate, she may discuss family planning. At the same time, she will be assessing any social needs, remaining constantly alert to the possibility of puerperal depression, child abuse or inadequate parentcraft .... On the basis of the first visit, information about the birth and any relevant facts available, the health visitor will assess how soon she should visit again (Health Visitors' Association, 1980).

Health visitors are trained nurses who have also obtained a midwifery qualification or have taken an approved course in obstetric nursing and have then undertaken a year's practical and academic training in which the psychological aspects of childbearing are emphasized. Because they must visit *all* mothers and their babies, health visitors are uniquely placed to promote health and prevent illness—emotional as well as physical. In most large cities, staff shortages dictate priorities and regular home visiting is exceptional. All mothers are seen at least once, but a single visit around the eleventh or twelfth day may not suffice for the detection of incipient puerperal mental disorder or of the risks of non-accidental injury. Postnatal depression and puerperal psychosis can afflict women of all social backgrounds. Therefore, the presence of florid symptoms, and then only in the most disadvantaged women, may be picked up by the busy health visitor, who, incidentally, is not required to have any experience or training in psychiatric nursing.

All parents are advised to register their newborn babies with their family doctors as soon as they return home and unless there are particular reasons for return to hospital out-patient clinics, mothers attend their family doctors around the sixth week postnatally for a health check and for contraceptive advice, if needed. Effectively, however, the mother is returned to the care of her family doctor when she leaves hospital. She is encouraged by the health visitor and her doctor to attend her local "well baby" clinic, where her child's health is checked at regular intervals and immunization is available. At any point a referral can be made to the community social worker or indeed by the family doctor to a psychiatrist.

On the face of it, such a system with repeated contacts between health care professionals and the mother and baby, seems geared to efficient detection treatment and prevention of puerperal psychiatric disorders. It is chastening to note, however, that surveys of maternal mental health in the community (e.g. Kumar and Robson, 1978a) indicate that the great majority of such problems remain unnoticed, or at least unremarked, by most health visitors and doctors.

Common Psychosomatic Reactions to Pregnancy

Emotional Reactions

In an early survey of pregnancy which touched upon the emotional health of expectant women, McDonald (1958) reported that 445 out of 3251 women who were interviewed described "marked anxiety or emotional shock" at some time between their last menstrual period and the twelfth week of pregnancy. No information was given about the ways in which anxiety or "shock" were evaluated, but such findings are nevertheless of interest at an impressionistic level. Most women are "booked in" in early pregnancy but it is unusual for there to be more than a cursory enquiry about their emotional condition. If asked, many mothers describe a lability of mood in early pregnancy which they often find hard to explain in terms of what is happening around them. Anxieties about the state and health of the foetus are almost universal, although there are some conflicting findings about whether pregnancy is a time of better (e.g. Hooke and Marks, 1962; Osborne, 1977) or worse psychological adjustment (Meares et al., 1972; Shereshefsky and Yarrow, 1973; Nilsson and Almgren, 1970). Discrepancies between investigators can be ascribed to different measuring scales and methods, variations in timing, in selection of subjects and to the lack of a proper comparison group or the use of a retrospective prepregnancy baseline. The general consensus, however, is that many pregnant women report that they are intermittently moody, edgy, irritable and at times tearful. Evidence for exaggerated and persistent mood changes characteristic of anxiety and depression will be presented in a later section.

Tiredness

The early months of pregnancy are a time when most women describe tiredness and lethargy, sometimes to the point of exhaustion; they are not, however, unwell in any medical sense and can recognize that the tiredness is related to their pregnancies.

Food Preferences and Aversions

Changes in appetite and food preferences are also very common but marked cravings and pica are rare (Trethowan and Dickens, 1972). It is much commoner for women to report aversions for various food and drinks than preferences, and the substances which figure most frequently as being unpleasant are coffee, tea, alcohol, tobacco smoke and fatty foods. Relative preferences are also mentioned but direct questions may be needed to elicit accurate descriptions of such changes. Many pregnant women describe a greater liking for foods such as biscuits or certain fruits and vegetables. It is tempting to see biological advantages behind such appetite changes and to regard them as a sign of some underlying tendency to avoid potentially harmful substances. However, many mothers continue to smoke and drink, and some still like coffee and fatty foods. There is no obvious coherence in the patterns of aversions and it would be of interest to try and relate reactions in pregnancy with earlier responses to novel foods and tastes. More systematic tests in pregnant women, e.g. of recognition of gustatory stimuli are needed.

Nausea and Vomiting

A majority of pregnant women experience some degree of nausea and a proportion may vomit, but hyperemesis is infrequent (Fairweather, 1968; Tylden, 1968). The physiological basis for nausea in pregnancy is not well understood and one fruitful line of study may be to investigate the mode of action of anti-emetic drugs of known efficacy. Recent controversies (see e.g. Donnai and Harris, 1978; Fleming *et al.*, 1981) over teratogenic potential of widely prescribed substances such as dicyclomine (Debendox) have led to marked reductions in their use.

Relationships have been sought between the presence and absence of somatic symptoms of pregnancy, such as vomiting, and a woman's "acceptance" of her foetus. Two propositions have been advanced: hyperemesis is a sign of "rejection" of the foetus or, alternatively, lack of nausea is an indication of denial of the pregnancy (Deutsch, 1945). The suggested psychological factors underlying hyperemesis have been derived mainly from individual case reports.

Studies of the extent and severity of normal vomiting and nausea in pregnancy (Uddenberg *et al.*, 1971; Wolkind and Zajicek, 1978) suggest an association between the absence of nausea in early pregnancy and the subsequent occurrence of emotional disturbance during pregnancy and after childbirth, but possible mechanisms remain obscure. Wolkind and Zajicek (1981) found that prolonged nausea and vomiting occurred more commonly in women who lacked support in their family relationships and they also found a link between prolonged nausea and a history of miscarriage or previous induced abortion. Their results supported Tylden's earlier (1968) suggestions that on the one hand prolonged nausea might be looked upon as a cry for help, and on the other, as providing some kind of protective influence against a pregnancy threatened by miscarriage.

Sexual Activity and Enjoyment

Libido is sharply reduced in the first trimester of pregnancy, together with a fall in the enjoyment of sexual intercourse and in its frequency. There is a further reduction in the third trimester of pregnancy. Many women describe fears that sexual intercourse will harm the foetus or that it may induce miscarriage (Kumar *et al.*, 1981, Robson *et al.*, 1981).

Psychoanalytic Views of Emotional Changes in Pregnancy

Any pregnancy is a time of profound physiological and pyschological change for an expectant mother, but a first pregnancy probably represents one of the greatest transitions in the life of women. The idea of pregnancy as a developmental or maturational crisis is an attractive one (see e.g. Benedek, 1959; Bibring, 1959; Rapoport *et al.*, 1977; Raphael-Leff, 1980; Pines, 1972). It is a time of acquisition of an additional and different identity, of both subtle and gross bodily changes, of major alterations in role, of emotional instability and of harking back to earlier developmental conflicts. Bibring *et al.* (1961), in an influential paper, note that

> the crisis of pregnancy is basically a normal occurrence and indeed even an essential part of growth, which must precede and prepare maturational integration . . . . The woman moves through a phase of enhanced narcissism early in the pregnancy, until quickening immediately introduces the baby as the new object within the self. The mother's relationship to her child, if it finally fulfills the maturational requirements, will have the distinctive characteristics of a freely changeable fusion—varying in degree and intensity—of narcissistic and object-libidinal strivings so that the child will always remain part of herself, and at the same time will always have to remain an object that is part of the outside world, and part of her sexual mate.

Many authors have commented on the complexities of the identifications which must be unravelled during pregnancy. Becoming a mother recalls a woman's relationship to her own mother—she identifies with her own mother or the one she wished she had had. In the preparation for caring for her own child may be seen the wish to be cared for herself as a child. A mother initially experiences the infant as an extension of herself and her ability to nurture the baby as well as to gradually give up total control will reflect the foundations for future relationships that were laid down in her own infancy.

An object relations approach to the mother–child identification emphasizes the quality of the early interactions and, in theory, no distinction is made between the capacity for parenting that is laid down in boy infants as opposed to girl infants. Careful observational investigations of mothers' interactions with their babies (e.g. De Chateau, 1976) show, however, that mothers treat boy and girl infants differently. Most societies favour male children and such biases are clearly evident in the more "traditional" psychoanalytic writings. There has, however, been a perceptible shift away from the views on sexuality and reproduction that were originally propounded by Freud. Most contemporary analysts would not wish to challenge the proposition that resolution of the Oedipal complex and the psychic differentiation of gender identity are closely bound up processes. Nor would they quarrel with the suggestion that within the accomplishment or otherwise of such processes lie the foundations for subsequent patterns of healthy or neurotic behaviour. Where feminists part company with Freudian orthodoxy is over concepts such as penis envy. Chodorow (1978) summarizes the female dilemma: "a baby and heterosexuality . . . are roundabout ways to get a penis—a real penis from fathers and men, a symbolic penis in the form of a baby." There is also much criticism of Helen Deutsch (1930) who extended Freud's ideas about female passivity and masochism, viz.

"In the deepest experience of the relation of mother to child, it is masochism in its strongest form which finds gratification in the bliss of motherhood."

Men are seen as the sexual aggressors and

Women would never have suffered themselves throughout the epochs of history to have been withheld by social ordinances on the one hand from possibilities of sublimation, and on the other from sexual gratifications, were it not that in the function of reproduction they have found magnificent satisfaction for both urges (Deutsch, 1930).

Within a remarkably short time it has become possible for women to regulate their reproductive lives and thus achieve selective emancipation from the maternal process. Social adaptation to a development of such significance is patchy and inconsistent—equal rights for women is still a slogan rather than a fact. Protagonists of the feminist view point (e.g. Cartwright, 1979; Oakley, 1980) argue powerfully that the confrontation between (usually) male obstetricians and their female clients is symbolic of much that men do to women while protesting the best of intentions. Expectant mothers are dehumanized and rendered powerless in the grip of a medical machine where individual accountability is sometimes hard to pin down. It is very hard to argue against those who both promote *and* assess the procedures which are part of obstetric management. However, the pendulum, or should one say the penis, can swing too far the other way. Raphael-Leff (1980), in the context of discussing group therapeutic methods for pregnant and parturient women, argues that "The *only* prerequisite for group leaders (other than general mental health) is that they should have experienced a full-term pregnancy" (my italics).

There is much that is thought-provoking that emerges from analytically oriented investigations, but there is also an endemic risk of generalizing from the particular, and from a highly selected and worked over particular at that. Thus the nausea and vomiting of early pregnancy *may* reflect a symbolic rejection of the parasitic foetus or it may have something to do with maternal physiology. Deutsch (1945) points to the symbolic significance of fecundity in food preferences—womb-shaped pears and cucumbers abound, but what about rejection of instant coffee or tea or preferences for dry bread? It seems important therefore to try and relate psychological changes to physiological events as well as to past experiential material.

Neurotic Reactions to Unwanted, Lost or Phantom Pregnancies

Only neurotic disorders that can be regarded as having some specific link with pregnancy will be considered here:
(1) Unwanted pregnancy and termination of pregnancy.
(2) Reactions to stillbirth.
(3) Pseudocyesis.

Unwanted Pregnancy and Termination of Pregnancy

There are great differences between countries in their attitudes to therapeutic abortion, varying from almost total prohibition to abortion on demand (see reviews by Cook and Dickens, 1978; David, 1981). Some Eastern bloc countries, which previously allowed virtually free access to abortion, have now tightened up their regulations and there are almost annual attempts in the British parliament to amend and restrict the provisions of the Abortion Act (1967). In general, however, many countries, and their medical professions, have radically altered their views about termination of unwanted pregnancy and the change has occurred within the relatively short space of the past 10 or 15 years. The ethical issues regarding the taking of an unborn life have not really been clarified and the moral dilemma posed by therapeutic abortion has, in some ways, been made more acute by medical advances, e.g. successful fertilization outside the uterus and the trend for younger and younger foetuses to survive as medical techniques have improved. The definition of the beginning of life and the distinction between abortion and some methods of contraception, e.g. with intra-uterine devices continues to exercise medico-legal minds. Thus while the fundamental issues about life and death have not changed in any substantive way, social, legal and medical attitudes and practice have. The reasons why such changes have occurred probably include an increasing awareness of over population, changes in sexual *mores*, probably linked with the dramatic developments in contraceptive methods in the past 20 years, an acceptance that an unwanted pregnancy is also a major psychological and social problem and that termination of pregnancy is a medically safe procedure, relatively speaking. Another important change has been the progressive emancipation of women and, with it, an acknowledgement of some, at least, of their rights as individuals to decide whether or not to carry a pregnancy to term.

Since the Abortion Act (1967) came into effect about 100 000 residents of England and Wales have obtained terminations of their pregnancies each year (Lewis, 1980). Table 1 shows how the annual numbers of live births seem to have varied largely independently of the numbers of terminations and in recent years, one out of every seven or eight pregnancies has been terminated under the provisions of the Abortion Act. The law in Britain requires two doctors to certify that they are "of the opinion in good faith" that one or more of the following conditions are met:

(1) The continuation of the pregnancy would involve risk to the life of the pregnant woman greater than if the pregnancy were terminated.
(2) The continuance of the pregnancy would involve risk of injury to the physical or mental health of the pregnant woman greater than if the pregnancy were terminated.
(3) The continuance of the pregnancy would would involve risk of injury to the physical or mental health of the existing child(ren) of the family of the pregnant woman greater than if the pregnancy were terminated.
(4) There is a substantial risk that if the child were born it would suffer from such physical or mental abnormalities as to be seriously handicapped.

The Act stipulates that the abortion must normally be carried out in an NHS hospital or other approved place. The gynaecologist who performs the abortion need not be one of the two doctors who have certified that abortion is indicated and a gynaecologist can object on conscientious grounds to performing the operation in which case the patient may be referred elsewhere. There is at present much disquiet about the way in which the certification procedure has been altered without consultation with the medical profession. This is seen as an underhand way of making it harder to terminate pregnancy on psychosocial grounds.

Between 1971 and 1977, 60% of women have regularly gone outside the NHS for their terminations. In some instances this has been because of marked regional variations in the provision of services in the NHS (Coles, 1975; Fowkes *et al.*, 1979) but there are some other important general differences. Women treated in the private sector have always had a quicker service and, consequently, a greater number of abortions in the NHS have been done at a later gestational stage. Thus only some of the delays can be explained on strictly clinical grounds. More single women and multiparous women obtain private sector abortions and a multiparous woman with two children who has her pregnancy terminated is much more likely to be simultaneously sterilized if she is treated in the NHS than in the private sector (36% v. 3% of such women respectively were sterilized in 1975). As Fowkes *et al.* (1979) observe, the time of abortion may not be the optimum occasion for a woman to make major decisions about her future ferility.

The Psychiatrist's Role

Whereas, ten years ago, a psychiatrist was typically asked to assess whether continuation of a pregnancy to term was likely to have disastrous consequences for the mother's mental health, questions nowadays are much more frequently asked about the extent of a subject's ambivalence and the possibility that, for her, abortion may be a maladaptive way of coping with intrapsychic and interpersonal problems. A recent survey (Kumar and Robson, 1978a, b, see also Table 2) revealed a very high association between either antenatal and postnatal depression and what may be regarded as a sign of fundamental ambivalence about the pregnancy. Almost every woman who had entertained the thought of obtaining a termination, however briefly, subsequently became depressed. Most of these women had desired and planned their pregnancies.

The decriminalization of abortion and the removal of the necessity to justify the termination on medical grounds has virtually eliminated the role of the psychiatrist in the decision process. Previously a doctor was required to be confident that not to terminate the pregnancy could result in the woman becoming a "physical or mental wreck" (B.M.J., 1938).

As a profession, psychiatrists have, in general, recognized that it is impossible to evaluate a person's physical and psychological health in isolation from social factors and have been in favour of liberalizing the laws in abortion. Repeated and regular contact with women in the sort of crisis caused by an unwanted pregnancy leads many doctors to acknowledge that there are very wide grounds for induced abortion. Thus, the aim is to prevent the humiliation and risk of illegal procedures and to move away from the need to subject healthy women to unnecessary and detailed psychiatric interviews. It is also important, however, to acknowledge that termination of a pregnancy cannot just be regarded as a minor event, a hiccup in the reproductive process without psychological significance for the parents "not to be" (Kumar and Robson, 1978b; and p.100).

Psychological Sequelae of Refused Abortion

Illsley and Hall (1976) draw attention to three reasons why studies of refused abortion should be interpreted with caution: subjects who are refused abortion may be more "stable" than those whose requests were granted; those refused may obtain abortions elsewhere, legally or illegally; follow-up is likely to be incomplete particularly when subjects associate the research staff with the people who originally refused the abortion.

In a study of women with mental illness who were refused abortion (Arkle, 1957) it was subsequently noted that while their mental states were little changed, many of the subjects (mental defectives, those with psychotic illnesses, psychopaths) were quite unable to look after their children or their homes. Where there is a history of relevant previous psychiatric disorder and a high risk of relapse, as in women who have previously had puerperal psychotic break- downs, it is important that the risks are fully explained so that the pregnant woman, and her partner if she wishes it, can reach a very difficult personal decision with the maximum amount of information made available to them. It is estimated that the risks of a recurrence of psychosis are a hundredfold greater in a subsequent pregnancy i.e. between 10 and 20% as compared with the general rate of 1–2 per 1000 deliveries (Paffenbarger, Chapter 2).

Among the adverse psychiatric sequelae which have been noted in studies of refused abortion are an increased risk of suicide (Whitlock and Edwards, 1968; Tylden, 1966; Visram, 1972) increased likelihood of depression (Höök, 1963; Pare and Raven, 1970) and persistent regrets about the refused abortion in a proportion of subjects. Problems in accepting the originally unwanted baby as well as subsequent repercussions in the child, e.g. antisocial behaviour and incidence of psychiatric disturbance have also been described (Forssman and Thuwe, 1966). A more recent study of refused abortion in Czechoslovakia (Dytrych *et al.*, 1975) is methodologically superior to previous investigations and the main findings were that the "unwanted" children had poorer school records than control subjects and their own families were more unstable. The children were disadvantaged but less markedly so than was found in the previous study in Sweden (Forssman and Thuwe, 1966).

Psychological Sequelae of Induced Abortion

Moderate to severe guilt feelings are commonly recorded after legal and illegal abortion (Ekblad, 1955; Simon and Senturia, 1966; Osofsky and Osofsky, 1972; Greer *et al.*, 1976) but, typically, such feelings are shortlived. Feelings of grief and guilt can, however, persist and in some cases they remain dormant until they are "reawakened" by a subsequent pregnancy (Kumar and Robson, 1978b). Severe mental illness, e.g. psychotic breakdowns analogous to puerperal psychosis are virtually unknown (Brewer, 1977) and most investigators have found that states of depression and anxiety lift once the pregnancy has been terminated. It has recently been suggested by Donnai *et al.* (1981) that adverse psychological sequelae are more likely to persist in women who have had "genetic" terminations of pregnancy following the diagnosis of foetal abnormality but the sample in this preliminary investigation was small (n = 12), and it was acknowledged that the data were anecdotal and open to bias. Nevertheless, this is an important observation which needs confirmation.

Much of the early research into the impact of abortion in women presenting with psychiatric disturbance is suspect because women often had to manifest a degree of disorder that was sufficient to convince doctors that abortion was indicated. As a general rule, women are more likely to experience psychiatric disturbances after an abortion if they already have a previous history of psychiatric disorder, but several studies have shown that the incidence of depression after legal abortion is low (Ekblad, 1955; Pare and Raven, 1970; Lask, 1975; Greer *et al.*, 1976). Many more women are depressed after childbirth (Pitt, 1968; Nilsson and Almgren, 1970; Kumar and Robson, 1978a) than after abortion, but such direct comparisons are complicated by the way in which the populations have selected themselves.

Reactions to Stillbirth

The reasons why investigators have shied away from researching such an obviously painful subject as stillbirth do not need to be underlined. Recent individual case reports (e.g. by Lewis, 1976 and Lewis and Page, 1978) may stimulate further systematic enquiries into the psychological sequelae of the death of the foetus *in utero*. There has been a steady fall in the numbers of stillbirths recorded each year (DHSS, 1979). In 1977 in England and Wales there were 5405 stillbirths, about a third of the number recorded in 1949. The ratio of still to live births is now, therefore, about 1:100. The difficulty of coping with stillbirth, particularly by staff, is now acknowledged, as is the fact that "denial" by staff exacerbates parental reactions to the stillbirth when there is a lack of a real baby to mourn. It is suggested that the loss be made as tangible as possible and the parents be encouraged to grieve the death of their baby. Further psychological support may be needed both afterwards and in the special circumstances of a subsequent pregnancy. Similar principles apply when babies are born with congenital malformations.

Pseudocyesis

The syndrome of false pregnancy is rare, and among the symptoms which it comprises are amenorrhoea or hypomenorrhoea, abdominal enlargement, breast changes, reported foetal movements, softening of the cervix and sometimes enlargement of the uterus, nausea and vomiting and weight gain (Bivin and Klinger, 1937; Moulton, 1942; Fried *et al.*, 1951). The diagnosis of pseudocyesis is based upon the presence of a firmly held belief by the patient that she is pregnant and the co-existence of one or more "physical" symptoms. The diagnosis is confirmed by the presence of an inverted umbilicus (in pregnancy there is effacement of the umbilicus), the absence of a foetus on ultrasound tests and the subsidence of the abdominal enlargement during anaesthesia. The differential diagnosis, of course, includes organic causes of abdominal enlargement. In a comprehensive review, Barglow and Brown (1972) note that there are differing views about the true nature of pseudocyesis—it has been looked upon as an illusion, a conversion symptom, a delusion, an hysterical identification, and as a manifestation of a fear of, or a wish for, pregnancy, a form of mourning, or, as a defence against psychotic breakdown. The symptoms (and signs) typically subside following psychotherapy and unless there is firm evidence of other overt psychological distrubance, medication with psychotropic drugs is not indicated.

Incidence of Depressive Neurosis and Anxiety States in Pregnancy

Pregnancy as an Aetiological Agent

This section examines the proposition that pregnancy is an important aetiological agent for the genesis of depressive neurosis and anxiety states. The unusual syndrome of pseudocyesis and the question of a specific relationship between unwanted pregnancy (continuing or terminated) and depression have already been discussed. The general impact of childbearing on maternal emotional health has also been reviewed and this section starts from the premise that the changes which accompany childbearing are so fundamental and far reaching, e.g. in terms of physiological and physical functioning, intrapsychic and interpersonal activity, social and occupational roles, that they may exert a destabilizing influence on maternal psychological equilibrium. Individual and anecdotal case reports will not be reviewed here and the emphasis will be on those studies which attempt systematically to examine if, and how, pregnancy can contribute to the occurrence of neurotic disturbance. A related hypothesis is examined first, that is, does pregnancy increase the risk of developing or experiencing a recurrence or exacerbation of a functional psychotic illness, such as schizophrenia or manic-depressive illness? It is possible that there may be both specific and general links between pregnancy and severe mental illnesses and some general factors may apply with equal force in the manifestation of neurotic disturbances.

Pregnancy, Schizophrenia and Manic-depressive Illness

There are two main sources of epidemiological evidence, both suggesting that the incidence of mental illness is actually diminished during pregnancy; the sources are studies of hospital admissions and research based on psychiatric case registers. Paffenbarger's (1964) study of admissions to mental hospitals during pregnancy and in the six months afterwards pointed to a sharp rise in the incidence of postpartum psychosis, but during pregnancy there was a "random timing of onset and ... preponderance of psychoneurotic illness." Pugh et al. (1963) found that admissions to mental hospital occurred less frequently during pregnancy than at times other than the puerperium and therefore the possibility must be considered that pregnancy in some way ameliorates existing, or prevents or postpones incipient, psychotic illnesses. Kendell et al. (1976) argued that the postpartum rise in the occurrence of psychiatric disorder was "too large to be accounted for by any pre-partum postponement of illnesses (or admissions)." Although inspection of their data shows some reduction during pregnancy of numbers of women "in treatment" in comparison with the 15 months before conception, there is nothing in the findings of Kendell et al. (1976, 1981) to suggest that pregnancy reduces the occurrence of new episodes of functional psychosis, nor of "affective illness" (depression plus anxiety states). It seems possible, therefore, to explain the slight fall in admissions to mental hospitals while women are pregnant on the grounds that obstetricians who are supervising antenatal care are unlikely to route mothers into mental hospitals unless such a course becomes absolutely necessary. The clinical threshold for such admissions may be raised because the woman is pregnant and is under medical supervision. It is also possible that the expectant mother derives benefit and support from the antenatal resources which she might otherwise have sought under a different aegis, i.e. the psychiatric services. Such speculations have not, up to now, been tested in any rigorous way.

There have also been some intriguing suggestions that schizophrenia is ameliorated during pregnancy (Baker, 1967; Horsley, 1972; Priest, 1978), but no evidence has been advanced in support of such statements. If, indeed, there is some substance to these observations, then research into any "protective" mechanisms during pregnancy could have some important general implications. It has been recognized for a long time that changes occur in the sensitivity of brain mechanisms to circulating hormone levels during pregnancy, but systematic studies of effects of pregnancy on biological mechanisms in psychotic illness have not been described.

Research into pre- versus postpartum manic-depressive illness has been reported, but in small numbers of patients (Bratfos and Haug, 1966; Brockington et al., Chapter 3) and it is not possible to tell for certain whether pregnancy has any beneficial effects on severe affective disorders. Targum et al. (1979) have described three women who were maintained on lithium therapy for manic-depressive psychosis and who discontinued medication in anticipation of conceiving and carrying babies to term. All three remained well during pregnancy, but two of them relapsed shortly after delivery. The general, and somewhat surprising conclusion, however, is that the major physiological and psychological changes of pregnancy do not *increase* the risks of severe mental illnesses; the evidence relating to pregnancy is mostly indirect and much less substantial than the data showing an increased incidence of mental illness after childbirth (Paffenbarger, Chapter 2).

Pregnancy and Neurotic Disturbance: Methodological Problems

Only depression and anxiety states are considered here; pseudocyesis, which can be regarded as a hysterical disorder, has already been discussed and there do not seem to have been any systematic investigations of possible links between pregnancy and other forms of hysteria, obsessive-compulsive neurosis or phobic states. Drug dependence cannot properly be regarded as a neurotic disorder and in any case there is no evidence to suggest that pregnancy is relevant as an aetiological agent. The special circumstance of unwanted pregnancy has already been discussed.

Most of the studies of maternal psychoneuroses in pregnancy have been primarily concerned with postnatal depression and the data in pregnancy were intended to serve as "base-line" for the postnatal findings. Measurements have often been made on single occasions in pregnancy or if information has been gathered in a serial fashion, this has sometimes been done in unstandardized ways. Samples have been highly selected or have selected themselves, and the criteria for diagnosing depression have often been poorly described. In the light of such marked differences in methods and in subjects, it is not at all surprising to find that there is very little firm evidence upon which to rest generalizations about the incidence or nature of antenatal depression.

Studies of hospital in-patient populations and of psychiatric services give a very biased picture of neurotic disorders because, for the most part, patients with minor psychiatric disturbance are managed exclusively by their family doctors. The most meaningful way of studying the prevalence, incidence and nature of neurotic disorder in pregnancy is by means of surveys of unselected pregnant women; unselected, that is, from a psychiatric point of view. Only a few investigators (Breen, 1975; Cox, 1979; Jarrahi-Zadeh *et al.*, 1969) have tackled the problem of finding a "control" or comparison group against which to place either single or serial observations of their pregnant samples. The selection of a meaningful comparison group poses interesting problems and, ideally, it would be best to have subjects serve as their own controls. Studying a group of women before they become pregnant is not a sensible proposition and following them for a long time after delivery may be of value, but of course their circumstances will have changed very considerably once they have an infant and then a toddler at home. Some investigators therefore find themselves obtaining pre-pregnancy "base-line" data in a retrospective fashion (e.g. Kumar and Robson, 1978a, b) but here, over and above the usual criticisms of retrospective enquiries, the investigators have to allow for the fact that they are studying mothers shortly after a very important event has occurred. Comparisons of mothers with fathers (e.g. Kendell et al., 1976) are beset with problems of sex differences, but they do offer one way of controlling for environmental changes which may have some impact on both partners.

The investigation of antenatal depression by Cox (1979) is one of the very few to incorporate a "control" group of non-pregnant subjects, in this case 89 women aged between 15 and 45 years, who were attending the health centre with a sick child. The women were selected if they were not pregnant or if they had not delivered a baby in the previous nine months, and they were matched for age, marital status and parity with the antenatal sample. Cox acknowledged the problems of matching a pregnant sample with mothers who had a sick child. Breen (1975) also used a non-pregnant comparison group (n = 20) in her survey, but here the women were as selected in their own way as the index group. The women were under 35 years of age, married for at least ten months and were brought into the survey through advertisements, contacts at work (research assistants, secretaries, wives of students etc). They differed in background and social class from the pregnant sample but most importantly, as Breen notes (p.64) "In any case these women were often different in the sense that many had decided not to have children at this time in their life, or even not to have children at all." The only other "control" group to be described was in the study of Jarrahi-Zadeh et al. (1969) where 21 white females of childbearing age were selected randomly (sic) from the secretaries of the Hospital and University and from students and faculty housewives.

Studies of Depression and Anxiety States in Pregnancy

In one of the largest surveys of pregnant and parturient women Tod (1964) interviewed 700 consecutive pregnant patients in his general/obstetric practice in London. Most women were seen between the tenth and twelfth weeks of pregnancy and thereafter at approximately monthly intervals. Following delivery, they were again seen at 10 days, at 2, 6, 12, 26 and 52 weeks postnatally. Tod did not describe the prevalence of neurotic disturbance in pregnancy as such, but focused in his report upon the women he subsequently assessed as suffering from postnatal depression ... "Where symptoms of pathological anxiety arise during pregnancy puerperal depression is to be expected." Tod (1964) also noted that, aside from the mothers who were obviously anxious and depressed and who were destined for puerperal depression, there were other pregnant women who appeared to be in the best of physical and mental health and "only exhaustive probing revealed their underlying distress." Thus, this prospective and influential study purported to reveal a virtually unitary relationship between pathological anxiety in pregnancy and postnatal depression. Some additional reasons for cautious interpretation of Tod's results are that he does not give any data about women who were thought to be anxious in pregnancy and who did not develop puerperal depression, and his assessment of the incidence of puerperal depression is low—2.9% of the total sample. Finally, he makes no comment about other concurrent psychiatric morbidity in his sample of 700 women. Studies of female attenders in general practice (Shepherd *et al.*, 1966) have revealed annual period prevalence rates for neurotic disorder of around 10–15%. Tod does, however, comment on the fact that the numbers of his depressed (anxious) group all had "previous inadequate personalities"; over half had a "previous psychiatric history", but it is not clear how these categories were defined.

Two other studies seem to support Tod's hypothesis that antenatal anxiety and postnatal depression are related. Dalton (1971) surveyed 500 women during pregnancy and presented her findings on 189 of the women who had replied to a minimum of seven questionnaires in pregnancy and the postnatal period. The general practitioner or obstetrician was asked to rate whether, at the first interview, the mother was "placid, normal or anxious." In all, there were 14 women who developed puerperal depression (defined as being of sufficient severity to require out-patient psychiatric treatment, n = 11, or drug therapy from their general practitioner, n = 3) and five of these women had been classed as being "anxious" at first interview. Of the remaining 175 subjects, 23 (13%) had originally been regarded as anxious. The difference in previous "anxiety" between the two groups of puerperal depressed versus non-depressed women was significant ($P<0.05$). A further difference was reported: the future puerperal depressives were more likely to become elated during the course of their pregnancies. The methodological deficiencies of this study, e.g. the large "drop-out" of subjects and poorly specified "clinical" criteria, are obvious causes for concern. Nevertheless the analysis can be taken a stage further than with Tod's (1964) data because Dalton does give rates for "depression during pregnancy" as well as for tiredness, irritability, headache, backache, nausea and vomiting during pregnancy. The criteria for severity and duration of "depression" are not specified. While anxiety was rated only in the first trimester by the family doctor or obstetrician on the somewhat idiosyncratic three point scale, "depression" and the other symptoms were rated throughout pregnancy and, overall, depression was noted in 67 subjects (37% of the sample), which is clearly greater than the incidence of puerperal depression of 7%. The definition of depression in pregnancy is unclear and it is reasonable to assume that the observers were recording mild, short-lived mood changes as well as clinical depressions. Such a suggestion is consistent with Dalton's comment that "during the puerperium a further 48 women (34% of the sample) were found to be mildly or temporarily depressed for which they did not require treatment."

A major deficiency of Dalton's study is the lack of specified and agreed criteria for clinically significant disturbance; it is not possible, therefore, to tell whether the 29 women who were rated as anxious at the first interview (15% of the entire sample) were suffering from debilitating anxiety states or whether, for example, they were temporarily concerned because of some obstetric problems. Women who suffered from puerperal depression were also noted to be more "elated" as pregnancy progressed; in all about 28% of the sample was described as being elated during pregnancy, but essential information is not provided about how the distinction between elated women and the others was made. The study by Dalton (1971) is important because she has gone on to link puerperal depression with hypotheses of endocrine dysfunction (Dalton, 1980). Such elasticity of clinical criteria can lead to biased categorization of clinical groups and thus at least one of the pillars supporting her hypotheses is unstable.

There is a third study which suggests a link between antenatal anxiety and postnatal depression (Meares *et al.*, 1976). One hundred and twenty-nine married women filled in questionnaires during pregnancy at an unspecified time and they were also briefly interviewed. At some time between six and 18 months after delivery they were sent postal questionnaires comprising visual analogue scales about the severity and persistence of depressive symptoms. The mothers were also asked whether they had had any treatment for depression. Forty-nine of the original sample (n = 129) responded to the postal enquiry and eight of these women were judged to have been depressed. They were more likely to have scored high on an anxiety (trait) questionnaire, the Taylor Manifest Anxiety Scale, and on a measure of "neuroticism" which was derived from a personality questionnaire (Eysenck and Eysenck, 1964, 1975). Meares *et al.* (1976) contrasted their own objective measures of anxiety with the unreliable and possibly insensitive measures used by Tod and by Dalton, but they concurred in finding an association between antenatal anxiety and postnatal depression. They drew attention to the possibility that "differing physiological conditions of pregnancy and the puerperium may induce anxiety and depression in the same individual." They concluded that "This association may have some implications for research into the biological basis of non-psychotic mental illness." Unfortunately, Meares *et al.* (1976) did not include any measure of depression during pregnancy. Neuroticism and depression are known to covary and it is possible that anxious and depressed women in pregnancy are more likely to reply to postnatal questionnaires, maintaining their previous involvement in the study. Had they filled in the visual analogue scales antenatally, it might at least have been possible to have looked for change scores. In conclusion, although the link between antenatal anxiety and postnatal depression is an attractive one, the evidence for it is dubious. Furthermore, the three studies by Tod (1964), Dalton (1971) and Meares *et al.* (1976) do not directly address themselves to the question of prevalence of clinically significant anxiety states at different times in pregnancy.

Several other investigators have enquired into psychiatric problems during pregnancy, but it is difficult to make direct comparisons between studies because of differences in the methods used and in the stages of pregnancy during which the subjects were studied. In Pitt's classic study (Pitt, 1968) of postnatal depression, over 300 women attending antenatal clinics around the 28th week of their pregnancies completed a questionnaire which aimed at evaluating depressive symptomatology. The questionnaire was repeated postnatally and change scores were used to arrive at estimates of the incidence of postnatal depression. The subjects were not given a clinical interview during pregnancy and in the absence of absolute scores from the questionnaire and of some means of validating them, it is not possible to draw any conclusions from this study on the prevalence of antenatal depression.

Jarrahi-Zadeh *et al.* (1969) investigated 86 upper and middle class, white American women, about half of whom were having their first babies. They were given a semi-structured clinical interview and also completed psychological tests and some rating scales in the last trimester of pregnancy as well at three days postpartum. These authors were struck by the amount of mild mood disturbance in pregnancy—"Approximately 50% of our normal clinic population reported that they were anxious, worried, depressed, experienced mood lability and/or had difficulty in sleeping while they were pregnant." Information about the severity, timing and duration of such symptoms was not provided, but Jarrahi-Zadeh *et al.* (1969) commented that "the stress of pregnancy and childbearing would seem to evoke neurotic symptoms in substantial numbers of a non-neurotic population." The lack of evidence for almost all component parts of their general statement makes it impossible to evaluate mental disturbance in this pregnant sample. Unfortunately, the "within measure" comparisons pre- and postpartum, suggesting a reduction in symptoms after delivery, cannot be extended beyond the third day when the second batch of tests was done.

Shereshefsky and Yarrow (1973) have reported a longitudinal investigation of 57 young, married, American, upper and middle class, highly selected primiparae. An unstandardized method of psychiatric classification gave the following results, 78% of the sample were normal or relatively healthy. The remaining 22% were diagnosed as neurotic (16%), borderline psychotic (3%), or personality disordered (3%); none of them were receiving or had actively sought treatment and by "gross criteria the women were essentially normal." In about 40% of the pregnant women they noted a tendency to moodiness or depressive attitudes, either occasionally or persistently. A larger proportion were irritable, tense or edgy, but the clinical relevance of such symptoms was not further evaluated. Anxiety was high in the first trimester, but subsided in mid-pregnancy and was then more intense as delivery approached. A similar study by Breen (1975) involved two interviews, antenatally at around the third to fourth month and the seventh month, and a third interview at 10 weeks after delivery. The 50 subjects who took part were primiparae who mainly came from the upper/middle socio-economic groups; they completed Pitt's (1968) screening questionnaire for depression pre- and postpartum, as well as a range of other tests. Response on the Pitt scale were subjected to principal components analysis, the subjects' replies seemed to cluster differently depending on whether the questionnaire was answered before or after delivery. Breen did not describe rates of occurrence of depression but it seemed that, whereas in pregnancy, changes in anxiety and confidence, in libido and in memory and energy were prominent, after delivery the picture had changed. "After birth of the child many women become more interested in sex, find they do not cry so easily and find they are more like their normal self."

Oakley (1980) also investigated about 60 primiparae during early and late pregnancy and at 1–2 months and 4–7 months postnatally. She did not comment specifically on the occurrence of antenatal neurotic disturbance, but she did argue that her findings suggested an inverse relationship between depression before and after birth. Uddenberg and Nilsson (1975) interviewed 95 women between the eleventh and twenty-first weeks of pregnancy and then four months after delivery. The degree of mental handicap was categorized according to criteria described by Uddenberg (1974) as severe, moderate or none. That the thresholds for moderate handicap were relatively low can be gleaned from the finding that 41% of the sample were rated as having had severe/moderate psychiatric disturbance in the previous year. However, a surprisingly large proportion (40%) of the sample had received psychotropic drugs in that year. Thirty-seven women (39% of the sample) were rated as having moderate/severe psychiatric problems during pregnancy and 22 of these subjects had both pre- and postpartum disturbance. A further 23 women had only postpartum problems. It does not seem, therefore, that the prevalence of mental disorder during the first half of pregnancy is very different from the period prevalence for the year before. Without details of the nature of the psychiatric disturbance it is not possible to assess how, if at all, pre- and postpartum mental disorders were related in the women studied by Uddenberg and Nilsson (1975).

An earlier, but more clinically oriented survey was described by Nilsson and Almgren (1970) who followed a very similar protocol to that of Uddenberg and Nilsson (1975). They comment that

> the high occurrence of mental symptoms and disturbances *during* pregnancy is remarkable, both in view of the long-standing general belief that psychological symptoms occur relatively infrequently during this period ... and since several authors have maintained that mental illness is considerably more common after partus than before."

The increase of mental disorder in pregnancy is less dramatic than is implied by Nilsson and Almgren (1970)—32.3% of their sample of 152 women were rated as experiencing moderate or pronounced psychiatric symptoms *before* pregnancy as opposed to 44.7% during pregnancy. Even allowing for difficulties in comparing counts of different symptoms, the increase is relatively small. However, half the women said they experienced a debut or a worsening of existing psychiatric symptoms during pregnancy with only 5% describing a reduction. The clinical relevance of such changes is unclear, because on mental state examination in early pregnancy only 9.2% of the sample were rated as showing definite signs of neurotic disturbance. The check list of psychiatric symptoms that was used by Nilsson and Almgren (1970) is unusual and it includes items such as globus hystericus, obsessive compulsive reactions, shortness of breath, as well as items more typically related with depression. In this study there was some evidence of a correlation between pre- and postpartum psychiatric problems, but the nature of the link (cf. Breen, 1975; Dalton, 1971; Oakley, 1980; Tod, 1964) was not specified.

Cox (1979) examined psychiatric morbidity in 263 pregnant Ugandan women by using a translated version of a standardized psychiatric interview (Goldberg *et al.*, 1970). The women were all seen at the time of their first antenatal visit and all attenders were seen, irrespective of parity, duration of pregnancy, age or domicile. A control group of non-pregnant women was also surveyed (see p.92). Cox (1979) found that 16% of his sample were suffering from clinically significant psychiatric disturbance—depressive neurosis 8.0%, depressive psychosis 2.7%, anxiety neurosis 3.4% and phobic neurosis 1.9%. The proportion of pregnant women with psychiatric morbidity exceeded that found for control women, but the difference only tended towards significance. There was more depression and anxiety in the pregnant women, but only anxiety was significantly greater in overall severity than in the non-pregnant women.

Wolkind and Zajicek (1981) have recently reported a prospective survey of pre-dominantly working class women who were about to have their first babies. Three samples of mothers were studied, once briefly in early pregnancy and then again in some detail in the seventh month; the samples consisted of 105 randomly selected married women, 81 unmarried women and 61 subjects who were selected according to two criteria of "vulnerability" i.e. a previous history of psychiatric disturbance or a history of separation in childhood from their parents, within the context of a disrupted family background. Clinical ratings of the prevalence of depression and/or anxiety in the previous month were categorized in terms of problems that were absent, dubious or definitely present. A semi-structured interview was used but few details are provided about the precise ways in which it was used and modified. Although individual symptom scores are provided for 94 women in the married group, it is not clear how these relate to the definition of a case; the main criterion seems to have been whether or not "the pattern of symptoms was severe enough to produce definite impairment of daily functioning and of relationships" and the single vignette suggests that a mild to moderate degree of disturbance might be consistent with a rating of definite problems.

The prevalence of definite problems in the unselected married women at the beginning of the third trimester was 14%, and a third of these women had reported psychiatric problems prior to pregnancy. Of 21 women in the vulnerable group who had a pre-pregnancy psychiatric history, 17 were found to have definite problems in late pregnancy. The authors therefore emphasize the important of a prior history of psychiatric disturbance not only in the occurrence of similar problems in pregnancy, but also postnatally and they point to the value of early identification of women "at risk".

The single mothers did not show an increased prevalence of psychiatric disorder in pregnancy; the women in this group were younger, came more often from disrupted homes, were more likely to belong to social classes 4 and 5 and to lack family support. Many of these features seem to fit well with the model of Brown and Harris (1978) in which severe contextual threat, together with the impact of an unwanted conception, might be expected to lead to a raised incidence of depression in pregnancy. Perhaps there was some element of selection in that only the "healthiest" women continued with their pregnancies and we are not told about their progress in the puerperium. Nevertheless the lack of a higher rate of depression in these subjects is surprising.

Kumar and Robson (1978a, b and in preparation) carried out a prospective survey of 119 primiparae in the first, second and third trimesters of pregnancy and then at intervals for a year postnatally. Retrospective information was obtained about any previous psychiatric history, psychiatric problems in the year and in the three months preceding conception. A comparison group of non-pregnant women was not used for the reason outlined earlier. Two other groups of women 38 primiparae and 39 multiparae, were investigated only postnatally in an attempt to control for the impact of participation in such a study on the incidence of postnatal depression. All the women in the main sample (n = 119) were interviewed by the psychiatrist who used a standardized method (Goldberg et al., 1970) at 12–14 weeks antenatally and again at 12 and 52 weeks postnatally. Some subjects were re-interviewed at other times if they met predetermined criteria. All the subjects were seen by a psychologist at 12, 24, 36 weeks in pregnancy and again at 1, 12, 26 and 52 weeks postnatally. There were very few refusals or "drop-outs" (see Kumar and Robson, 1978a, b), but the sample was skewed towards higher socio-economic status (about three-quarters of the women came from the white collar and higher social grades). They were all married or stably cohabiting and spoke good English (selection criteria). Their mean age was 28 years, range 18–40 years.

Figure 2 shows a sharp and significant rise in the incidence of depression and anxiety in the first trimester of pregnancy and a similar rise in the three months after delivery. Table 2 summarizes some of the factors that are associated with either antenatal or postnatal depression and it can be seen that the patterns of associations are rather different. There was very little overlap between the women who became depressed before and after delivery, supporting earlier suggestions of a lack of relationship between antenatal and postnatal psychiatric problems. It is possible, however, that participation in the study had some preventive effect on postnatal depression in particular for women who had manifested problems such as depression during pregnancy.

No significant increase was seen in antenatal anxiety states or general symptoms (cf. Dalton, 1971; Meares et al., 1976; Tod, 1964), but most subjects expressed fears of varying intensity and persistence about the health of their babies. Worries about the foetus were exacerbated in women who were also

Fig. 2. The prevalence and incidence of neurotic disorder during pregnancy and for up to a year postnatally is shown. The incidence of depression is significantly increased in the first trimester of pregnancy and also at 12 weeks postnatally. A subject is counted as a "new" case of depression only if she was not rated as depressed at the immediately previous occasion. Figures in parentheses refer to "new" cases. Data from survey by Kumar and Robson (in preparation).

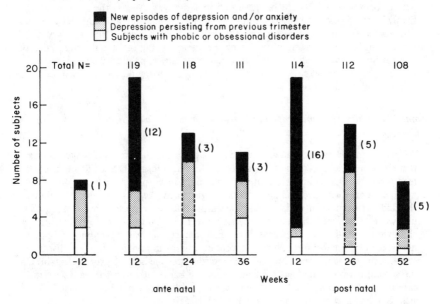

depressed in early pregnancy and both these factors were significantly linked with a history of previous induced abortion (Kumar and Robson, 1978b). Fears were often of some damage or harm to the foetus and they were frequently couched in terms of guilt and fears of retribution. Such prolonged and delayed reactions following terminations of pregnancy were reminiscent of delayed and suspended grief reactions, lying dormant until reawakened by another pregnancy. Some case histories illustrate the nature of such early depressive reactions and it is possible that some of the women who become depressed during pregnancy may derive benefit from supportive counselling. The nature of the association between prior abortion and depression in pregnancy is being investigated in more detail. The antenatal part of the survey also shows that a few women became depressed in the second and third trimesters and in each case this followed a major event such as bereavement (see Table 2).

Clinical accounts (from Kumar and Robson, 1978b):

Case History

A woman in her late twenties had obtained a legal abortion two years previously and she denied having had any immediate physical or emotional complications. The present pregnancy had been planned, and while she reported feeling under strain beforehand, after conception she became irritable, forgetful, tired and run-down. She felt miserable and pessimistic and was intermittently weepy; she blamed herself for being unreasonable and for not coping as well as others. She brooded about the future, about the responsibility of having a baby; it was "not a toy to be put away". She did not "feel" pregnant and expressed the profound worry that having aborted a perfect baby this one would be deformed in some way. Yet, at the same time, she firmly believed that she had been right to have had an abortion although her husband had wanted the first baby. This time she wanted a boy but could only think of girls' names. She broke down and wept during the interview, but resisted the suggestion of referral for psychotherapy. By the third trimester she emphatically denied any difficulties, present or past, and continued to maintain a fragile façade until she was delivered of a healthy baby at term.

Some Examples of Comments made by Women who were not rated as Clinically Depressed

(1) A woman who had had an abortion in a private clinic three years ago now said that she would really like to be hypnotized in order to forget it. She felt she could go mad if she thought about it too much. She might have to pay for it.

(2) A woman who had had an abortion 11 years ago (illegally by a doctor) said that she had not been greatly distressed afterwards. She had repressed her feelings. She had worried whether she might not be able to have children and now whether her child would be all right. She occasionally had an irrational fear of retribution. She had not talked of these feelings before and wept during the interview. She then miscarried at about the sixteenth week and some six months later she became pregnant again. On the second occasion she had few fears about the baby, although she had worried in case she miscarried again. This time it was a "good" pregnancy because she had felt sick. She had had no irrational fears like the last time.

(3) A woman who had had two illegal abortions 11 and 12 years ago had had to keep them secret from the family. She had no intention of marrying the fathers and both were unexpectedly traumatic experiences, after which she felt very guilty and depressed; she had "lost" something and used to find herself looking at young babies in prams. After the break-up of an important relationship three years later, she had become depressed and had made a suicidal gesture. She was now miserable at times, but coping reasonably well. She said spontaneously that she worried a lot about the baby's health. She was afraid that some punishment was due for the fact that she had had terminations before. If there was something wrong (with the baby) she would feel directly responsible. It was a case of crime and punishment; she would have to pay. She felt she had murdered her previous babies. She was a lapsed Catholic.

In summary, therefore, the incidence of depression does seem to be raised, particularly during the early stages of pregnancy. The view of pregnancy as a "maturational crisis" receives support from the survey findings linking antenatal depression with prior termination and with present ambivalence about going to term (see Table 2). The suggested association between antenatal anxiety and postnatal depression (Tod, 1964; Dalton, 1971; Meares et al., 1976) still requires confirmation. In conclusion, one important reservation about such surveys must be emphasized—the information has almost always been derived from women who attend antenatal clinics. It may well be the defaulters who are most psychologically disturbed and in need of help.

Table 2.   The presence of depression in the first trimester of pregnancy or three months postnatally was found to be associated with a number of variables. Such variables may be categorized as "predisposing" or as "life events" (i.e. premature delivery or bereavement). In some cases, e.g. infrequent sexual intercourse or anxieties about the health of the foetus, the association may be a consequence of maternal depression. Examples of items which did not associate with maternal depression are listed in the Footnote to Table 1. Data from survey by Kumar and Robson (in preparation).

Associations with depression and anxiety in primiparae		
	Antenatal	*Postnatal*
Age (30 + years)		x
Personality (Neuroticism—EPQ)	xxx	
Prior psychiatric disturbance	xx	
Childhood separation from father		x
Marital conflict (a/n)	xxx	xx
Dissatisfaction leisure activity (a/n)		x
Poor relationship with mother (a/n)		x
Husband: prior psychiatric disturbance		xxx
Infrequent sexual intercourse p/n		x
Subfertility (2 years +)		xx
Thought about T.O.P. this pregnancy	xxx	xx
Prior T.O.P.	xxx	
Anxieties about foetus	xxx	
Mixed feelings and worries about baby		xxx
Still smoking at end of pregnancy	xx	
Premature baby (<2 kg)		x
Bereavement	xxx	

x = $P<0.05$;   xx = $P<0.01$;   xxx = $P<0.001$
(a/n: antenatal — p/n: postnatal — T.O. P: termination of pregnancy)
Footnote. Individual factors which did not associate with maternal depression included—social class, employment status, domestic or financial problems, chronic illnesses and individual life events apart from bereavement and birth of a premature baby.

Postnatal Depression

Incidence and Nature of Postnatal Depression

A very important study of postnatal depression was reported by Pitt (1968) and his finding of an incidence rate of about 11% for neurotic depression within six weeks of delivery has been broadly confirmed by many investigators. Salient details of Pitt's enquiry have already been mentioned and it is important to note here that he was recording incidence (new cases) and not prevalence. All subjects showing an increase of six or more points on Pitt's screening questionnaire which was administered twice, around the twenty-eight week of pregnancy and the sixth week after delivery, were interviewed as potential depressives. Unlike many other researchers both before and since, Pitt (1968) took care to list the criteria that he, as a psychiatrist, used to define the presence of puerperal depression:

(1) Subjects should describe depressive symptoms.
(2) These symptoms should have developed since delivery.
(3) These symptoms should be unusual in their experience, and to some extent, disabling.
(4) The symptoms should have persisted for more than two weeks.

In addition a clinical check list, giving a severity score (Hamilton, 1960) was also used, but details are not published other than to note that the mean Hamilton rating of puerperal depressives (distinguished by means of Pitt's questionnaire and the clinical interview) was clearly and significantly higher, by 10 points, than for the rest of the sample. These results support the reliability of Pitt's scale, which is very similar in its content to other questionnaires aiming to measure depressive symptomatology. In fact Pitt only succeeded in interviewing 27 of the 33 depressed patients, in six the diagnosis was based on postal enquiry, but any effect on his overall conclusions is likely to be marginal.

The clinical account of depression is worth quoting because it encapsulates practically all the important features of postnatal depression.

It was chiefly after return home that depression was almost always evident, chiefly as tearfulness, despondency, feelings of inadequacy and inability to cope—particularly with the baby. ("Every other woman seems to be blooming".) Mood was often labile, and any diurnal variation took the form of greater distress in the evenings. Guilt was mainly confined to self-reproach over not loving or caring enough for the baby. Suicidal ideas were present only in women admitted to psychiatric hospital, and feelings of actual hopelessness were not frequent. Yet many felt quite changed from their usual selves, and most had never been depressed like this before.

Depression was almost invariably accompanied and sometimes overshadowed, by anxiety over the baby. Such anxiety was not justified by the babies' health; none was seriously ill, and most were thriving. Feeding worries were the commonest. Babies who would not sleep and kept crying were found hard to love, with consequent guilt and anxiety. Overt hostility to the child, though, was rare. Two mothers had great difficulty in accepting their babies as really theirs. A few, while able to satisfy their babies' physical needs, feared spoiling them. Multiparae tended to worry over the older children's jealousy of the new arrival. Anxiety was also often manifest in hypochondriasis. Somatic symptoms abounded and formed the basis of fears of ill-health .... Unusual irritability was common, sometimes adding to feelings of guilt. A few patients complained of impaired concentration and memory. Undue fatigue and ready exhaustion were frequent, so that mothers could barely deal with their babies, let alone look after the rest of the family and cope with the housework and shopping. Sometimes there was a loss of normal interests. Anorexia, occasionally associated with nausea was present with remarkable consistence. Sleep disturbances, over and above that inevitable with a new baby, was reported by a third of the patients, taking the form of getting off to sleep, and nightmares, more often than of early morning waking. (Pitt, 1968)

It is hard to think of a better clinical description of a depressive syndrome in or out of the context of childbearing. On the grounds that only two patients showed "the classical picture of depressive illness, with suicidal ideas, worsening of depression in the morning and early morning waking" Pitt decided to describe postnatal depression as "Atypical". Further reasons were the prominence of neurotic symptoms and the generally milder nature of the disturbance. In many ways the label is an unfortunate one because the depressions are very typical of the sorts of common affective disturbances that are mainly dealt with by general practitioners. At the time when Pitt published his findings, the controversy over the endogenous-reactive dichotomy with respect to depressive disorders was in full swing. Although the dust has now mostly settled without the issue being fully resolved, postnatal depression has reawakened the "illness" versus "reaction to events" argument. This issue will be taken up later (p.111) in relation to "biologically" oriented observations by Dalton (1980). Bonham-Carter *et al.* (1980) and Hayworth *et al.* (1980) on the one hand, and research with a psycho-social bias by other workers such as Almgren and Nilsson (1970), Breen (1971), Brown and Harris, (1978), Kumar and Robson (1978a, b), and Oakley (1980) on the other.

Pitt (1968) also followed up 28 of the women who had been depressed following childbirth, by a postal enquiry when their babies were a year old. Twelve of the women seemed to have made little or no improvement but he was unable to find any special features which distinguished between the women who had improved and those who had not.

The study by Pitt has been described in some detail because it can be regarded as the main work against which to compare other investigations. Other estimates of the incidence of postnatal depression have ranged between 2.9% (Tod, 1964) to 16% (Meares *et al.*, 1976). Some reasons for such differences may be the marked variations in the size of samples studied, the composition of the samples and the methods used for detecting and defining postnatal depression.

Tod's (1964) study has already been mentioned in the discussion of antenatal depression and given his large, unselected sample of consecutive attenders for antenatal and postnatal care and his knowledge of the women as their general practitioner, it is difficult to reconcile his very low estimate of the incidence of postnatal depression with that of Pitt and other workers. Tod drew a clear distinction between the evanescent mild forms of depression seen three or four days after delivery, which he regarded as normal accompaniments of pregnancy and parturition, and the pathological reactions, where some women became "seriously depressed after the birth of the baby". The clue may lie in the words "seriously depressed" which fit the case vignettes given by Tod; in three of the five instances described, referral to a psychiatrist was made, in the other two antidepressants were prescribed. All the women were seen on several occasions during the year after delivery and it is surprising that Tod does not comment on the occurrence or otherwise of less severe but none the less handicapping depressive states.

At the other end of the scale, Meares *et al.* (1976) report an incidence of about 16% for postnatal depression, but the reliability of their findings is open to question. The time interval for recording puerperal depression ranged between six and 18 months after delivery, by which time their sample had reduced itself from 129 to 40. Depression was assessed by postal response on visual analogue scales and by positive replies to questions about treatment for depression.

Nilsson and Almgren (1970) reported that in their longitudinal survey of 152 women, 19% of the sample had "clear mental disturbance" postpartum, (i.e. pronounced psychiatric symptoms, large number of symptoms of a serious nature). Elsewhere, they commented that in about two-thirds of the women their symptoms had begun or had become worse in the two months following delivery; such a "correction" would bring the estimate of "incidence" closely in line with that by Pitt (1968). Clinical evaluations of post-partum mental state revealed a point prevalence of 10.7% and mild neurotic signs in 22.0% of the sample. Unfortunately, it is not possible to evaluate these findings in more detail because the authors did not specify their clinical criteria for depression more fully. Nevertheless, the findings of this important Swedish survey are broadly consistent with other studies.

The results of several other studies of maternal mental adjustment can be culled for information on the incidence of post-natal depression. Thus Dalton (1971) found that 14 out of 189 (7.5%) women became depressed, a depression of sufficient severity to require out-patient psychiatric help or drug therapy from the general practitioner. Six months after delivery a psychiatrist saw 11 of the 14 women and confirmed the diagnosis. Shereshefsky and Yarrow (1973) reported that three of their study population (n = 57) developed severe psychiatric disorders within six months of childbirth—the disorders represented "the broad spectrum of mental disturbance which have been described in the post-partum period." The case summaries indicate that two of the women were hospitalized with psychotic reactions. In spite of the intensive nature of this study the authors do not report or discuss milder variants of postnatal psychopathology such as those described by Pitt (1968).

Breen's (1971) sample of 50 primiparae completed the "Pitt" scale in the seventh month of pregnancy and at 10 weeks after delivery, but in this study *any* increase in the score was regarded as suggestive of disturbance. Ratings of difficulties with their babies were also made, as well as of obstetric difficulties, Taking results for these three "criteria of adjustment" together, Breen defined an "ill-adjusted" group of 18 women (36% of the sample) who had evidence of disturbance on two or possibly all three measures. Such observations are of great interest in a more descriptive analysis of maternal reactions, but the significance of the overall "ill-adjusted" group in terms of post-natal depression is unclear. Oakley (1980) also studied a somewhat similar sample of just over 50 primiparae; she assessed their mental states in pregnancy and at four to nine weeks and 17-27 weeks after delivery. Oakley used questions which were derived from a structured clinical interview, the Present State Examination (Wing *et al.*, 1974) to evaluate depression and found that 15% of her sample fitted specified criteria for clinical depression—"a depressed state occurring at any time from hospital discharge to five months post-partum, characterised by two or more symptoms and lasting at least two weeks."

Paykel *et al.* (1981), who studied 120 women attending post-natal clinics around the sixth week post-partum, also used a semi-structured clinical interview (Paykel *et al.*, 1970). They found 21 cases of depression (17%) with an onset after delivery, two thirds starting in the first week. The scale (Raskin *et al.*, 1970) that was used for rating depression examined three aspects of the syndrome, verbal reports, observed behaviour and secondary symptoms,; it had been widely used in trials of the efficacy of psychotropic drugs. Unfortunately, Paykel *et al.* (1980) do not give concordance figures for the scale with their clinical interview ratings and this is a potentially serious problem. Although both interviewers "underwent training in the use of the rating instruments", neither had any clinical psychiatric experience. Both were students on a course of human biology and general nursing training. This issue is raised not because of a predilection for demarcation disputes, but because there are problems in interpreting clinical data which may be unrecognized or misunderstood even by trained psychiatrists, who are not a notably agreement-prone group at the best of times. Yet very important generalizations can stem from studies such as the one by Paykel *et al.* (1980) (see section on associations with postnatal depression).

Playfair and Gowers (1981) have reported a survey of 618 mothers, which was carried out by 64 general practitioners working in the British Isles. Thirteen symptoms of depression were rated as present or absent during pregnancy and postnatally and associations between raised symptom scores between the eight and twentieth week after birth and a range of factors were tested. Seventeen of the mothers (2.75% of the sample) required referral to a psychiatrist some time after delivery and in five cases the breakdown was thought to be primarily psychotic. Of the remaining 12 women, nine had substantially elevated symptom scores for depression at the time of the postnatal interview. Taking the presence of six or more symptoms as a criterion, 62 mothers (10% of the sample) were regarded as suffering from post-natal depression. Predictors of such depression were found to be: a history of puerperal depression, a history of miscarriage, raised symptom scores for depression during pregnancy, severe postpartum blues and the presence after the birth of stressors such as marital difficulties, housing problems or ill-health of the mother. Other less clearly related variables were a history of dysmenorrhoea, the partner's socio-economic status and a positive history of psychiatric disorder in his case.

The study by Playfair and his general practitioner colleagues is especially important because it encompassed a large number of subjects. The aim was to search for predictors of postnatal depression as judged by observers using "their ordinary standards of clinical assessment." It is possible, however, that the fact of participating in the study influenced these standards and it might have been preferable to have included more rigorous evaluations of the severity and persistence of the individual symptoms. Similarly, the ways in which potentially associated factors were assessed was not specified. The benefits of having observers with prior knowledge of their patients are counter-balanced by the possibility of bias when two supposedly independent sets of ratings are made by the general practitioner.

The final study of relevance was by Kumar and Robson, 1978a, b (see also Table 2 and Fig. 2). The clinical interviews were all conducted by a psychiatrist who had been trained in the use of a semi-structured interview schedule (Goldberg *et al.*, 1970). The incidence of depression in this study was found to be around 12%, which is very close to Pitt's finding. The depressed women in this survey differed, however, in that the depressions did not persist in clinically significant form for the whole year. Pitt (1968) based his findings on postal reports of symptoms at a year and his conclusions must be regarded as tentative. Repeated clinical interviews give more reliable information (Kumar and Robson, 1978a, b), but it is possible that the different resources and social backgrounds of the two samples may have contributed to the divergent findings on the persistence of postnatal depression. Furthermore, intensive participation in a longitudinal survey of mental health may of itself bring about some reduction in manifest neurotic disturbance.

What can one conclude about the incidence of depression after childbirth? Is there really such a thing as postnatal depression? Most of the surveys described here have been based upon relatively small numbers of subjects—a few hundred at best. Paffenbarger's elegant epidemiological analysis of puerperal psychosis culled mental hospital admission statistics in Hamilton County, Ohio, over 18 years—an analogous investigation of neurotic disorders would require identification of "cases" by means of interviews and questionnaires of a similarly large population of subjects and the time and resources needed challenge the imagination. Comparisons of "point prevalences" in pregnant and non-pregnant samples of women are unreliable unless there are sufficient numbers of subjects and comparable methods of assessment are used. The best evidence for postnatal depression therefore comes from longitudinal surveys which make several measurements in the same subjects before and after delivery, as well as a retrospective assessment of the time before conception. About 10–15% of the women in several of the studies reviewed here, manifested a "new" episode of depression by two or three months after delivery and the question about raised incidence postnatally can be answered positively. What is not at all clear, however, is when postnatal depression becomes ordinary depression on the time scale after delivery, and whether there are any special clinical or other features which distinguish postnatal depression from episodes of depression at other times unrelated to childbirth.

Personal, Social and Biological Correlates of Postnatal Depression

Personal History and Personality

In the review of the psychoanalytic literature on pregnancy and motherhood (p.82) the suggestion was made that maternal puerperal depression was more likely to occur in those women who had themselves had disturbed relationships with their parents in early childhood. It was also argued that the period of transition to motherhood was also a time for regression and reopening of past developmental conflicts. Such suggestions receive some support from the study by Frommer and O'Shea (1973) and from the results of a survey of primiparae by Kumar and Robson. Table 2 shows that women who became depressed post-natally had reported separations of four weeks or longer from their fathers before the age of 11 years and they had also described concurrent difficulties in their relationships with their mothers (cf. Brown and Harris, 1978). Of the 14 women who mentioned in early pregnancy that they had considered asking for a termination of their pregnancies, 13 were found to be depressed either during pregnancy of after delivery. Contemplating termination, even though many of the women had planned and wanted their pregnancies, can be looked upon as a sign of profound ambivalence, which is witnessed by the high rate of occurrence of depression, either in early pregnancy, or after the baby is born. These results provide some tangible support for psychoanalytically based view of pregnancy as a maturational crisis.

It is important to note that the information about parental relationships and about attitudes to the pregnancy was obtained during pregnancy and the postnatal psychiatric assessment was carried out without knowledge of these data. Nevertheless, the numbers of subjects in this study are small and the results of other prospective studies should help resolve discrepancies. For example, Nilsson and Almgren (1970) were unable to find a link between postpartum depression and maternal childhood disturbances.

In the study of Kumar and Robson (Table 2) primiparae who were aged 30 or more years or who gave a history of subfertility were also more likely to become depressed after delivery; such women usually had untroubled pregnancies. With regard to the predisposing effects of a previous history of psychiatric disorder, Pitt (1968) found that women with a history of psychiatric disturbance were not more likely to become depressed after delivery and the study by Kumar and Robson (see Table 2) supports this observation. However, many women were depressed during pregnancy and it is possible that participation in a longitudinal survey of emotional changes facilitates the resolution of psychological problems. There is some evidence from the survey by Kumar and Robson (1978a, b) to support the suggestion that participation in clinical research can be therapeutic. Investigation of the two subsidiary groups who were not interviewed during pregnancy (n = 38 primiparae and n = 39 multiparae) suggested that they were indeed more prone (28%) to become depressed postnatally.

Playfair and Gowers (1981) found that women who described previous postnatal depressions were more likely to be rated as depressed 2–5 months after delivery and Paykel et al. (1980) have reported a positive correlation between postnatal depression and previous treatment for psychiatric problems, but they were unable to demonstrate any links with the subject's own childhood relationships with her parents (cf. Frommer and O' Shea, 1973). The depressed women in Paykel's study were younger than the non-depressed subjects, 24 years v. 28 years. Measurements of personality are relevant to the subject of depression but concurrent assessments of personality and of clinical status are open to the criticism that the measures may covary. Thus Kumar and Robson found that raised scores on a measure of neuroticism (Eysenck and Eysenck, 1975) which were obtained during pregnancy correlated significantly with clinical ratings of depression made around the same time, but failed to do so with ratings of post-natal depression made several months later in the same sample of subjects (Table 2).

Social and Environmental Influences

Several groups of investigators have reported that the incidence of postnatal depression does not seem to be influenced by the subject's socio-economic status (Pitt, 1968; Nilsson and Almgren, 1970; Kumar and Robson, 1978a, b, Table 2; Paykel et al., 1980). Brown and Harris (1978) have, however, found that working-class women who are exposed to other social pressures (e.g those with young children at home and lacking supportive confiding relationships) are more at risk than comparable middle-class women for developing depressive disorders. These findings bear directly on the question of psychiatric morbidity in pregnant and parturient women and the results of the important survey by Brown and Harris (1978) will be discussed in some detail later. Some other conclusions which have emerged from surveys by Nilsson and Almgren (1970), Paykel et al., 1980 and Pitt (1968) are that parity does not by itself seem to influence the incidence of postnatal depression, but it may be worth testing for possible interactions between social class and parity (cf. Brown and Harris, 1978). A very similar incidence of postnatal depression was found in two relatively large prospective surveys, done 10 years apart, one in a predominantly working-class sample of multiparae and primiparae (Pitt, 1968) and the other in a predominantly middle-class sample of primiparae (Kumar and Robson, 1978a).

Marital conflict was not specifically examined by Pitt (1968) but a lack of support in the marriage or the presence of disharmony have been found to correlate with the occurrence of postnatal depression (Kumar and Robson, 1978a; see also Table 2; Nilson and Almgren, 1970; Paykel *et al.*, 1980 Playfair and Gowers 1981). Kumar and Robson rated the nature and severity of marital difficulties during pregnancy, i.e. many months before the onset or otherwise of postnatal depression. However, as with practically all the surveys that are reviewed here, the information was obtained primarily from one source, the mother, and future surveys will hopefully improve the reliability of the data by gathering information from several sources. Henderson (1981) has recently made the very important observation that there may not be always an actual lack of social support when individuals become depressed but rather that they perceive the available support as being deficient. Conclusions about aspects of the social correlates of depression cannot be regarded as anything more than very tentative until more comprehensive studies are done. In their survey, Brown and Harris (1978) commented that they collected information from a close relative of 50 of their sample of psychiatric patients (n = 114) but they do not provide detailed corroborative data about, for example, the supportiveness (confiding) in marital relationships. Such data were apparently not obtained in their community sample (n = 458) from which they draw most of their conclusions.

The main thrust of the work by Brown and Harris (1978) has been to clarify the part played by social and environmental factors in the aetiology of depressive disorders. They found that women who became depressed were more likely to have experienced "severe" life events in the recent past and that certain factors, either in isolation or in combination, enhanced the womens' vulnerability to life events—the prototypical woman "at risk" was working class, with young children at home and therefore not employed, with a poor relationship with her spouse and having lost her mother before she was 11 years of age. The presence of a strong confiding relationship mitigated the effects of the other "vulnerability" factors. The derivation of Brown and Harris's interactional model for vulnerability factors and provoking agents has been criticised on methodological grounds (Tennant and Bebbington, 1978) and in the context of this review of childbearing some further comments may be appropriate, especially in the light of their general conclusion (p.141) that "As things turned out in our series there is *no* evidence that childbirth and pregnancy *as such* are linked to depression." It is important to note that the series referred to is the sample of 114 psychiatric in- and out-patients and *not* the community sample from whom the profile of vulnerability factors was obtained (i.e. working class, young children at home, poor confiding relationships, loss of mother).

Psychiatric patients who were pregnant or had recently given birth were however contrasted with comparable women drawn from the "normal" segment of the community sample (n = 382) but unfortunately Brown and Harris (1978) do not report on relevant comparisons concerning childbearing between the patients and the remaining 76 women in the community who were rated as being "cases" of depression, or between the community "cases" and the normal women.

It was found that the proportion of psychiatric patients who were pregnant or had given birth in the previous nine months was twice as great as in the normal women 17/114 v. 37/382. Five of the childbearing psychiatric patients had very bad marriages and five lived in grossly inadequate housing; one more was unmarried and one had a miscarriage; in contrast only six of the 37 pregnant "normal" women had such problems ($P < 0.01$). Brown and Harris therefore concluded "while the numbers are small, the results clearly suggest that it is the meaning of events that is usually crucial: pregnancy and birth, like other crises, can bring home to a woman the disappointment and hopelessness of her position....". These conclusions would have been more persuasive had Brown and Harris obtained or described similar results from comparisons of cases and normal women in the community sample.

In the absence of published results of such comparisons the reader is unable to separate out the factors which may have been relevant to the onset of depression as distinct from those which may have contributed to an individual becoming a psychiatric patient with the diagnosis of depression. Patients of psychiatric hospitals comprise a very small and selected segment of the population with manifest psychiatric problems and generalizations to the wider context that are based upon patients must therefore be hedged with *caveats*. There is little doubt that severe ongoing problems can contribute to the occurrence of depression but Brown and Harris seem to suggest an exclusive and almost unitary relationship viz. "The high rate of depression associated with childbirth and pregnancy was *entirely* [their italics] due to those rated severe: only pregnancy and childbirth associated with a severe ongoing problem played an aetiological role." In fact, nearly a third (5/17) of their very small sample did not describe a severe threat associated with pregnancy and birth, and in the remaining 12 women the authors do not go beyond juxtaposing social adversity and childbearing and assigning "meaning" to such an association in very general terms. In order to try and maintain objectivity of their data, which, in this case, went back over a period of nine months, these workers restricted their convention for rating severe contextual threat to factors such as poor housing, acute financial shortage or very poor health of the mother. Such factors are obviously relevant to psychiatric patients and are undoubtedly meaningful irrespective of the nature of the crisis—be it birth or bereavement. The threat posed by childbirth may transcend the level of meaning to which Brown and Harris confine themselves. They acknowledge that their approach "has a devastating disadvantage: it treats essentially all similar types of 'event' such as births as alike ...... The birth of a child does not mean the same thing for all women." A woman's age, her developmental and psychosexual history, her obstetric history and her desire for the pregnancy, her personality, her occupation and plans for the future, the quality of her marriage, her past medical and psychiatric history are but some of the variables which may determine how much of a threat having a baby is to her. The failure of Brown and Harris to find links between the incidence of depression and childbearing *as such* does not, therefore, necessarily imply that such links do not exist. Their inability to demonstrate more specific and more subtle associations may reflect their intentionally restricted methodology and the incompleteness of their comparisons.

Biological Correlates of Postnatal Depression

Brockington *et al.* (Chapter 3) and Hamilton (Chapter 1) discuss the part played by biological mechanisms in the genesis of puerperal psychotic disorders, particularly of the affective type (cf. Kadrmas *et al.*, 1979) and Stein (Chapter 5) reviews research into biological correlates of the transient mood changes that are seen in the "blues". Investigations of disorders of neuroendocrine or neurotransmitter systems in postpartum depression are either negative (e.g. Nott *et al.*, 1976) or are unrelated to parturition *per se* (e.g. Bonham Carter *et al.*, 1980; Hayworth *et al.*, 1980). It has been suggested that fluctuations in mood in the puerperium may be linked with changes in plasma concentrations of cortisol (Handley *et al.*, 1980) or fluctuations of urinary cyclic AMP (Ballinger *et al.*, 1979) but aside from the need to replicate such findings, there is still no certainty that they can provide insights into mechanisms underlying *pathological* mood states.

Dalton (1980) has recently written a potentially influential account of postnatal depression which is firmly cast in the medical model, e.g.

> Depression is an illness . . . Postnatal depression has some characteristics which are different from those usually found in typical depression, and so it is known as "atypical" (meaning not typical) (sic). This is an important distinction . . . . because the commonly prescribed drugs are effective for typical depression, but special types of drugs are more effective for atypical depression.

She picks out the following symptoms as being characteristic of postnatal depression—irritability, hypersomnia, worsening of tiredness and dysphoria in the evenings, increased appetite and possibly even cravings with weight gain, dizziness and vertigo and, if it is present, she regards galactorrhoea as pathognomonic of postnatal depression. This syndrome is undoubtedly atypical in that it differs from the clinical pictures of depression in the puerperium that have been obtained from several surveys, e.g. Kumar and Robson, 1978a; Paykel *et al.*, 1980; Pitt, 1968; Nilsson and Almgren, 1970). The treatment recommended by Dalton is energetic—she advises preventive measures in women who have a family history of postnatal depression and suggests that progesterone should be given by daily injections from the onset of labour for the next eight days. Subsequently the hormone may be taken by suppositories for a month and the early results of a survey of the efficacy of such preventive measures are described as "most gratifying". If patients are seen before menstruation has begun it is suggested that progesterone should be combined with monoamine oxidase inhibitors. The reason for choosing monoamine oxidase inhibitors is that postnatal depression is not typical depression because it does not respond to tricyclic antidepressants. In addition, if a mother is not breast feeding she can be given bromocriptine to suppress lactation. If perchance the depression is untreated and menstruation has recommenced, the treatment becomes that of the premenstrual syndrome.

The therapeutic claims which are advanced by Dalton do not have the backing of controlled clinical investigations. Individual case reports are presented but the nature of depression is such that spontaneous remissions and placebo reactions must be distinguished from responses to pharmacotherapy. It is powerful treatment indeed, to give daily hormone injections and potentially dangerous antidepressant drugs which require dietary restrictions. Hopefully, such measures will not be generally adopted without some formal evidence of their efficacy, even in highly selected, atypical patients.

Priorities for Future Research

There is an outstanding need to develop reliable and rapid techniques for evaluating psychiatric disorders in childbearing women. Studies which have been based upon established methods—e.g. the clinical interview schedule of Goldberg et al. (1970) can at least be directly compared. Even so, investigators (e.g. Cox, 1979; Kumar and Robson, 1978a, b) are obliged to make some arbitrary decisions about rating procedures. How does one assess tiredness and loss of energy during early pregnancy and how should sleep disturbance be evaluated in a mother who is breast-feeding a six-week-old baby "on demand"? Some form of simple, self-administered scale is also needed for use in antenatal and postnatal settings to pick out potential cases of women with depression and anxiety. Existing questionnaires contain questions which are dissonant with the woman's pregnant or parturient state and, on the other hand, questions about her mental state which take account of her condition are lacking.

Improvements in methodology will inevitably lead to a better distinction between "cases" and "non cases" and between conditions such as puerperal psychosis, postnatal depression and the "blues." Operational methods are, however, no better than the clinical observations from which they are derived. One of the deficiencies of the research so far into maternal mental disorders, has been the lack of corroborative data from spouses or relatives. The absences (almost by definition) of defaulters at clinics in the findings of the surveys which have been reviewed is also a matter of concern.

Some of the problems of mounting epidemiological enquiries into the incidence and prevalence of neurotic disturbance have already been discussed and one way of obtaining sufficient numbers is to try and "nest" an investigation of disorders of childbearing women in a wider enquiry of neurotic disturbance in the community (cf. Brown and Harvis, 1978). Meanwhile, the results of more recent longitudinal surveys, based upon comparable methods (e.g. Kumar and Robson, symposium communication, Manchester 1980; Nott, personal communication; Rugg and Elliott, symposium communication, Manchester 1980) may confirm existing findings of a link between childbearing *per se* and neurotic disturbance. The nature of such a link and the relationships, if any, between the blues, postnatal depression and puerperal psychosis are incompletely understood. More studies are needed which combine the psychosocial and biological approaches but they require extra resources and the demands made of patients may strain their compliance.

Much clearer guidelines are needed about the indications and contraindications for prescribing psychotropic drugs for pregnant and lactating women. The information about mutagenic and teratogenic actions of some drugs is sparse but compelling—analogous findings relating to behavioural teratogenicity may also be important, but the data are patchy and the research is not coordinated in any obvious way. Studies of "treatment" should extend beyond physical treatments and there are very few investigations of the efficacy of counselling as a preventative procedure for postnatal depression (e.g. Gordon *et al.*, 1959; Shereshefsky and Yarrow, 1973). Half a million births each year allied to an incidence of about 10% for postnatal depression add up to a substantial potential problem. Virtually nothing is known of the consequences, if any, of neurotic disturbance in childbearing women.

References

Adelstein, A.M., Macdonald Davies, I.M. and Weatherall, J.A.C. (1980). Perinatal and infant mortality: social and biological factors 1975-77. Studies on medical and population subjects No. 41. (O.P.C.S.) HMSO, London.

Arkle, J. (1957). Termination of pregnancy on psychiatric grounds. *Br. med. J.* **1**, 558-560.

Baker, A.A. (1967). *Psychiatric Disorders in Obstetrics.* Oxford, Blackwell.

Ballinger, C.B., Buckley, D.E., Naylor, G.J. and Stansfield, D.A. (1979). Emotional disturbance following childbirth: clinical findings and urinary excretion of cyclic AMP (adenosine 3'5' cyclic monophosphate). *Psychol. Med.* **9**, 293-300.

Barglow, P. and Brown, E. (1972). Pseudocyesis. *In Modern Perspectives in Psycho-obstetrics*, (ed. J.G. Howells) pp. 53-67. Oliver and Boyd, Edinburgh.

Benedek, T. (1959). Parenthood as a developmental phase: A contribution to libido theory. *J. Amer. Psychoanal. Assoc.* **7**, (no. 3) 389-417.

Bibring, G. (1959). Some considerations of the psychological processes in pregnancy. *Psychoanalytic Study of the Child,* **14**, 113-121.

Bibring, G.L., Dwyer, T.F., Huntington, D.S. and Valenstein, A.F. (1961). A study of the psychological processes in pregnancy and of the earliest mother-child relationship. *Psychoanalytic Study of the Child* **16**, 9-72.

Bivin, G.D. and Klinger, M.P. (1937). *Pseudocyesis.* Principia Press, Bloomington, Indiana.

Bonham Carter, S.M., Reveley, M.A., Sandler, M., Dewhurst, J., Little, B.C., Hayworth, J. and Preece, R.G. (1980). Decreased urinary output of conjugated tyramine is associated with lifetime vulnerability to depressive illness. *Psychiatry Research (Amsterdam)* **3**, 13-21.

Bratfos, O. and Haug, J.O. (1966). Puerperal mental disorders in manic-depressive females.*Acta Psychiat. Scand.* **42**, 285-294.

Breen, D. (1975). *The Birth of a First Child.* Tavistock, London.

Brewer, C. (1977). Incidence of post abortion psychosis: a prospective study. *Br. med. J.* **1**, 476-477.

British Medical Journal (1938). Charge of procuring abortion: Mr. Bourne acquitted. **2**, 199-205.

Brown, G. and Harris, T. (1978). *Social Origins of Depression.* Tavistock, London.

Cartwright, A. (1979) *The Dignity of Labour.* Tavistock, London.

Central Statistical Office (1981). Social trends, vol. 11, HMSO, London.

Chard, T. and Richards, M. (eds) (1977) *Benefits and Hazards of the New Obstetrics.* Spastics International Medical Publications. Heinemann, London.

Chodorow, N. (1978). *The Reproduction of Mothering.* University of California Press, Berkeley & Los Angeles.

Coles, R. (1975). A retrospective study of patients seeking pregnancy advice, January 1971 to June 1974 *J. Biosoc. Sci* **7**, 357-366.

Cook, R.J. and Dickens, B.M. (1978). A decade of international change in abortion law: 1967-1977. *Amer. J. Publ. Hlth.* **68**, 637-644.

Cox, J.L. (1979). Psychiatric morbidity and pregnancy: a controlled study of 263 semi-rural Ugandan women. *Br. J. Psychiat.* **134**, 401-405.

Dalton, K. (1971). Prospective study into puerperal depression. *Br. J. Psychiat.* **118**, 689-692.

Dalton, K. (1980). *Depression after Childbirth.* Oxford University Press, Oxford.

David, H.P. (1981). Abortion policies. In *Abortion and Sterilization,* (ed. J.E. Hodgson) pp.1-38. Academic Press, London and New York.

De Chateau, P. (1976). The influence of early contact on maternal and infant behaviour in primiparae. *Birth & Family Journal* **3:4**, 149-155.

Deutsch, H. (1930). The significance of masochism in the mental life of women. In *The Psychoanalytic Reader: An anthology of essential papers with critical introductions,* (ed. R. Fliess) pp. 195-207. International Universities Press, New York.

Deutsch, H. (1945). *The Psychology of Women, vol. II—Motherhood.* Grune and Stratton, New York.

DHSS (1977). Health and Personal Social Services Statistics for England—1976. HMSO, London.

DHSS (1979). Report on confidential enquiries into maternal deaths in England and Wales—1973-1975. HMSO, London.

Donnai, D. and Harris, R. (1978). Unusual fetal malformations after antiemetics in early pregnancy. *Br. med. J.* **1**, 691-692.

Donnai, P., Charles, N. and Harris, R. (1981). Attitudes of patients after "genetic" termination of pregnancy. *Br. med. J.* **282**, 621-622.

Donnison, R. (1977). *Midwives and Medical Men.* Heinemann, London.

Dytrych, Z., Matejcek, Z., Schuller, V., David, H. and Friedmann, H. (1975). Children born to women denied abortion. *Fam. Plann. Perspect.* **7**, 165-171.

Ekblad, M. (1955). Induced abortion on psychiatric grounds: a follow-up study of 479 women. *Acta Psychiat. Scand. Suppl.* **99**, 1-238.

Eysenck, H. and Eysenck, S.G.B. (1964). *Manual of the Eysenck Personality Inventory.* London University Press, London.

Eysenck, H. and Eysenck, S.G.B. (1975). *Manual of the Eysenck Personality Question-*

naire. Hodder & Stoughton, London.

Fairweather, D.V. (1968). Nausea and vomiting during pregnancy. *Obs. Gyn. Ann.* **7**, 91-105.

Fleming, D.M., Knox, J.D.E., Crombie, D.L. (1981). Debendox in early pregnancy and fetal malformation. *Br. med. J.* **283** (ii) 99-101.

Ford, C.S. (1945). *A Comparative Study of Human Reproduction*. Yale Univ. Publications in Anthropology, No. 32: New Haven.

Forssman, H. and Thuwe, I. (1966). One hundred and twenty children born after application for therapeutic abortion refused. Their mental health social adjustment and education level up to the age of 21. *Acta Psychiat. Scand.* **42**, 71-88.

Fowkes, F.G.R., Catford, J.C. and Logan, R.F. (1979). Abortion and the NHS: the first decade. *Br. med. J.* **1**, 217-219.

Fried, P.H., Rakoff, A.E., Schopbach, R.R. and Kaplan, A.J. (1951). Pseudocyesis: a psychosomatic study in gynecology. *J. Amer. med. Ass.* **145**, 1329-1334.

Frommer, E.A. and O'Shea, G. (1973). Antenatal identification of women liable to have problems in managing their infants. *Brit. J. Psychiat.* **123**, 149-156.

Gintzler, A.R. (1980). Endorphin-mediated increases in pain threshold during pregnancy. *Science* **210**, 193-195.

Goldberg, D.P., Cooper, B., Eastwood, M.R., Kedward, H.B. and Shepherd, M. (1970). A standardized psychiatric interview for use in community surveys. *Br. J. Prev. Soc. Med.* **24**, 18-23.

Gordon, R.E., Gordon, K.K. and Englewood, N.J. (1959). Social factors in the prediction and treatment of emotional disorders of pregnancy. *Amer. J. Obstet. Gyn.* **77**, 1074-1083.

Greer, H.S., Lal, S., Lewis, S.C., Belsey, E.M. and Beard, R.W. (1976). Psychosocial consequences of therapeutic abortion. King's termination study III. *Br. J. Psychiat.* **128**, 74-79.

Hamilton, M. (1960). A rating scale for depression. *J. Neurol. Neurosurg. Psychiat.* **23**, 56-62.

Handley, S.L., Dunn, T.L., Waldron, G. and Baker, J.M. (1980). Tryptophan, cortisol and puerperal mood. *Br. J. Psychiat.* **136**, 498-508.

Hayworth, J., Little, B.C., Bonham Carter, S.M., Raptopoulos, P., Priest, R.G. and Sandler, M. (1980). A predictive study of post-partum depression: some predisposing characteristics. *Br. J. Med. Psychol.* **53**, 161-167.

Health Visitors Association (1980). *Health Visiting in the 80's*. H.V.A., London.

Henderson, S. (1981). Social relationships, adversity and neurosis: an analysis of prospective observations. *Br. J. Psychiat.* **138**, 391-398.

Höök, K. (1963). Refused abortion: a follow-up study of 249 women whose applications were refused by the National Board of Health in Sweden. *Acta Psychiat. Neurol. Scand. Suppl.* **168**.

Hooke, J.F. and Marks, P.A. (1962). MMPI Charactistics of pregnancy. *J. Clin. Psychol.* **18**, 316-317.

Horsley, S. (1972). Psychological management of the pre-natal period. *In Modern Perspectives in Psycho-Obstetrics*, (ed. J.G. Howells) pp.291-313. Oliver & Boyd, Edinburgh.

Illsley, R. and Hall, M.H. (1976). Psychological aspects of abortion. A review of issues and needed research. *Bull. W.H.O.* **53**, 83-106.

Jarrahi-Zadeh, A., Kane, F.J., Van de Castlf, R.L., Lachenbruch, P.A. and Ewing, J.Q. (1969). Emotional and cognitive changes in pregnancy and early puerperium. *Br. J. Psychiat.* **115**, 797-805.

Kadrmas, A., Winokur, G. and Crowe, R. (1979). Post-partum mania. *Br. J. Psychiat.* **135**, 551-534.

Kendell, R.E., Wainwright, S., Hailey, A. and Shannon, N. (1976). The influence of childbirth on psychiatric morbidity. *Psychol. Med.* **6**, 297-302.

Kendell, R.E., Rennie, D., Clarke, J.A. and Dean, C. (1981). The social and obstetric correlates of psychiatric admission in the puerperium. *Psychol. Med.* **11**, 341-350.

Kitzinger, S. (1979) *The Good Birth Guide.* Fontana Paperbacks, William Collins, Glasgow.

Kitzinger, S. and Davis, J.A. (eds) (1978). *The Place of Birth.* Oxford University Press, London.

Kumar, R. and Robson, K. (1978a). Neurotic disturbance during pregnancy and the puerperium: preliminary report of a prospective survey of 119 primiparae. *In Mental illness in Pregnancy and the Puerperium*, (ed. M. Sander) pp.40-51. Oxford University Press. London.

Kumar, R. and Robson, K. (1978b). Previous induced abortion and antenatal depression in primiparae: preliminary report of a survey of mental health in pregnancy. *Psychol. Med.* **8**, 711-715.

Kumar, R., Brandt, H.A. and Robson, K.M. (1981). Childbearing and maternal sexuality: a prospective survey of 119 primiparae. *J. Psychosom. Res.* **25**, 373-383.

Lask, B. (1975). Short-term psychiatric sequelae to therapeutic termination of pregnancy. *Br. J. Psychiat.* **126**, 173-177.

Lewis, E. (1976). The management of stillbirth: coping with an unreality. *Lancet* **ii**, 619-620.

Lewis, E. and Page, A. (1978). Failure to mourn a stillbirth: an overlooked catastrophe. *Br. J. med. Psychol.* **51**, 237-241.

Lewis, T.L.T. (1980). Legal abortion in England and Wales 1968-78. *Br. med. J.* **1**, 295-296.

MacFarlane, A., Chalmers, I. and Adelstein, A.M. (1980). The role of standardization in the interpretation of perinatal mortality rates. *Health Trends,* **12**, 45-50.

MacIntyre, S. (1977). The management of childbirth: a review of sociological research issues. *Soc. Sci. Med.* **11**, 477-484.

McDonald, A.D. (1958). Maternal health and congenital defect: a prospective investigation. *New Eng. J. Med.* **258**, 767-773.

Mead, M. and Newton, N. (1967). Cultural patterning of perinatal behaviour. *In Childbearing—its Social and Psychological Aspects.* (eds S.A. Richardson and A.F. Guttmacher). Williams & Wilkins.

Meares, R., Grimwade, J., Bickley, M. and Wood, C. (1972). Pregnancy and neuroticism. *Med. J. Aust.* **1**, 517-520.

Meares, R., Grimwade, J. and Wood, C. (1976). A possible relationship between anxiety in pregnancy and puerperal depression. *J. Psychosom. Res.* **20**, 605-610.

Moulton, R. (1942) Psychosomatic implication of pseudocyesis. *Psychosom. Med.* **4**, 376-389.

Nilsson, A. and Almgren, P.E. (1970). Paranatal emotional adjustment. A prospective investigation 165 women. *Acta Psychiat. Scand. Suppl.* **220**, 65-141.

Nott, P., Franklin, M., Armitage, C. and Gelder, M.G. (1976). Hormonal changes and mood in the puerperium. *Br. J. Psychiat.* **128**, 379-383.

Oakley, A. (1980). *Women Confined—Towards a Sociology of Childbirth.* Martin Robertson, Oxford.

Osborne, D. (1977). Comparison of MMPI Scores of pregnant women and female medical patients. *J. clin. Psychol.* **33**, 448-450.

Osofsky, J.D. and Osofsky, H.J. (1972). The psychological reaction of patients to legalised abortion. *Amer. J. Orthopsychiat.* **42**, 48-60.

Paffenbarger, R.S. (1964). Epidemiological aspects of parapartum mental illness. *Br. J. Prev. Soc. Med.* **18**, 189-195.

Pare, C.M.B. and Raven, H. (1970). Follow-up of patients referred for termination. *Lancet* **1**, 653-658.

Paykel, E.S., Klerman, G.L. and Prusoff, B.A. (1970). Treatment setting and clinical depression. *Arch. Gen. Psychiat.* **22**, 11-21.

Paykel, E.S., Emms, E.M., Fletcher, J. and Rassaby, E.S. (1980). Life events and social support in puerperal depression. *Br. J. Psychiat.* **136**, 339-346.

Pines, D. (1972). Pregnancy and motherhood: interaction between fantasy and reality. *Br. J. med. Psychol.* **45**, 333-343.

Pitt, B. (1968). Atypical depression following childbirth. *Br. J. Psychiat.* **114**, 1325-1335.

Playfair H.R. and Gowers J.I. (1981). Depression following childbirth—a search for predictive signs. *J. Roy. Coll. Gen. Practitioners* **31** 201-208.

Priest, R.G. (1978). Introduction *In Mental Illness in Pregnancy and the Puerperium*, (ed. M. Sandler) pp.7-8. Oxford University Press, London.

Pugh, T.F., Jerath, B.K., Schmidt, W.M. and Reed, R.B. (1963). Rates of mental disease related to childbearing. *New Eng. J. Med.* **268**, 1224-1228.

Raphael-Leff, J. (1980). Psychotherapy with pregnant women. *In Psychological Aspects of Pregnancy, Birthing and Bonding*, (ed. B.L. Blum) pp.174-205. Human Sciences Press, New York.

Rapoport, R., Rapoport, R.N., Strelitz, Z. and Kew, S. (1977). *Fathers, Mothers and Others.* Routledge & Kegan Paul, London.

Raskin, A., Schulterbrandt, J., Reatig, N. and McKeon, J. (1970). Differential response to chlorpromazine, imipramine and placebo. A study of sub-groups of hospitalized depressed patients. *Arch. Gen. Psychiat.* **23**, 164-173.

Robson, K.M. and Kumar, R. (1980). Delayed onset of maternal affection after childbirth. *Br. J. Psychiat.* **136**, 347-353.

Robson, K.M., Brant, H.A. and Kumar, R. (1981). Maternal sexuality during first pregnancy and after childbirth. *Br. J. Obst. Gyn.* **88**, 882-889.

Shepherd, M., Cooper, B., Brown, A.C. and Kalton, G.W. (1966). *Psychiatric Illness in General Practice.* Oxford University Press, London.

Shereshefsky, P.M. and Yarrow, L.J. (eds) (1973). *Psychological Aspects of a First Pregnancy and Early Post-natal Adaptation.* Raven Press, New York.

Simon, N.M. and Senturia, A.G. (1966). Psychiatric sequelae of abortion: review of the literature 1935-1964. *Arch. Gen. Psychiat.* **15**, 378-389.

Social Services Committee (1980). Perinatal and neonatal mortality. Vol. 1, Second report from the Social Services Committee Session 1979-1980. HMSO, London.

Stott, D.H. (1957). Physical and mental handicaps following a disturbed pregnancy. *Lancet* **i**, 1006-1012.

Stott, D.H. (1961). Mongolism related to emotional shock in early pregnancy. *Vita. Hum.* **4**, 57-76.

Targum, S.D., Davenport, Y.B. and Webster, M.J. (1979). Post-partum mania in bipolar manic-depressive patients withdrawn from lithium carbonate. *J. nerv. ment. Dis.* **167**, 572-574.

Tennant, C. and Bebbington, P. (1978). The social causation of depression: a critique of the work of Brown and his colleagues. *Psychol. Med.* **8**, 565-575.

Tod, E.D.M. (1964). Puerperal depression, a prospective epidemiological study. *Lancet* **ii** 1264-1266.

Trethowan, W.H. and Dickens, G. (1972). Cravings, aversions and pica of pregnancy. *In Modern Perspectives in Psycho-Obstretrics*, (ed. G. Howells) pp. 251-268. Oliver & Boyd, Edinburgh.

Tylden, E. (1966). Suicide risk in unwanted pregnancy. *Medical World*, January, 25-28.

Tylden, E. (1968). Hyperemesis and physiological vomiting. *J. Psychosom. Res.* **12**, 86-93.

Uddenberg, N. (1974). Reproductive adaptation in mother and daughter. A study of personality development and adaptation to motherhood. *Acta Psychiat. Scand. Suppl.* **254**.

Uddenberg, N. and Nilsson, L. (1975). The longitudinal course of paranatal emotional adjustment. *Acta Psychiat. Scand.* **52**, 160-169.

Uddenberg, N., Nilsson, A. and Almgren, P.E. (1971). Nausea in pregnancy: psychological and psychosomatic aspects. *J. Psychosom. Res.* **15**, 269-276.

Visram, S.A. (1972). A follow-up study of 95 women who were refused abortion on psychiatric grounds. *In Psychosomatic Medicine in Obstetrics and Gynaecology*, (ed. N. Morris) pp.561-563., Karger, S. Basel.

Whitlock, F.A. and Edwards, J.E. (1968). Pregnancy and attempted suicide. *Comprehen. Psychiat.* **9**, 1-12.

Wolkind, S. and Zajicek, E. (1978). Psycho-social correlates of nausea and vomiting in pregnancy. *J. Psychosom. Res.* **22**, 1-5.

Wolkind, S. and Zajicek, E. (1981). *Pregnancy — a psychological and social study*. Academic Press, London and New York.

5

The Maternity Blues

G. Stein

Introduction

Transient mild depression in the first few days after delivery is so common and apparently benign that it has only recently begun to be the subject of scientific investigations. Episodes of weeping and depression occur in 50–70% of recently delivered women (Yalom et al., 1968; Pitt, 1973); and the phenomenon has been called the maternity blues (Victoroff, 1952) or the third day blues (Moloney, 1952). The phrase "the maternity blues" while evocative and now in common usage perhaps fails to convey that many women are also elated at this time. Hamilton (1962) has coined the term "the transitory syndrome" to capture the evanescent nature of postpartum mood changes.

The maternity blues are often heralded by brief episodes of weeping beginning on the third or fourth day after delivery. Many other symptoms may occur, including feelings of irritability, anxiety, headache, confusion, forgetfulness and depersonalization, as well as elation. In some women such symptoms may last for only a day or two but among others some disturbance is present almost every day for a week or more. Pitt (1973) regards the blues as a "trivial fleeting phenomenon" which is very different from postnatal depression.

This review will begin with a consideration of the nosological status of the blues, followed by a clinical description of the psychological changes, their timing, and the range of their severity. Various definitions and methods of measuring the blues will be described, and then a detailed description of some of the more common symptoms will be given. Factors that correlate with the severity of the blues reaction will be considered and possible relationships with premenstrual tension will be reviewed.

In the second part of this chapter recent biochemical investigations into the origin of these symptoms will be described. Changes in endocrine function, body

119

weight, electrolyte excretion, and monoamine metabolism during the early puerperium have all recently been reported, and even though no single biochemical cause has so far emerged much promising work is presently in progress.

Nosological Status: Illness, Syndrome, or Normal Reaction?

Women who experience the maternity blues do not regard themselves as ill, nor do their relatives or attendants. Kraupl-Taylor (1980) has suggested that whether a condition is deemed to be an illness depends on the degree of therapeutic concern it arouses, and the maternity blues manifestly fail to elicit such feelings. Scadding (1967) provided a more comprehensive definition of illness as "A specified common set of characteristics by which living organisms differ from the norm of their species in such a way as to place them at a biological disadvantage." As the blues occur in over half the population at risk and do not appear to be associated with any particular biological disadvantage they also fail to qualify for Scadding's definition. Nevertheless a specified common set of mental changes do occur in the early puerperium and even if they are regarded as a normal reaction and not as an illness these psychological phenomena are of interest and merit detailed investigation. Knowledge of the biological correlates of mental changes in normal women at this time may lead to a better understanding of pathological reactions such as the psychoses that also start soon after delivery.

Clinical Description

The Typical Picture

Until recently, information about the maternity blues was mainly derived from brief descriptions in obstetric text books, which usually confined themselves to accounts of episodes of weeping and dysphoria occurring on the third or fourth day. For example Bourne (1975) wrote:

> It is said that every new mother should experience the blues. This is a period of fairly acute depression which starts for no apparent reason and disappears for no reason. It usually lasts for 12 to 24 hours generally between the third and sixth day after delivery. She may feel rather miserable and will certainly burst into tears at the slightest provocation, or even without provocation. Most midwives and doctors consider that an attack of the blues is almost essential to relieve tension after delivery. If a woman does not experience this so acutely she will almost certainly have a good cry for no apparent reason.

While this account attempts to reassure by providing some sort of an explanation for the phenomenon viz. "an attack of the blues", it does not do justice to some of the more severe mood changes that occur, or to the complexity of the syndrome. Many early studies, for example by Hamilton (1962), Robin (1962) and Pitt (1973) were based on single interviews with either midwives or patients and they generated useful checklists of symptoms that were extensively used and adapted by subsequent investigators. However, it was not until Yalom *et al.* (1968) examined their subjects each day that the wide variety of the mental phenomena of the early puerperium became apparent. Others such as Davidson (1973), Nott *et al.* (1976) and George (1981) have had alternate day contact, while Kane *et al.* (1968) interviewed his patients for the first three postpartum days only, and so probably missed the bulk of the disturbance. More recently Ballinger *et al.* (1979), Handley *et al.* (1977, 1980) and Stein (1980) examined their patients daily, and it would seem in a such rapidly fluctuating condition that daily contact with the subjects provides the best method of assessing mental changes.

Two examples of "typical day four maternity blues reactions" are given below, the description being based on daily clinical interviews. The first case fits the accepted stereotyped concept of a single fourth day weep.

On the first day a mother was mildly euphoric but was also weeping four and nine hours after delivery. On the second day she was content and complained only that she was very thirsty and on the next day she was well. On the fourth day she was quite well in the early morning but later in the day reported, "I felt rough all day, depressed and near to tears. I felt irritated with the baby. Two hourly demand feedings has been quite a lot (for me). I also have a headache and was feeling worse at six in the morning". She remained well thereafter.

The next case history illustrates a reaction that is rather more severe and intense. As well as the mother being weepy and depressed, she also manifests irritability and a marked fluctuation of symptoms. The dysphoria, even though relatively mild, interferes with the mother's feelings towards her baby, the nursing staff, and her husband on different days. Her mood is worse in the evenings and the whole episode seems to have lasted 17 days, which is longer than usual. In this case, an event, namely the departure of the husband at the end of visiting hours, precipitated the weeping.

On the first day a mother reported that she felt strange but she was neither depressed nor elated. On day 2: she was quite well in the morning but, in the evening she was weepy. "I felt miserable and a bit sensitive, up and down, low and weepy. I felt I didn't want her, I wanted my husband for moral support, the tears just kept rolling down". On day 3: she said, "I felt well in the morning but when my husband left after visiting I felt low and irritable and wept, but then I woke in the middle of the night and felt quite fine". On the fourth day she said, "In the evening, after my husband left I wept, my nipples were very sore and I asked one of the nurses to get some cream for me but she didn't return for over an hour and when she did I was so angry I snapped at her, but then I felt so bad about losing my temper that I drew the curtains around my bed and wept". On day 5: she said "I had my first taste of forgetfulness today". (The patient had forgotten to complete the forms for the research.) "Also I have quite a bad headache". On day 6: she was a little weak, but not as bad as previous days. On the seventh day she was well and left hospital. She later said she had remained depressed for a further ten days "I would have felt suicidal if it had gone on any longer, but then I went out one night with a friend and it just lifted".

The Spectrum of Symptoms

What symptoms should be included in the maternity blues? Moloney (1952) developed a brief checklist of four symptoms: fatigue, despondency, tearfulness and an inability to think clearly. Hamilton (1962) distilling the observations of ten district midwives, listed the following symptoms in order of frequency: fatigue, crying, anxiety, confusion, headaches, insomnia, hypochondriasis, and hostility to the husband. Pitt (1973) utilized these symptoms as the basis of his maternity blues rating scale, and administered his checklist to 100 women on their eighth postnatal day. In a similar type of study Stein (1979) administered the Moos Menstrual Distress questionnaire (1968) to 24 women on their seventh postpartum day. The Moos questionnaire lists 47 symptoms and as both these studies give an approximate estimate of the prevalence during one week for individual symptoms, their results can be compared. Pitt's figure is given first and Stein's figure is given second for each symptom: Insomnia 62%, 79%; Weeping 50%, 66%, Depression 54%, 38%; Anxiety 50%, 51%; Headache 33%, 35%; Confusion 36%, 21%; Fatigue 44%, 54%; Pitt gives figures for hypochondriasis 24%; Antagonism to the husband 2%; Stein provides figures for Elation 91% Feeling of unreality 50%; Restlessness 50%; Tension 37%; Irritability 33%; Forgetfulness 29%; Anorexia 29%; Poor concentration 29%; Dreaming and nightmares 21%; Guilt, Self-dislike, Dissatisfaction all 12%; Faintness 21%; Pessimism 4%.

Just because a particular psychological change occurs during the postnatal period does not necessarily mean that it is a part of the blues syndrome. All the symptoms listed occur more or less frequently in the general population, and for a particular symptom to be included as a part of the blues it is necessary first to establish that it began, or was exacerbated in the early puerperium and secondly, to demonstrate a coherent pattern of change. There is still no concensus about the symptoms which should or should not be included, for example both Robin (1962) and Ballinger et al. (1979) regard "emotional lability" as an important component of the blues but neither Pitt (1973) nor Stein (1980) include it in their checklists.

Timing of the Episode

Detailed daily examination of women in the postnatal period reveals that episodes of dysphoria can occur on almost any day in the first week and for several weeks after delivery. When is the incidence of the blues highest? When do the blues stop being the maternity blues and merge into postnatal depression?

There are no simple answers to either of these questions but as most studies of the maternity blues cease on the seventh, eighth or tenth day, the implication is that these episodes are uncommon after the tenth day. However weeping and depression may persist for several weeks (Melges, 1968; Pitt, 1973) and one of the cases described earlier in this chapter reported that her depressed mood lasted 17 days. Thus the definition of the temporal limit of blues is arbitrary.

There is also no agreement as to when symptoms are most frequent or severe; thus Gelder (1979) has reported that symptomatic disturbance is greatest on day 1, and indeed the symptom of crying may be most frequent then (Stein, 1980). Moloney (1952) coined the term "the third day blues" and Pitt (1973) also reported the peak incidence on the third day. Handley *et al.* (1977) in their first study and George (1981) observed a peak on the fourth day. Haas (1952) has written "it is known to every clinician that about the fifth or sixth day of the lying in period, many women get nervous, depressed, and demanding. This mood is somewhat similar to pre-menstrual tension." Both Robin (1962) and Stein (1976) identified the sixth day as the peak day while Yalom *et al.* (1968) found a general increase in symptoms from the 5th to 10th day, but no clear cut peak and Handley *et al.* (1980) similarly found no specific time in the first five days when symptoms were markedly increased, although there was a non-significant trend for symptoms to be increased around the fourth day. How can such discrepant findings be reconciled?

Careful analysis of the reports of individual symptoms reveals that these do not necessarily have the same time course. Figure 1 shows the frequency with which individual symptoms were reported in a study of 37 normal women in their first week (Stein, 1980). Some symptoms such as exhaustion, anorexia, and poor concentration are most frequent on the first day and then gradually improve, while others such as depression, irritability, restlessness, and dreaming are more noticeable between the fourth and sixth days post-partum. Crying is frequent on the first day but it occurs again later, and the second bout is usually rather more prolonged. The pattern that is obtained is shaped by the structure and content of the rating scale and the emphasis it places on particular symptoms. A scale that measured weeping, exhaustion, and poor concentration might show that the maximum disturbance occurred on the first day but the use of scales focusing on irritability and depression might well point to a greater disturbance on the fourth or subsequent days.

A further reason for the confusion over the timing of the blues episode may relate to the fact that whereas most women have an abrupt beginning and end to their disturbances, a minority manifest symptoms every day. Pitt (1973) described all his cases has having a "peak" of symptoms, but Yalom *et al.* (1968) found that of their 39 subjects, 26 (66%) had the blues, and of these only 10 (22%) had "acute depressive episodes". In a study of 37 women, Stein (1980) also found that of 28 women who had the blues, 17 had an acute episode while 11 showed a rather more diffuse pattern. Handley *et al.* (1980) summated the scores of patients who had acute episodes on different days and combined them with the scores of patients who had a more diffuse pattern; this may explain why they found the average symptom scores to be relatively evenly distributed over the first five days.

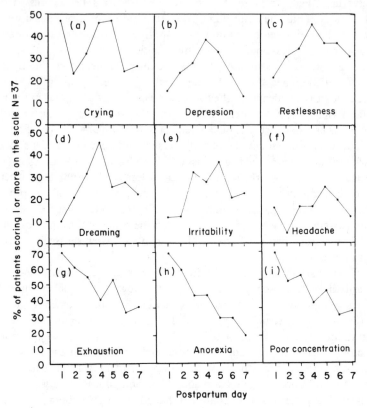

Fig. 1. The pattern of mental symptoms in the first postpartum week. Symptoms (a)-(f) show a day 4-5 peak, while symptoms (g)-(i) show a gradual diminution with no day 4 peak.

The Severity of the Blues

One shy non-complaining subject described a ten minute period on the fourth day when she felt close to tears and was upset after her two year-old son left the ward. Had she actually wept she would have been thought of as having the blues. Harris (1980) includes the feeling of being about to weep, though not actually shedding tears in his criteria for the blues. Most other investigators have disregarded such mild, but very common shifts in mood. At the other extreme, some women clearly suffer a great deal and their families may be affected as well. The following account is an example of a severe episode of the blues in a 26-year-old midwife who had just had her first baby.

"About three hours after the baby was born, he seemed cold and a bit slow. I jumped up and rubbed his back and he was OK and just opened his eyes. I was glad I had jumped up because that told me my instincts were still there even though I felt detached. Around 11 p.m. (22 hours after delivery) I became very emotional and got angry with the baby and felt very aggressive. I am a controlling sort of person but I just couldn't control the baby and I was upset and felt like shaking him. I said to the baby 'be quiet' and I prayed that he would be, and felt I would need a lot of support. I wept a great deal and then afterwards had a heavy sleep". On the second day she was still in a very emotional state, weeping for most of the day. She described her fears of becoming psychotic as her own mother had done after her fifth child. She also related with distress how she had recently read in a newspaper about a young mother who had thrown herself out of the window of another hospital shortly after delivery and killed herself. "You identify with that sort of situation, don't you?" During the second and third nights she experienced a visual hallucination on waking up. "I saw a cat's face with big green eyes in front of me. I said to myself you will have to get rid of this rubbish and it went away. I can do that". She recalled as a child she had had similar visual experiences during episodes of fever. On the third day she was talking non-stop with great pressure and anxiety for over an hour, once again expressing fears of going insane as her mother had done. "Do husbands reject women who go psychotic? Will my husband reject me if I go mad?" On the fourth day she was rather calmer. She wept when her husband visited because he bought her laxative tablets instead of granules. She expressed relief that the cause of her weeping was seemingly trivial. On the fifth day she was upset at her husband's visit. "He talked about work the whole time. I can see it will be work first, baby second, and me third. I still find I can't write letters even though I'm normally a good letter writer." On the fifth and sixth nights she had disturbing dreams. "I was having a laparoscopy and it was being done by Dr. A. I'd eaten a banana but I didn't tell him about the one I had secretly eaten before that". During the sixth and seventh days, however, she was feeling well. After discharge said that she had sexy dreams for about 2 weeks, but had experienced no subsequent depression.

In very rapid succession, this mother expressed feelings of detachment, acute anger, a panic attack, depression with suicidal thoughts, fears of insanity with visual pseudo hallucinations, and she was weepy throughout. She had had an episode of depression lasting six months a few years previously. Her mother had had a puerperal psychosis after her fifth child and the patient herself had experienced transient hallucinations during febrile episodes as a child; all these factors may have contributed to the severity of her disorder. In the author's series four out of seventy cases had such severe and complex reactions. Thus not all women conform with the stereotype of "a trivial fleeting phenomenon" (Pitt, 1973). It is a matter of some debate whether women with such severe reactions have a condition that is distinct from the blues, and should therefore be classified separately, or whether they may legitimately be placed at one end of a continuum of blues reactions (Nott *et al.* 1976).

What is a "Case" of the Blues?

When daily scores on various blues symptoms are summated and then converted into global ratings a unimodal distribution seems to emerge (Nott *et al.*, 1976;

Ballinger *et al.*, 1979; Stein, 1979; Handley *et al.*, 1980). The validity of such global, composite scores of severity may be challenged, they are derived from ratings of various symptoms which happen more or less to coincide. Furthermore, the ratings do not always clearly distinguish between incidence, severity or duration of individual symptoms. However, if such global scores are taken as an index of severity, then their unimodal distribution suggests that there is no clear distinction between a "case" and a "non-case" of the blues.

Kendell (1975) has argued that the presence of a clear boundary between a case and a non-case of a syndrome is central to the definition of that syndrome. With the blues no such clear cut-off has been found and because different authors have used different levels of severity to define their cases they have produced a wide range of estimates of incidence of the blues. Thus, at the lower extreme Oppenheim (1962) reports an incidence of 15%. Handley *et al.* (1980) who counted only severe cases gave a figure of 39%, most published series gave an overall incidence between 50–70%, 50%, Pitt (1973), 60% Davidson (1972), 66% Yalom *et al.* (1968), 70% Harris (1980a), 76% Stein (1980) and finally Robin (1962) provides a figure of 80%. These differences probably reflect the varying ways in which a case is defined and only when a definition has been agreed can real differences in incidence from place to place or among any particular subgroups be ascertained. Yalom *et al.* (1968) regarded an episode of weeping as the hallmark of the blues and both his group and Pitt have used this measure to define their cases. The criterion of weeping is simple and readily understood by patients and their attendants. On the other hand its simplicity does little justice to the psychological complexity of the syndrome. Davidson (1973) defined his cases in terms of the number of episodes of crying; "Mild blues" meant less than three cries or three sad days or a combination of both, and "severe blues" meant more than two cries or two sad days or a combination of both. Handley *et al.* (1980) used an even more complicated definition of "severe blues" as a score above the 80th percentile on any of three depression scales: the Beck Depression Scale (1961), the MAACL (Zuckerman and Lubin, 1965) and a Visual Analogue Scale. This last definition may be useful in a specific research project since it ensures that all the cases so defined not only have the blues, but are also probably experiencing a fairly severe episode as well. On the other hand, such a definition has little use outside a research setting. Until the syndrome is more completely understood it may be prudent to adhere to a "belt and braces" policy, i.e. to use both a rating scale and a simple criterion which is assessed at interview, namely the presence of a single episode of weeping in the first ten postpartum days. Tears of joy just after the delivery or upon the first meeting with the baby are, however, best discounted.

Measurement

At present there is no standard method for measuring the blues. Ideally a scale for measuring the maternity blues should be relatively brief as women do not tolerate detailed interviewing at this time, be suitable for self-rating, cover both depression and anxiety and be both reliable and valid in the post partum situation. Two scales have been specifically devised for the assessment of the maternity blues, namely those of Pitt (1973), and Stein (1980). Pitt utilized the eight symptoms described by Hamilton (1962) as being the most frequent and these were weeping, depression, insomnia, headache, anxiety, confusion, fatigue, hypochondriasis and antagonism to the husband. Stein (1980) devised a list of 13 common symptoms: weeping, depression, exhaustion, restlessness, anxiety, tension, anorexia, dreaming, headache, irritability, confusion, forgetfulness and poor concentration. Certain of the frequently occurring symptoms were specifically excluded, namely elation and depersonalization (because they were unrateable by the subjects themselves) and insomnia (because this may be due to the baby's restlessness rather than the maternal mental state). The scale provides an overall severity score each day, as well as an average score for the whole week, and it is useful in following the time course of individual symptoms.

So far, only one investigator (George, 1981) has attempted to use the Present State Examination (Wing, *et al.*, 1974). This is an exhaustive interview covering the whole range of psychiatric symptomatology and is not suitable for daily use; it was devised mainly to assess psychiatric illness and its validity in cases of puerperal dysphoria is uncertain. No single scale is ideally suitable for all purposes and the selection of the scale used must depend on the purpose of the research. If the breadth of syndrome is to be explored a scale such as the Menstrual Distress Questionnaire may be suitable, but if the severity of depression is of greatest interest a scale such as the Beck may be more appropriate.

A brief non-intrusive daily clinical interview is useful, partly to aid the maintenance of rapport, but also because some women will not record their symptoms on forms, while others may have completed their form early in the day but during the evening may experience a severe weepy episode which would be missed if self-rating were the only source of data.

The Individual Symptoms of the Blues

Weeping

According to Yalom *et al.* (1968) weeping is the hallmark of the blues, and is present in 50–70% of women. It is most frequently present in the first few hours after delivery when almost all women will have a very brief cry which lasts for a minute or two, most commonly with feelings of elation, and patients describe "tears of joy" or happiness at this time. A small minority, however, may be acutely depressed or feel strange or depersonalized soon after delivery and their weeping then has a more distressing character.

A second, more prolonged and severe weep frequently occurs between the third and tenth day and this second episode is less readily explained. Yalom *et al.*

(1968) have described how women are inordinately vulnerable to very minor rebuffs during this period. Crying occurs if any adverse comment is made or if husbands arrive late for visiting. Exaggerated empathy may occur, such as weeping over a newspaper story or a television programme. The tears usually occur in the setting of a change of mood which need not necessarily be depression. Anxiety, elation, irritability and depersonalization may all be associated. Although weeping may occur at any time of the day it is most frequent mid-morning and again between 6 to 8 p.m. in hospital populations, and the association with visiting hours suggests that social interactions may have an important role in triggering these episodes.

Most women are able to provide a reason for their weeping, but the diversity of their explanations suggests that they are secondary to some other underlying cause. After the episode many women recognize the frailty of their explanations. The reason given usually refers to an event that has occurred during the day, often something that has happened an hour or two prior to the disturbance, and it has the character of a rationalization. Sometimes the same event, e.g. a difficulty in feeding, will precipitate profuse crying on one day but on another occasion may have no adverse effect at all, suggesting that the vulnerability to weep is present only at certain times. Common reasons that mothers give for their tearfulness include feelings of rejection by their husbands, nurses or doctors, minor ailments in themselves or their babies. Mothers may be anxious about their babies being jaundiced or ill in other ways. Illness in the baby usually takes precedence over all other possible causes for maternal anxiety and weeping. Among multiparae Kitzinger (1977) has described how the weeping is often focused around the mother's other children at home. Robin (1962) has also cited recent ward disturbance as a possible cause of the weeping, but some women are unable to provide any reason. Irrational episodes of weeping lasting for a day or two, associated with exaggerated affect, are not uncommon in thyrotoxicoses (Labhart, 1974), Cushing's disease (Starkman *et al.*, 1981), premenstrual states (Dalton, 1964) and in some cases of idiopathic oedema (Edwards and Bayliss, 1976) suggesting the possibility of an underlying endocrine or metabolic cause.

Surprisingly, painful or difficult labours rarely figure in the patient's explanation of her blues episode, although many years later the trauma of a difficult labour will be vividly recalled when the episode of the blues has long since been forgotten. Helen Deutsch (1945) has suggested that such episodes of weeping are caused by a woman's sudden awareness of her new responsibility. Occasionally patients do allude to such an awareness, but then almost incidentally and by and large most women are preoccupied with practical problems during their first few postpartum days.

What then is the cause of this increased tendency to weep? Is it environmentally determined or is it caused by some underlying endocrine or metabolic disorder? The phenomenon of postnatal weeping has been reported both in the USA, Europe, the West Indies (Davidson, 1972) and in Tanzania (Harris,

1980b) with an approximate incidence of 50–70% and is therefore unlikely to be a purely cultural phenomenon. Davidson (1972) studied a group of Jamaican multiparae and favoured a socio-economic explanation for the blues. In order to account for an association with increased parity he argued that subjects who had more children than they either wanted or could cope with were more likely to experience the blues. Such an explanation would not hold for mothers in the UK where the blues do not appear to be associated with increased parity.

Depression

The world "depression" may refer to a mood, a symptom, or an illness; here it is used to denote a symptom. While may women experience small ups and downs of their mood or get "fed up", a substantial minority describe more definite depressive feelings, associated with low self-esteem, self-criticism and guilt, pessimism and sometimes suicidal, violent or bizarre thoughts.

For example, a 29-year-old primagravid mother said on the fourth day "I feel excited and happy, my parents have come up from Wales; for the first time caring about the baby makes sense, and I am able to ask things without having to ask all the time". But on the fifth day she reported "I feel depressed and guilty because I have not even fixed up a G.P. which I know I should have done. I am frightened and feel inadequate now that all the more competent mothers have left the ward. I am frightened I shall run amok and harm someone elses baby". On day six she was better though still weepy, but felt quite normal on day seven. Five years earlier she had had a fifteen month depressive illness for which she consulted her G.P. There was no other obvious reason why she should have developed this depressive mood swing.

A woman, who had had two previous stillbirths, had developed mild hypertension and had become mildly irritable and depressed in the last month of pregnancy. The baby was prematurely delivered by caesarian section. She was content for the first three days but on the fourth day she said:

"I'm depressed, I keep thinking someone will say I have a large normal baby and I'll be able to cope. If I had a bit more sleep I'd be OK. I'm slow, I'm wrapped up in concrete or mud, I have to fight my way through it. I couldn't just lie there like my cousin did, she had six months of postnatal depression–I'd rather walk off a bridge. I feel I'm just made of jelly and cannot relax and I can't concentrate and I keep reading the same paragraph in the newspaper. On the sixth day she said, "Yesterday was terrible, I was crying all day. I feel guilty that I can't cope with the baby. He has difficult moments. He is very demanding as he is so tiny, I'm hopeless, I'll never cope on my own. I shouted at my husband "I'm a pathetic sort of depressive" I'd like to get out of this trough of not being able to do anything. Everything is very negative at the moment and I can't make my mind up on anything. Sometimes stupid things whiz around my head like adoption, just walk out and leave it all, any avenue of escape, I'm at a standstill and I can't get better".

The patient lost her appetite, slept poorly and felt worst in the morning. She remained in this depressed state on the fourth, fifth and sixth days and then intermittently for the next month but thereafter was quite well. Many factors may have contributed to this patient's depression. She had had two previous stillbirths, and now had hypertension, a caesarian section, and a premature baby.

In addition she had had a six month depressive illness soon after getting married during which she ate excessively to comfort herself and would not go out of the house. A final factor that may be relevant was the presence of a positive family history of postnatal depression. This case illustrates the difficulty to distinguishing a severe case of the "maternity blues" from postnatal depression.

Ballinger *et al.* (1979) found that more intense depressive symptoms were common among women with a previous "history of nerves" and Stein (1980) found that women with a previous history of a depressive episode of two or more months' duration, were significantly more likely to experience depression in the early puerperium. Riley (1980) identified seven out of the 21 women she studied as having "previous psychiatric vulnerability" by which she meant they had some previous psychiatric history, even though the details were not specified, and she found that the "vulnerable" group tended to have higher blues scores although the association did not reach statistical significance.

Elation

While earlier accounts of the blues have emphasized distressing symptoms such as weeping and depression, elation also occurs very frequently. The majority of women are very happy and relieved that labour is over but the question of the distinction between happiness and elation as a normal reaction as opposed to a (borderline) pathological one has not been properly addressed.

"Elation" is most frequent on day one (Klaus *et al.*, 1975; Ballinger *et al.*, 1979; Macfarlane, 1979; Stein, 1981) and is present in around 80% of subjects at that time, but this figure falls to 40% on day four. Hofer (1975) has suggested that elation which occurs soon after delivery, has a psychogenic basis. A successful and safe childbirth is a happy event and Klaus *et al.* (1975) has reported that elation is also often present among others present at the birth.

Among some women however the mood remains persistently elated, and at around the same time other women are experiencing their blues episodes, they may experience an intensification of their elation. Robin (1962) has described how some women become giggly, over-excitable and garrulous at the time most women are experiencing "the blues".

> For example, a woman was very happy and appeared euphoric for the first 2 days. On day three she said "I feel high, I feel I could get on a pair of roller skates and skate down the corridor. I am an organizer and I am just filling up my diary. I feel we must go to the races and have lots of social engagements". On day four she said her appetite was enormous, and ate two breakfasts, two lunches and two suppers. On the next day she was drinking champagne and on the sixth day she reported the following mood swing at around 7 p.m.
>
> I suddenly felt very emotional, not miserable, just choked up with baby, and was very happy. I didn't cry but a lump came to my throat. An hour later when I was feeding her I felt very attached with very close feelings, very much more intense than usual. Afterwards I slept heavily and when I woke up I found my thirst and appetite were very much less. Following discharge she then reported two or three weeks of exhaustion, but no subsequent depression.

Ballinger (1979) has estimated that around 8% of her subjects had such an elated reaction when the degree of happiness and high spirits appeared to be outside the euthymic range, but it is doubtful if any of her subjects could properly be described as hypomanic. Klerman (1981) in a recent review of states of mania has commented on the sparseness of the psychiatric literature on those states of elation that are outside the normal euthymic range but are not within the hypomanic range. He uses the term neurotic elation to describe this and suggests that this may be the same mood that some analysts have described as a "manic defence". Klerman describes how cyclothymic individuals may pass into and out of these states of mild persistent non-psychotic elation and only rarely report such changes whereas the discomfort of the depressive phases is all too obvious to the individual. Puerperal elation does not have the character of a manic defence but it would be of interest to ascertain whether the more persistent elated reactions were more common among those subjects who had a premorbid cyclothymic personality.

Lability of Mood

This means the presence of both depression weeping, and elation in the same patient, often on the same day, with changes from one state to another. Robin (1962) and Ballinger *et al.* (1979) consider such lability to be an important symptom of the maternity blues. Robin stated that "Sixteen of the 25 patients complained of emotional lability saying they were "giggly' 'excited' or 'oversensitive' or 'cried at nothing', 'laughed at nothing' or were 'up and down'." Ballinger has (1979) suggested that the stress of delivery may be associated with an increased level of arousal and that this may explain the fluctuating mood state. Lability of mood is sometimes associated with acute organic reactions or chronic brain syndromes and may be a symptom of mania. It has often been noted in puerperal psychosis.

Headache

Headache is very frequent during the first post partum week. Pitt provides a figure of 33% (based on a single interview on day 8), Hamilton of 30% (based on interviews with midwives) and Stein of 35% (based on daily clinical interviews). The headache takes a characteristic and relatively constant form and it usually persists for most of the day. It is generally bilateral frontal and is occasionally associated with photophobia, but rarely with nausea, vomiting or any of the visual prodromata of migraine. Patients can usually distinguish their postnatal headaches from migraine, they they may be related in some way. Dalton (1980) has described how women who have a history of migraine, but have not had an attack for many years, may experience headaches between the third and seventh post partum days. In a study of 40 patients, Stein (1981b) found that such headaches were more common among women with a previous or family history of migraine.

Eight subjects reported severe premenstrual headache and six of them also developed a postpartum headache. The headaches are infrequent on days one and two but reach a peak between days four to six after delivery. Thus, on the fifth day, women with a history of migraine were eight times more likely to develop a headache, compared with those without a history of migraine (Stein, 1981b). Patients were weighed daily and the headache was found to occur at the time weight loss commenced. Shottdstead et al. (1955) have shown that episodes of migraine are often preceded by weight gain, and that weight loss and a diuresis may follow the attack.

Confusion and Forgetfulness

The presence of confusion in a psychiatric syndrome is of the greatest interest because it usually points to an organic aetiology. Thus Pitt (1973) reported that 36% of women with the blues complained of feeling confused and he therefore argued in favour of an organic basis for the syndrome. However, the complaint of confusion does not necessarily imply that cognitive function is impaired when objective tests are applied. Thus Kane et al. (1968) who also described postpartum forgetfulness, poor recent memory and distractability, found only slight impairments in 137 women tested with the Porteus Maze and the Trail Making tests. Cognitive function was, if anything, rather worse in late pregnancy than after delivery. Decrements could only be detected post-natally among women who had some dysphoria. Similar findings have been reported by Yalom et al. (1968) using the digit-span test, the 30 second time estimation test and other tests of concentration. Thus, even though the complaint of confusion is frequent, objective evidence of cognitive impairment is lacking and does not support the hypothesis of an acute brain syndrome. However, the observation that mild degrees of impairment were only present among the dysphoric group is of interest in the light of recent studies of cognitive function in depression (Weeks et al., 1980).

Irritability

Irritability is a frequent and sometimes troublesome symptom which is often associated with depression. The target of patient's irritability is often her husband (Hamilton, 1962); but it may be the hospital staff or other members of the family such as other children.

> A woman on day 5 said "I felt irritable with my daughter. She wouldn't go home and she kept wanting to touch the baby and said she was going to stay here. She is half a baby herself, and I don't know how to handle her".
>
> Another woman expressed some irritation at both the nurses and her baby, "I was so tired, and the baby played up between feeds, and I gave her some water and that helped, then the nurses came round and said "you have to do this, and you have to do that". I just want to go home".

Irritability of this severity is common. Occasionally the reaction can be considerably more intense as the following example illustrates.

> The patient was a 29 year old who had one live child, but had had a previous stillbirth after which she had been depressed and stayed in bed for a year. Apart from mild hypertension the present pregnancy has been uneventful. The patient became very bad tempered and irritable on day five postpartum and later said, 'I was very angry about the caesarian section, I was crying all day even my poor husband couldn't say the right thing and I snapped at my daughter. I waited 10 years to have the baby but I couldn't enjoy it, I knew if I could have a night's sleep I'd be OK—do you know what the nurse said, she said to me "did you want to be a mother?"—I just blew my top!'
>
> "The patient in the next room had been barrier nursed, when I realized that she had something contagious I went beserk, and I created such a stink. I was quite livid and I wanted to hit the staff. They fumigated the room and then I made a statement to the staff nurse, I wanted to scream at them and I wanted to discharge myself. A nurse came near me and I said I was going to hit her, I threatened to jump out of the window if the agency nurse came near me. Then they gave me a valium pill and I was calmer after that, and they gave me two sleeping tablets later on". This patient was irritable for only two days and did not experience any subsequent postnatal depression.

Women sometimes discharge themselves from postnatal wards on days four and five, and they are typically angry and depressed with much hostility directed against the hospital staff. Severe degrees of irritability and temper are often associated with weeping, insomnia, and depression.

Depersonalization

Feelings of unreality and depersonalization are frequent and may occur either shortly after the birth or during an episode of the blues a few days later (Stein, 1979; George, 1981). Many women are surprised when they feel distant or strange after delivery and may even express some guilt about feeling detached. Episodes of depersonalization occurring between days four to seven are often more severe. One frightened woman said "I kept going off into a trance, I felt miles away. I told the nurse I would end up across the road in the mental hospital. Another patient reported on the fifth day "I felt sleepy and depressed and cried. I also felt a bit funny as if I was getting the gas and air again, and was irritable with it." Some patients experience only a part of their body as being depersonalized, e.g. "my breasts feel alien to me".

Depersonalization is frequent in normal subjects, especially during fatigue or minor toxic states. In the maternity blues depersonalization is distressing only if there is associated dysphoria. If elation is present, the patients sometimes laugh about their strange feelings.

Negative Feelings towards the Baby

The feelings a woman has for her new born infant show considerable variation, and not all mothers immediately experience warm and loving feelings (see

Robson and Powell in Chapter 6). Robin (1962) and MacFarlane (1979) have described how many women are distressed by their lack of warm maternal feelings in their first few postpartum days. In a detailed study of this phenomenon, Robson and Kumar (1980) examined 119 primigravidae and found that as many as 40% of women described a lack of affection immediately after delivery. They found an association with amniotomy and painful labour and speculated about a possible physiological basis for the delayed onset of maternal affection. Transient decline in maternal feelings as measured on a linear analogue scale has also been found to correlate with the severity of depression in some patients (Stein, 1981).

Insomnia

Sleep disturbance, excessive dreaming, nightmares, visual pseudo hallucinations particularly on waking and heavy sleeping following mood swings are all frequently reported. Women sleeping with their babies, were found to sleep for a little over five hours per night as measured by sleep charts scored by night nurses (Stein, 1979). When mothers slept without their babies in a sleep laboratory, Karacan et al. (1969) found that they slept for a little over six hours for the first three postpartum nights. Normative data on women who were not hospitalized and not pregnant have been provided by Thune (1968) and the average amount of time spent asleep by women in the 20–30 age group was 7 hours 40 minutes, suggesting that there is a reduction in the total amount of time women sleep in the postnatal period if they are in hospital.

Vivid dreaming particularly on nights four to six is common and around 20% of the patients have nightmares which wake them from their sleep. Gordon (1977) has commented.

> In these disturbing post partum dreams, old conflicts with members of their immediate family are relived and feelings and incidents repressed for years are brought to the surface of consciousness. These upsurges of dormant disharmony, recrimination and fantasy can be very frightening and are bound to disturb the mother's initial adjustment to her child.

Vivid pseudo hallucinations occur in around 10% of women on nights four, five and six, mainly on waking. Sometimes the baby is seen in a grossly distorted form, for example one patient said, "I saw a little elephant gift, it looked like the baby's head decapitated, the head was coming out of the table, it was a very distressing experience". Another patient reported, "There was a horrible dwarf; he had run to the room; I said you are in the wrong place you should be in a mental hospital."

Many factors may be responsible for postpartum insomnia, painful perineal scars, sleeping in a strange environment in hospital, the presence of the baby and feeding at night, as well as the presence of other patients and their babies. Insomnia may also be associated with depressive illness or hypomania, and sleep is usually disturbed postoperatively. Certain aspects of the sleep disturbance, particularly the dreaming and nightmares and hypnopompic hallucinations which occur towards the latter half of the first week appear to be rather more intimately related to the affective changes and weeping. On the other hand, the generally poor sleep of this period appears to occur in all women almost independently of the other affective changes. These subjective changes are reinforced by the results of EEG studies. Karacan *et al.* (1969) studied 13 women in late pregnancy and during the first three nights postpartum. They showed that REM sleep and stage 4 sleep were considerably diminished and that stage 4 sleep rebounded on nights 2 to 3, REM sleep returning somewhat later. A correlation with hormone changes has also been reported by Nott *et al.* (1976) who found that the greater the fall in blood concentrations of progesterone after delivery the less likely were women to report sleep disturbance. Analgesic and anaesthetic drugs also affect sleep and most hospital patients are given hypnotic drugs. Drug induced changes in sleep patterns may therefore be as important as some of the mechanisms that are discussed above.

Other Symptoms

Exhaustion is common and generally refers to physical tiredness which is worst just after delivery and then gradually decreases over the next few days, suggesting it is a response to the stress of labour and delivery (Fig. 1). Mothers sometimes complain of mental exhaustion in association with low spirits.

Restlessness and mild agitation are common and some women can be seen pacing around their beds or taking walks in the ward corridor, being unable to settle. This pattern is often seen in women who are either euphoric or among those who are depressed and agitated (see Fig. 1).

Thirst is almost always present immediately after delivery and is sometimes very intense, and as a group, postpartum women drink rather more than other women in hospital (Stein, 1981a). At the onset of the blues episode most women report a reduction of thirst. Moos (1968) considers thirst to be an important symptom of the premenstrual syndrome, which also abates at the onset of menstruation.

Anorexia is often present after delivery and for the first day or two but this gradually diminishes, although when the blues episode is severe women sometimes go off their food for one or two days.

Breast congestion is also frequent around day four but lactation is often successfully established on days one and two although the switch from colostrum to milk may not occur until days three or four. At around the same time as breast congestion is maximal, around one third of women develop ankle swelling, and this often occurs when there has been no ankle swelling during pregnancy. Oedema has been associated with mental change in both the premenstrual syndrome (Moos, 1968) and the rate condition of periodic oedema (Edwards and Bayliss, 1976). The synchonous appearance of oedema, breast congestion, diminished thirst all suggest the possibility of some disturbance in mechanisms of fluid balance around the fourth day.

Clinical Correlates of the Blues

Although many clinical correlates of the blues have been found, few of these have been reported by more than one group. One exception, which has been repeatedly described is the association between the blues and mental symptoms in late pregnancy (Davidson, 1972; Nott, 1976; Handley *et al.*, 1980; Stein, 1980; Harris, 1980). Anxiety in the first trimester (Davidson, 1972), a previous history of neurotic depression (Ballinger, 1979; Stein, 1980) and previous post-natal depression (Yalom *et al.*, 1968; Stein, 1980) appear to be associated with rather more severe maternity blues. This is consistent with the findings of Jacobsen *et al.* (1965) that anxiety and depression in the first postpartum year correlate with their presence both before and during pregnancy.

While the overall social and psychological impact of the birth of the first child is usually greatest, only Yalom *et al.* (1968) and Nott (1976) have found an increased incidence of the blues among primiparous subjects. Other investigators have found no links with parity (Pitt, 1973; Ballinger *et al.*, 1979; Stein, 1980; Handley *et al.*, 1980); Breast feeding difficulties have been linked (Pitt, 1973) but as a high incidence has also been found among bottle feeders (Harris, 1980a) this association may reflect an altered perception of the problems encountered with normal feeding rather than a true association. It has been suggested that hospitalization contributes to the disorder and hospital personnel often figure prominently in the content of the patients' mood disorder. However the incidence of the blues found in home based studies is around 60–70% making it unlikely that hospitalization plays a causal role (Yalom *et al.*, 1968; Harris, 1980).

Apart from a possible suggestion of an association with the length of labour (Yalom *et al.*, 1968) no obstetric variable has been found to correlate with the blues (Nott, 1976; Ballinger, 1979; Stein, 1980; Handley *et al.*, 1980); Social Class, housing difficulties, and personality as measured by the Eysenck Personality Inventory (Pitt, 1973; Nott, 1976) are also not correlated. Harris (1980b) has examined the blues phenomenon in Tanzania and found it occurred in around 70% of subjects. They presented with complaints of aches and pains rather than with anxiety and depression, suggesting that cultural factors may influence the manner in which the blues presents, but not the overall incidence.

Relationship to Premenstrual States

A number of associations between the menstrual cycle and the maternity blues have been reported. The blues may be more severe among women with premenstrual tension (Nott *et al.*, 1976; Ballinger *et al.*, 1979) in those with a shorter duration of menstrual flow and those with a younger age of menarche (Yalom *et al.*, 1968) and menstrual irregularities (Handley *et al.*, 1980). Women with premenstrual headache are more likely to develop postnatal headache (Stein, 1981) and during a postpartum depression many women may experience an exacerbation of their depression during their premenstrual phase (Hamilton, 1962).

The symptom profiles of the maternity blues and of premenstrual tension do however resemble each other. Reid and Yen (1981) in a recent review of premenstrual states list the following symptoms: fatigue, depression, irritability, increased thirst and appetite, headaches, breast swelling and abdominal bloating, oedema of the extremities, constipation as well as an exacerbation of certain diseases such as acne. Almost all these symptoms occur in the blues as well, although the tendency for weeping to occur is considerably more prominent in the blues. Both Dalton (1964) and Moos (1968) have shown that the premenstrual syndrome is a very complex phenomenon even though it is rather poorly defined. Moos found eight symptom clusters corresponding to: pain, loss of concentration, reduced activity, autonomic symptoms, water retention, negative affect and increased arousal.

He found that each of these symptom clusters had its own particular relationship to the cyclical hormonal changes but that the combination symptoms varied from patient to patient. Some might have negative affect, others fluid retention, and yet others combinations of these clusters, but there was a tendency for patients to have the same pattern in successive cycles. On this basis he postulated the presence of many different subtypes of the premenstrual syndrome. The definition of different subtypes of the premenstrual state has been useful in searching for causal factors, e.g. in determining which patients experienced the specific symptom of depression premenstrually. Analogous analysis of the symptoms of the blues have not yet been described.

Biological Aspects

Certain clinical features of the maternity blues suggest the possibility of an underlying biological cause. Firstly the phenomenology of the blues is of a highly fluctuant mood change and this resembles the mental state found in other disorders such as Cushings disease and thyrotoxicosis. Secondly the absence of social, personality, or obstetric correlates mitigates against a primary environmental or psychological cause. Finally the mood swing appears to occur after a relatively fixed interval following delivery and also occurs at a time of many other rapid biological changes. So far no single biological cause has yet emerged, but about a dozen investigations that attempt to link early postpartum mood changes with one or other biological parameter have been reported. These investigations have focused on hormones, somatic changes, particularly body weight, and alterations in monoamine metabolism, and these studies will be reviewed in this section.

Sex Hormones

Large changes in the levels of oestrogen and progesterone occur in women during puberty, pregnancy, the puerperium, and at the menopause. Although psychiatric morbidity may be increased at all these times, they are also times of important role change as well, so the endocrine changes are likely to be only one of many contributory factors. Cyclical mood changes occurring premenstrually cannot readily be explained as a purely social phenomenon and there is a small but definite group of women who become depressed on oral contraceptives (Herzberg et al., 1970). Progesterone itself has sedative propeties (Gyermark et al., 1967), and the sudden reduction after delivery might be expected to lead to a state of arousal. Steiner (1979) has pointed out that the fall in the level of progesterone after delivery is larger than at any other time in a woman's life. It has for long been a part of medical and nursing mythology that this hormonal change is the cause of postpartum mental syndromes and indeed patients who weep severely with fourth day blues are usually consoled by the nursing staff who tell them their "hormones are responsible."

Nott et al. (1976) have described a detailed and careful methodology for examining the relationship between hormone changes and the maternity blues. They selected 27 women and carefully excluded all those with a previous psychiatric history, social, financial, marital, medical or obstetric problems. Mood was assessed frequently both antenatally and postnatally using a self-rating scale for depression that has the advantage of covering anxiety symptoms as well (Snaith, 1971), the Pitt Maternity Blues Scale (1973) and the Lorr mood scale (1966). Mood was assessed on alternate days when blood was taken for the estimation of oestrogen, progesterone, follicle stimulating hormone, luteinising hormone and prolactin. Patients were divided into a symptomatic group and an asymptomatic group and no difference was found in the levels of any of the hormones measured, or in their rate of change. However, four weak correlations with individual symptoms were found, and these were (1) higher pre-delivery oestrogen levels with greater irritability (2) the greater the progesterone drop the more likely were subjects to rate themselves as being depressed and (3) the less likely they were to report sleep disturbance and (4) the lower oestrogen levels post partum the greater the sleep disturbance that was reported. These four associations were out of a total of 30 possible correlations that were tested and so it is quite possible that some of these might have occurred by chance. Because of these associations and because of their difficulty in defining their cases, Nott et al. (1976) suggested that further research in this area should seek to link biological changes with individual symptoms rather than with a poorly defined global "maternity blues syndrome."

In contrast with Nott et al. (1976), George (1980) has reported a significant association between the severity of the maternity blues and plasma concentrations of prolactin. Prolactin is an important reproductive hormone which is secreted in bursts during suckling and the older terms of "lactational psychosis" and "milk fever" have for long implied a mysterious link between breast feeding and mental illness even though the literature is quite consistent in saying there is none (Paffenbarger 1964; Kendell *et al.*, 1981). George (1980) examined 38 women and took blood for prolactin on days 2, 4 and 6 postpartum and he used the Present State Examination (Wing *et al.*, 1974) to assess the mental state. The appropriateness of a complex interview schedule which is used mainly for the assessment of schizophrenia, for a fluctuating and minor mood disorder such as the blues, is questionable. However, he found significant correlations between prolactin levels and anxiety, tension and depression, although by day 6, the correlation with depression no longer held. Further work is needed to clarify the associations between mood states and and prolactin levels. Patients with prolactinomas do not have obvious affective changes nor does treatment with bromocriptine result in mood disorder.

Cortisol

Of all the endocrine changes associated with psychiatric illness, elevated plasma cortisol found in some cases of depression has been the most consistently reported finding (Gibbons, 1964, Carroll, 1972); The 24 hour output of cortisol is increased as measured by urinary free cortisol (Carroll, 1976). More subtle changes in the hypothalamo-pituitary-adrenal axis have also been described, thus the diurnal variation of plasma cortisol is altered (Sachar *et al.*, 1973) and there is an increased resistance to dexamethasone suppression (Browne *et al.*, 1979). All these changes revert to normal as the depression subsides.

In a recent study of 35 cases with Cushings' disease, Starkman *et al.* (1981) reported that the frequency of occurrence of the following symptoms was: fatigue 100%; irritability 86%; memory impairment 83%; depression 83%; insomnia 69%; anxiety 66%; crying 63%; restlessness 60%; dreaming and nightmares 31%; increased appetite 34%; decreased appetite 20%; elation–hyperactivity 11%; depersonalization 3%. The duration of depression was typically of one or two days, which is very similar to that of the blues, and furthermore unexplained unprovoked crying spells were also common. A minority of patients (11%) had an elated-excited dysphoria and this figure is remarkably similar to that reported by Ballinger *et al.* (1979) for an elated blues reaction. Nightmares are also common in Cushings' disease. Starkman *et al.* (1981) found that the more severe cases had higher ACTH levels and relatively lower cortisol levels and that adrenalectomy abolished the abnormal mental symptoms. Because of the symptomatic resemblance between Cushings' disease and the maternity blues the possible role of cortisol in the genesis of the maternity blues is worthy of detailed scrutiny.

During pregnancy there is a gradual increase in plasma cortisol and urinary free cortisol (Cope, 1973). At the end of pregnancy, plasma cortisol is raised some two and a half times. Most of this increase is in the form of bound cortisol because transcortin, the cortisol binding globulin, is also increased in pregnancy (Doe et al., 1964). There is nevertheless a modest but definite increase in free plasma cortisol in late pregnancy (Daly and Elstein, 1972). As in depressive illness, diurnal variation of plasma cortisol is diminished (Bourke and Roulet, 1970) possibly because the placenta itself manufactures an ACTH like substance (Gennazini et al., 1975). The level is raised during labour and on the first day postpartum but thereafter falls rapidly.

Only one group (Handley et al., 1977, 1980) have so far published their findings of cortisol in the blues. In their first study, a high plasma cortisol on the first day after delivery appeared to be linked with elation. This finding was however not replicated in their second and larger study but they did find that an elevated plasma cortisol at 38 weeks of pregnancy was associated with more severe postpartum blues. This may be an important discovery because it provides a possible endocrine explanation for the repeated clinical finding that severe blues are more prevalent among those with mood changes in late pregnancy. Handley et al. (1980) also reported a seasonal variation for plasma cortisol in late pregnancy which also occurs in non-pregnant subjects (Giordano and Radivoyevitch, 1970) with highest values in the winter and spring. An excess of cases in the spring was also found although this has not been reported by others. On the other hand the incidence of depression and suicide rises in the spring, and a spring excess for the puerperal psychoses has also been reported (Grundy and Roberts, 1975).

Thyroid Dysfunction

Transient thyroid dysfunction has frequently been reported after childbirth particularly among women with an autoimmune predisposition to develop thyroid disease. Hypothyroidism is considerably more common than thyrotoxicosis and the condition usually resolves some five to ten months after delivery (B.M.J. Editorial, 1975). Most of the reported cases of both thyrotoxicosis and postpartum hypothyroidism during the postnatal period present with anxiety, depression. It may be that some cases of postpartum anxiety are due to hypothyroidism but it is equally possible that those cases reported in the literature are women with postpartum depression who happened to have fallen under the wing of enthusiastic physicians and endocrinologists who went on to detect mild degress of thyroid dysfunction in some of them. No firm link between the thyroid abnormalities and the mental state in these women has been established. Thus How and Bewsher (1977) advocated screening all postnatal women for hypothyroidism because they suspected that there might be a large pool of subclinical postnatal hypothyroidism which was responsible for considerable misery. A controlled study of thyroid function in postnatal depressives and in blues cases has not yet been done.

Body Weight

The complex relationship between psychiatric illness and weight changes is reviewed in detail elsewhere (Crisp and Stonehill, 1976). During pregnancy weight is gained and lost rapidly in the postpartum period. Dennis (1965) was the first to describe the pattern of postpartum weight loss, he showed that the rapid weight loss did not usually start until the third or fourth day postpartum and that weight was either static or was gained in the first three postpartum days. Once the weight loss started, however, it was very quick with losses of 0.5–1.5 kg per 24 hours being quite frequent Dennis and Blytheway, 1965; Sheikh, 1971; Stein, 1980, 1981a).

The relationship of weight changes to postpartum mood disorder has been the subject of two recent studies (Stein, 1980, 1981a). In the first of these studies, 37 normal postpartum women were weighed each morning for the first seven postpartum days. Patients with toxaemia or Caesarian section were excluded. There was no direct correlation between the severity of the mood changes and the rapidity of the weight loss, but a striking finding was the temporal coincidence between the onset of rapid weight loss and episodes of weeping. The patients were divided into three groups according to their mood pattern, those with no mood changes, those with some changes each day and a third group of just over half the patients who had an abrupt onset to their weeping and mood disorder. Weight patterns in all three groups were similar, but among those with an abrupt onset of mood disorder there was weight loss of 0.5 kg per 24 hours on the day of the mood swing and this continued for the next two days whereas prior to the onset of the mood swing weight was relatively static (Fig. 2).

In a second study Stein (1981) compared the weights of 31 normal puerperal women with seven non-pregnant control subjects admitted to a metabolic ward in an attempt to examine how normal daily weight fluctuations differed from those found postpartum. Weight losses greater than 0.5 kg did not occur in the control subjects but were very frequent postpartum. The timing of even greater weight losses (1 kg or more/day) which occurred in about a quarter of the puerperal subjects seemed to follow a similar pattern to the psychological symptoms such as depression and crying, both of which were prominent between the fourth and the sixth days after delivery. Although mood and weight changes were uncorrelated in individual patients, the weight changes may be relevant links. Thus, Dennis (1965) and Sheikh (1971) have shown that when stilboesterol is used to suppress lactation, weight loss is attenuated particularly around days five and six postpartum. There are anecdotal reports suggesting that when stilboestrol is used for this purpose, the severity of the blues reaction

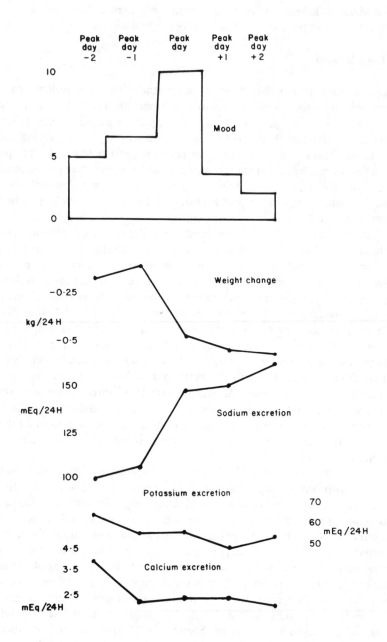

Fig. 2. Weight and electrolyte excretion in 17 women with an abrupt mood swing. Data arranged around the peak day histogram denotes mood. Rapid weight loss and a rising sodium excretion but no change in potassium or calcium occur on the peak mood day.

is also diminished (Hamilton, 1962). Secondly the postpartum weight pattern resembles the postoperative pattern and Stengel (1958) has drawn attention to the similarities between post-partum and post-operative psychoses. Finally the size and speed of the post partum weight changes is very similar to that found in some rapidly cycling manic depressive patients, as they switch from one phase to another (Jenner *et al.*, 1967).

Electrolyte Changes

Stein (1981) collected 24 hour urine samples from 31 postpartum women from days 2 to 7 postpartum. Mood was rated with a maternity blues scale and the Wakefield depression scale (Snaith, 1971), and a control group of seven non-pregnant female undergraduates completed a similar protocol in a metabolic ward. Sodium excretion correlated well with body weight changes thus confirming earlier observations (Stein *et al.*, 1979; Dieckmann and Pottinger, 1955). The excretion of sodium rose between days 2 and 6 postpartum, whereas potassium did not. Calcium excretion was lower in the postpartum subjects than in the controls and tended to fall over the first postpartum week. The day of greatest mood disturbance was found to coincide approximately with the onset of more rapid weight loss and sodium excretion showed a tendency to rise at this time (Fig. 2).

Which hormonal system is responsible for the changes in body weight and sodium excretion postpartum? Vasopressin, which was measured in the urinary samples, was found not to correlate with either weight, sodium or mood changes (Stein *et al.*, 1980). The regulation of sodium excretion in pregnancy is poorly understood (Lindheimer *et al.*, 1977) but it seems that the most important regulating mechanism is the renin angiotension system. Plasma renin activity and aldosterone are considerably raised during pregnancy and Dennis *et al.* (1965) have suggested that their postpartum fall is related to the weight loss. Furthermore, rapid weight changes of a similar type have been found among women who have been taking diuretics and developed an idiopathic oedema-like syndrome (Macgregor *et al.*, 1979) and these have been shown to correlate highly with changes in plasma renin. Additional evidence implicating the renin angiotension system comes from the observations on thirst which has now been shown in most mammalian species to be regulated by brain renin-angiotension systems (Anderson, 1976). Many patients report an abatement in their thirst at the same time as they have a lowering of their mood and the start of their weight loss, on the third or fourth postpartum day.

An abnormal mental state has been associated with both severe hypo- and hypercalcaemia, and restoration of normal calcium balance usually results in an alleviation of the psychiatric symptoms but disturbances in calcium metabolism have only rarely been found among psychiatric inpatients (Crammer, 1977). During pregnancy, because of increased demands of the foetus, the mother is in a state of negative calcium balance, but ionized plasma calcium is nevertheless held within remarkably tight limits (Pitkin and Gebhart, 1977). After delivery a small number of babies develop hypocalcaemia and investigation of these mothers has shown that some have mild transient hyperparathyroidism. Riley (1979) has discussed the possible role of mild transient hyperparathyroidism in the genesis of postpartum mental disorder. She studied possible relationships between plasma ionized calcium and puerperal psychoses (Riley, 1980). In her first study she examined 18 women admitted to a mental hospital with puerperal psychoses. Twelve of the eighteen patients had a family history of psychiatric illness and the remaining six did not. Mental status was assessed using the Foulds personal illness questionnaire (Caine et al., 1967) and she found that plasma ionized calcium was slightly elevated in the psychotic women but it was highest among the six cases with no family history of psychiatric illness. She also found a significant correlation between the change in plasma ionized calcium and changes in mental status. The validity of using a self rating technique for the assessment of psychotic patients is questionable. Nevertheless, Riley suggested that metabolic factors, such as an increased plasma calcium were of relevance in women without a genetic loading for mental illness.

In her second study of 21 women with the maternity blues, mood was assessed with the mood adjective affective check list (Zuckerman and Lubin, 1965). There were seven women with a previous history of some psychiatric disturbance although the nature of this was not specified. No gross elevation of plasma calcium was detected although it did tend to rise slightly between days 4–8 when mood disturbance was also maximal. Only among those with no previous psychiatric history did she find a significant association between the change in mood and plasma ionized calcium. She postulated that a mild degree of transient hyperparathyroidism was responsible for these changes, but it should be noted that plasma calcium levels were in the normal range and the mental symptoms only appear in hyperparathyroid states when there is a relatively gross elevation of plasma calcium. Furthermore urinary calcium is low in the puerperium, whereas in mild hyperparathyroidism it would be expected to be high.

Cyclic AMP

Cyclic AMP (Adenosine 3'5' cyclic monophosphate) is thought to be the second messenger in many hormonal interactions with their appropriate target cells. Cyclic AMP excretion has been reported to be increased in mania, and decreased in depression (Abdulla and Hamadah, 1970). Lowered levels of cyclic AMP have been found in both neurotic and psychotic depression and rise following treatment (Naylor et al., 1974; Sinanan et al., 1975) and in short cycle manic depressives a rythmical fluctuation in cyclic AMP in phase with the mood changes has been demonstrated (Naylor et al., 1974).

Ballinger et al. (1979, and personal communication) have investigated cyclic

AMP in relation to emotional disturbance following childbirth. An initial study of urinary excretion of cyclic AMP (Ballinger *et al.*, 1979) suggested that change in excretion of cyclic AMP following delivery was related more to mood change than to mood state at any particular time. Women who indicated a mood change in excess of 20 mm on a visual analogue rating scale between days 2 and 4 following delivery showed a significant rise in excretion of cyclic AMP and this relationship was most marked for those subjects who became "elated".

The urinary excretion of cyclic AMP is sensitive to exercise (Eccleston *et al.*, 1970) and renal function (Broadus, 1977) which complicates the interpretation of changes in urinary excretion of cyclic AMP following delivery. In a subsequent study (Ballinger *et al.*, personal communication) changes in plasma and whole blood cell cyclic AMP as well as urinary excretion of cyclic AMP were studied both during pregnancy and following delivery in relation to mood change. Those subjects who indicated a change in mood in excess of 20 mm on the visual analogue scale in the direction of becoming elated following delivery, showed a parallel rise in cyclic AMP and they also showed a significant fall in haematocrit. The changes in cyclic AMP and haematocrit following delivery resemble those observed in short cycle manic depressives (Buckely *et al.*, 1980). It has also been suggested by Paul *et al.* (1971) that a rise in cyclic AMP may act as a trigger for the onset of the metabolic changes of hypomania as patients switch from depression to mania. The findings in relation to cyclic AMP therefore add some further biochemical evidence for the presence of a "switch" process around the fourth postpartum day.

How can the weight, electrolyte, cyclic AMP, and plasma calcium changes be put together into a coherent hypothesis? None of these changes appear to be the direct cause of the mood disorder but a similar picture has been described at the onset of episodes in patients with short cycle manic depressive psychosis; rapid weight loss, increased sodium excretion and a rise in packed cell volume have been reported (Crammer, 1959; Jenner, 1967). Naylor (1976) has demonstrated that cyclic AMP excretion fluctuates in a cyclical fashion with mood and Jenner (1967) has shown that changes in sodium appetite also occur in these patients. More recently Carmen (1979) has reported a small rise in plasma calcium at the onset of the switch process. It remains to be seen whether the biological events which coincide with the onset of the blues are in any way related to the changes which are associated with cyclical switches in affective disorder.

Monoamines

The frequent presence of affective changes during the blues episode inevitably poses the question "To what extent does the blues syndrome resemble affective disorder both clinically and biochemically?" The main clinical distinction between the mood swings of the blues and of affective disorder is not in their character—both may be intense, but in their lability and duration. Thus depressive episodes of the blues last a few hours or a day or two at the most, while in affective disorder the mood changes can persist for several months. The extent to which the blues resemble affective disorder biochemically is not known. If alterations in monoamine metabolism cause affective disorder, then, possibly, changes in the same monoamines are responsible for the maternity blues.

Following the suggestion by Schildkraut (1965) that noradrenaline was a key substance in the pathogenesis of depression, Treadaway et al. (1968) examined catecholamine metabolism in relationship to the maternity blues. These workers examined 21 patients and rated their mood and personality using the MMPI, Clyde Mood Scale and the MAACI. They also collected 24 hour urine samples and measured catecholamine excretion both during pregnancy and postpartum. Their hypothesis was that greater degrees of mental disturbance might be associated with raised catecholamine excretion, but this turned out not to be the case. Instead they found a correlation between lowered levels of noradrenalin and mood during pregnancy but no significant changes postpartum, although there was a postpartum increase in normetanephrine excretion.

As well as noradrenalin, serotonin is now also thought to play a role in the pathogenesis of depression (for review see Eccleston, 1981) and the precursor of brain serotonin is tryptophan, particularly the unbound free tryptophan in plasma (Gessa and Tagliamonte, 1971). Even though the role of free plasma tryptophan in depression is presently controversial with some reporting a reduction (Coppen et al., 1973), while others find it unchanged (Niskanen et al., 1976), tryptophan metabolism has been investigated in the maternity blues.

Stein et al. (1976) examined 18 women, and took a single blood sample on the sixth postpartum day and estimated free and total tryptophan. Mood was assessed daily using a self-rating scale which had our symptoms, depression, weeping, irritability and insomnia and each symptom was rated on a four point scale. A significant association was found between lowered levels of free plasma tryptophan and the symptoms of depression and weeping. The study was small and could be criticised on the use of a scale without proven validity and reliability and the fact that the biochemistry was based on a single sample. Nevertheless, Handley et al. (1977) confirmed these findings in a similar small study of 18 patients; they took daily estimations of free and bound tryptophan and used the Hildreth mood scale (1946). Both free plasma tryptophan and cortisol were found to correlate significantly with depression. Handley et al. (1980) subsequently published a larger study of tryptophan metabolism during the puerperium. They examined 71 patients and used a complicated definition of the blues, namely, scoring on the eightieth percentile or more on any one of three depression scales as described earlier. Tryptophan was estimated at 38 weeks of pregnancy, for each of the first five postpartum days and again at six weeks postpartum. Total tryptophan was low during late pregnancy, rose rapidly on days one and two, fell slightly on days three and four and then gradually returned to normal. The rise in total tryptophan between late pregnancy and day one postpartum was absent in about one third of the women and absence of this rise was significantly associated both with the presence of severe maternity blues, and with depression at six months postpartum. Lowered tryptophan on day one correlated with the presence of depressed mood in the first five postpartum days. Free plasma tryptophan, like cortisol was found to vary seasonally, with lowest values in the winter and spring. It was only during these seasons that the previous findings (Handley *et al.*, 1977) of an association between mood and free plasma tryptophan could be replicated, and during the summer months no such correlation existed. If low free plasma tryptophan were the cause of the disorder, Harris (1980a) argued that therapy with L-tryptophan should cure the blues. The administration of L-tryptophan is known to raise plasma tryptophan (Aylward and Maddock, 1976). Harris (1980a) conducted a double blind placebo controlled study in 55 bottle-feeding multigravida and found no difference in either the incidence or severity of the blues between the treated and control groups. He concluded that the alterations in tryptophan metabolism were not causative. Handley *et al.* (1980) have suggested that the abnormalities in tryptophan may represent a defect in membrane transport, which is ultimately responsible for the blues, although the nature of this defect is obscure.

Monoamine Oxidase (MAO)

The discovery of a group of drugs that were sometimes effective therapeutic agents in depression, that also blocked the action of the enzyme monoamine oxidase led to speculation that this enzyme might also be involved in the pathogenesis of depression. MAO activity is largely genetically determined (Nies *et al.*, 1973; Murphy *et al.*, 1976), and is higher in females than males (Robinson *et al.*, 1971). A number of studies have been done on MAO levels in depression and schizophrenia but there is little firm evidence that they are altered in either of these disorders.

The menstrual cycle influences platelet MAO with the highest activity occurring just prior to ovulation and the lowest in the post ovulatory period, and hence studies of MAO activity in relation to post partum endocrine and mood changes may be of interest.

George and Wilson (1981) studied the mental states of 38 women using the Present State Examination (Wing *et al.*, 1974) on days two, four and six postpartum, and he also estimated platelet MAO activity on these days. Only eight PSE symptoms were present in an appreciabale frequency—depression, worries, tension, loss of concentration, obsessionalism, depersonalization, and listlessness. MAO activity correlated with depression throughout the study and with loss of concentration and obsessionalism on days 2 and 4 but not on day 6. George pointed out that platelets have a life of about 10 days and such correlations therefore reflect both pre- and postpartum events. He considered that both the mood and

MAO changes were probably caused by the same underlying (unspecified) hormonal changes. In contrast to the endocrinological investigations where correlations between mood and hormone levels have proved to be elusive, links between mood and both tryptophan and MAO have been found. It must be emphasized that the presence of a correlation does not imply a causal link, but it does suggest that further exploration into monoamine metabolism and the blues may be profitable.

Conclusions

Most women look back on the blues as an episode that was briefly unpleasant and difficult to explain. A few may have been severely distressed over a longer period and it is in such cases the distinction between the blues and postnatal depression becomes blurred. Some of the women in whom the blues blend into clinically significant depression may have been depressed at other times in the past and psychosocial factors predisposing to the blues and to postnatal depression and discussed in earlier sections of this chapter and in Chapter 4 of this book.

The ways in which internal and environmental factors might contribute to emotional disturbances during the weeks and months following delivery were of great concern to Marcé (1858), who also drew attention to transient, almost psychotic reactions that sometimes occur in the early puerperium. What is the relationship between the more severe blues and these transient psychotic phenomena, and with the puerperal psychoses? Are there some common triggering mechanisms? Both the blues and psychotic reactions usually start abruptly after a delay of two or three days (Karnosh and Hope, 1937; Hamilton, 1962; Melges, 1968) and psychotic illness is often preceded by a blues-like pro-drome of a day of severe weeping and mood change (Hamilton, 1962). However, the blues are very frequent while the psychoses are uncommon, and the rarity of the psychoses means that prospective studies of possible links with the blues are probably not practicable.

Research into psychiatric disorders has been held up by the lack of agreed criteria for defining clinical conditions. As a result researchers have turned to operational definitions in order to distinguish between "cases" and the rest (see Wing et al., 1981). Such definitions and relevant criteria are already available for the purpose of research into puerperal psychoses and postnatal depression but they do not exist in relation to the blues. This review has shown how far apart are the criteria that have been applied to the blues; they extend from a single weep (even of joy) on the first day or feeling like crying without doing so, to scores above predetermined thresholds on one of more clinical rating scales measuring dysphoria. The complexity and changing nature of the maternal mood state also makes for difficulties when attempts are made to collect symptoms and signs into a coherent syndrome. The distinguishing characteristics of a condition that is rare stand out from the rest of the population almost by definition. A similar exercise involving two-thirds of the population is somewhat more difficult to envisage. However, metabolic studies of the blues are unlikely to generate results that can be meaningfully compared until investigators agree about whom to select as subjects or "cases".

Descriptive accounts of the blues in the literature such as those of Robin (1962), Yalom *et al.*, (1968), Davidson (1972) and Pitt (1973) have perhaps been most informative and from them it has been possible to discern two components of the blues each of which may have a separate cause. Firstly there is a distinct episode, which has an abrupt onset and offset, is associated with weeping, lasts from one to three days and generally occurs between the third and tenth day, although sometimes the episode is rather less distinct and there is a fluctuating degree of disturbance each day. The second component is a group of mainly affective neurotic symptoms including depression, irritability, tension, anxiety, confusion, headache, depersonalization, restlessness and insomnia, that occur during the episode. These symptoms occur in varying combinations with differing severity in individual patients. It is unlikely that a single cause can explain why one patient may develop headache and depression on the third day, while another may feel irritable and depersonalized on day six. Dissecting the syndrome into its component parts may be helpful in attempting to elucidate its cause. Thus headache, for example, appears to be more frequent among those with a migraine diathesis, while depression is more frequent among those with previous depression. The maternity blues may resemble the premenstrual syndrome in that individual differences in the symptom profile may be determined by previous genetic or environmental influences, but the physiological changes in the early puerperium in some way result in their manifestation.

Two different formulations have appeared in the literature to explain the phenomenology of the blues. On the one hand, Moloney (1952) suggested they were minor depressive episodes, while Kane (1967) and Pitt (1973) have favoured an explanation of an acute organic reaction, but against this is the lack of any objective evidence for cognitive impairment (Kane, 1968; Yalom *et al.*, 1968; Gelder, 1979). Affective reactions, whether mild or severe, are usually thought of as having both environmental and endogenous causes. Is there any evidence that psycho-social stresses are responsible for the blues? Despite a great deal of diligent searching there does not appear to be any evidence linking the blues with the events of labour and delivery, nor with social class, marital status or other personal or environmental factors. Such a conclusion is hardly surprising given the almost universal prevalence of the blues and it leads to the suggestion that some biological factor is responsible. It may, however, be possible to delineate "subtypes" of the blues which are small and cohesive enough to show reliable associations with putative environmental influences.

Even though the maternity blues do not constitute an illness, many parties are interested to seek an explanation for them. Women themselves may perhaps be better reassured in the knowledge that their weeping and mood swings have a rational explanation. Paediatricians concerned with bonding behaviour are becoming increasingly interested in the maternal mental state in the early neonatal period. Psychiatrists, while attempting to explain the blues for their own sake, hope that some light may be thrown onto the aetiology of the more severe postpartum mental syndromes, and also in discovering any possible links between mental events and biological changes.

References

Abdulla, Y.H. and Hamada, K. (1970). Adenosine monophosphate in depression and mania. *Lancet* **i**, 378-381.

Anderson, B. (1976). The regulation of water intake. *Physiol. Rev.* **58**, 582-683.

Aylward, M. and Maddock, J. (1973). Plasma tryptophan levels in depression. *Lancet* **i**, 936.

Ballinger, C.B., Buckley, D.E., Naylor, G.J. and Stansfield, D.A. (1979). Emotional disturbance following childbirth and the excretion of Cyclic AMP. *Psychol. Med.* **9**, 293-300.

Beck, A.T., Ward, C.H., Mendelson, M., Mock, J. and Erbaugh, J. (1961). An inventory for measuring depression. *Archs. Gen. Psychiat.* **4**, 561-71.

Bourke, C.W. and Roulet, F. (1970). Increased exposure of tissues to Cortisol in late pregnancy. *Brit. Med. J.* 657.

Bourne, G. (1975). Pregnancy. Pan Books London.

British Medical Journal Editorial (1977). Thyroid disease and pregnancy. *Brit. Med. J.* **2**, 977-8.

Broadus, A.E. (1977). Clinical cyclic nucleotide research. *In Advances in Cyclic Nucleotide Research* Vol. 8 (eds P. Geig and G.A. Robinson) pp.509-549. Raven Press, New York.

Browne, W.A., Johnstone, E. and Mayfield, D. (1979). The 24 hour dexamethasone suppression test in a clinical setting and its relationship to diagnosis and response to treatment. *Am. J. Psychiat.* **136**, 543-547.

Buckley, D.E., Naylor, G.J., Stansfield, D.A. and Brown, R.A. (1980). Cyclic AMP Levels in blood cells from a short cycle manic depressive subject. *Brit. J. Psychiat.* **136**, 584-590.

Caine, T.M., Foulds, G.A., and Hope, K. (1967). Manual of the Hostility and Direction of Hostility Questionnaire, H.D.H.Q. University of London Press, London.

Carmen, J.S., Post, R.M., Runkle, D.C., Bunney, W.E., Wyatt, R.J., (1979). Increased serum calcium and phosphorous with the switch into manic or excited psychotic states. *Brit. J. Psychiat.* **135**, 55-63.

Carroll, B.J. (1972). The hypothalamo-pituitary adrenal axis in depressive illness. *In Depressive illness: some research studies* (ed. B. Danis et al.). Thomas: Springfield. Illinois.

Carroll, B.J., Curtis, G.C., Davies B.M., Mendels, J. and Sugarman, A.A. (1976). Urinary free cortisol in depression. *Psychological Medicine* **6**, 43−50.

Cope, C.L. (1973). *Adrenal Steroids and disease*, Chapter 33, pp. 649-667. Pitman Medical, London.

Coppen, A., Eccleston, E. and Peet, M. (1973). Total and free plasma tryptophan concentration in the plasma of depressed patients. *Lancet* ii, 1415-16.

Crammer, J.L. (1959). Water and sodium in two psychotics. *Lancet* i, 1122-1126.

Crammer, J.L. (1977). Calcium metabolism and mental disorder. *Psychological Medicine* 7, 557-560.

Crisp, A.H. and Stonehill, E. (1976). *Sleep, Weight, and Nutrition.* John Wiley, London.

Dalton, K. (1964). *The Pre-menstrual Syndrome.* Heinemann London.

Dalton, K. (1980). *Depression after Childbirth.* Oxford University Press, London.

Daly, J.R. and Elstein, M. (1972). Hypothalamo-pituitary adrenal function during oral contraception. *J. Obstet. Gynaecol.* 79, 544.

Davidson, J.R.T. (1973). Post partum mood changes in Jamaican women and a discussion on its significance. *Brit. J. Psychiat.* 121, 659.

Davis, J. and Kitzinger, S. (1977). *The Place of Birth.* Oxford University Press, London.

Dennis, K.J. and Blytheway, W.R. (1965). Changes in body weight after delivery. *Brit. J. Obstet. Gynaecol.* 95, 127.

Deutsch, H. (1945). *The Psychology of Women.* Grune and Stratton, New York.

Dieckmann, W.J. and Pottinger, R.E. (1955). Aetology of eclampsia—pre-eclampsia. *Am. J. Obstet Gynaecol.* 70, 822-860.

Doe, R.P., Fernandez, R. and Seal, U.S. (1964). Measurement of corticosteroid binding globulin in man. *J. Clin. Endocrinol.* 24, 1029.

Eccleston, D., Loose, R., Pullar, I.A. and Sugden, R.F. (1970). Exercise and the urinary excretion of Cyclic AMP. *Lancet* ii, 612-613.

Eccleston, D. (1981) Monoamines in depression. *Brit. J. Psychiat.* 138, 257-259.

Edwards, O.M. and Bayliss, R.I.S. (1976). Idiopathic oedema of women. A clinical and investigation study. *Quat. J. Med.* 45, 125-44.

Gelder, M.G. (1978). Hormones in post partum depression. *In Mental Illness in Pregnancy and Puerperium.* (ed. M. Sandler). Oxford University Press London.

Gennazini, A., Fraile, F., Hurliman, J. and Fiorritti Felber, J.P. (1975). Immuno-reactive ACTH and Cortisol plasma levels during pregnancy. Detection and partial purification of corticotrophic like placental hormone. The human chorionic corticotrophin HCC. *Clinical Endocrinology* 4, 1.

George, A.J., Copeland, J.R.M. and Wilson, K.C.M. (1980). Prolactin in the maternity blues. *Brit. J. Pharmalol* 70, 102-103.

George, A.J. and Wilson, K.C.M. (1981). Monoamine oxidase activity and the puerperal blues *J. Psychosom. Res.* 25, 409-414.

Gessa, G.K. and Tagliamonte, A. (1971). Serum free tryptophan and the control of brain tryptophan and 5HT concentration. *In Serontonin New Vistas* (eds E. Costa, G. Gessa and M. Sandler) No. 10. p.109. Ravens Press, New York.

Gibbons, J.L. (1964). Cortisol secretion rate in depressive illness. *Archs. Gen. Psychiat.* 10, 572-575.

Giordano, N.D., and Radivoyevitch. M. (1970). Seasonal variations of plasma cortisol in Haemophilia A. *Lancet* i, 249.

Gjessing, R.R., (1976). *Contributions to the Somatology of Periodic Catatonia.* (eds F.A. Jenner and L.R. Gjessing). Oxford University Press, London.

Gordon, B. (1977). *In The Place of Birth, Chapter 13.* (eds J.A. Davis and S. Kitzinger) pp.201-215. Oxford University Press, London.

Grundy, P.F. and Roberts, C.J. (1975). Observation on the epidemiology of post partum mental illness. *Psychol. Med.* 5, 286-290.

Gyermark, L., Genther, S. and Fleming, N. (1967). Some effects of Progesterone and related steroids in the nervous system. *Int. J. Neuropharmacol.* 6, 191.

Haas, S. (1952). *The Psychology of Physical Illness.* Churchill, London.

Hamilton, J.A. (1962). *Post Partum Psychiatric Problems.* The C.V. Mosby Co., St. Louis.

Handley, S.L., Dunn, T., Baker, J.M., Cockshott, C. and Gould, S. (1977). Mood changes in the puerperium and plasma tryptophan and cortisol. *Brit. Med. J.* **2**, 18-22.

Handley, S.L., Dunn, T.L., Waldron, S. and Baker, J.M. (1980). Tryptophan, cortisol and puerperal mood. *Brit. J. Psychiat.* **136**, 498-508.

Harris, B. (1980a). Prospective trial of L-Tryptophan in the maternity blues. *Brit. J. Psychiat.* **137**, 233-235.

Harris, B. (1980b). Maternity blues. *Brit. J. Psychiat.* **136**, 520-521.

Herzberg, B.N., Johnson, A.L. and Brown, S. (1970). Depression and oral contraceptives. *Brit. Med. J.* **3**, 142-144.

Hildreth, H.M. (1946). A battery of feeling and attitude scales for clinical use. *J. Clin. Psychol* **2**, 214-21.

Hofer, M. (1975). Introduction. *In Parent Infant Interaction*, pp.1-3. Ciba Symposium 33. Elsevier North Holland.

How, J. and Bewsher, P.D. (1978). Thyroid disease in pregnancy.*Brit. Med. J.* **2**, 1568-69.

Jacobsen, L., Kaij, L. and Nilsson, A. (1965). Post partum psychiatric disorders in an unselected sample. Frequency of symptoms and predisposing factors. *Brit. Med. J.*, 640-643.

Jenner, F.A., Gjessing, L.R., Cox, J.R., Davies Jones, A., Hullin, R.P. and Hanna, S.M. (1967). A manic depressive psychotic with a persistent 48 hour cycle. *Brit. J. Psychiat.* **113**, 895-910.

Kane, F.J., Harman, W.J., Keeler, H.M. and Ewing, A.J. (1968). Emotional and cognitive disturbace in the early puerperium. *Brit. J. of Psychiat.* **114**, 99-102.

Karacan, I., Williams, R.L., Hursch, C.J., Macauley, M. and Heine, M.W. (1969). Some implications for the sleep pattern for post partum emotional disorder. *Brit. J. Psychiat.* **115**, 929-932.

Karnosh, L.J. and Hope, J.M. (1937). Puerperal psychoses and their sequelae. *Am. J. Psychiat.* **94**, 537.

Kendell, R.E. (1975). *The Role of Diagnosis in-Psychiatry*. Blackwell, Oxford.

Kendell, R.E., Rennie, D., Clark, J.A. and Dean, C. (1981). Social and obstetric correlates of psychiatric admissions in the puerperium. *Psychol. Med.* **11**, 341-350.

Kitzinger, S. (1971). *A Woman's Experience of Birth at Home*. (eds J.A. Davis and S. Kitzinger) pp.135-155. Oxford University Press, London.

Klaus, M.H., Trause, M.A., Kennel, J.H. (1975). Does human maternal behaviour after delivery show a characteristic pattern. *CIBA Foundation Syposium* **33**, 69-85.

Klerman G.L. (1981). States of mania. *Comprehensive Psychiat.* **22**, 11-20.

Kraupl-Taylor F. (1980). The concepts of disease. *Psychol. Med.* **10**, 419-424.

Labhart, A. (1974). Clinical Endocrinology, p.182. Springer-Verlag, Heidleberg.

Lindheimer, M.D., Katz, A.I., Nolten, W.E., Oparil, S. and Ehrich, E.N. (1977). Sodium and mineral—corticoids in Normal and Abnormal Pregnancy. *Advances in Nephrology from the Necker Hospital. Chicago* **7**, 33-59.

Lorr, M., Daston, P. and Smith, I.R. (1967). An analysis of mood states. *Educational and Psychological Measurement* **27**, 89-96.

Macfarlane, A. (1979). *The Psychology of Childbirth* Fontana Open Books, London.

Macgregor, G.A., Markandu, N.D., Roulston, J.R., Jones, J.C. and De Wardener, H.E. (1979). Is idiopathic oedema idiopathic? *Lancet* **I**, 397.

Marcé, L.V. (1858). *Traité de la folie des femmes enceintes, des nouvelles accouchees et des nourrices.*

Melges, F.T. (1968). Post partum psychiatric Syndromes. *Psychosom. Med.* **30**, 95.

Moloney, J.C. (1952). Post partum depression or third day depression following childbirth. *New Orleans Child and Parent Digest.* **6**, 20-32.

Moos, R.H. (1968). The development of a menstrual distress questionnaire. *Psychosom Med.* **30**, 853-867.

Murphy, D.L. (1976). Clinical, genetic and drug influences on the activity of Enzyme Platelet Monoamine Oxidase. *In Monoamine Oxidase and its Inhibition.* Ciba Symposium No. 39 Elsevier North Holland.

Naylor, G.J., Stansfield, D.A., White, S.F. and Hutchinson, F. (1974). Urinary excretion of Adenosine 3'—5' Cyclic Monophosphate in depressive illness. *Brit. J. Psychiat.* **125**, 275-279.

Nies, A., Robinson, D.S. and Harris, L.S. (1974). Comparison of MAO substrates activities in twins, schizophrenics, depressives and controls. *In Neuropsychopharmacology of Monoamines and their regulatory enzymes* (Ed. E. Usdin) pp.59-70. Raven Press, New York.

Niskanen, P., Huttunen, M., Tamminem, T., Jaaskaleinem J. (1976). The daily rhythm plasma tryptophan and tyrosine in depression. *Brit. J. Psychiat.* **128**, 67-73.

Nott, P.N., Franklin, M., Armitage, C. and Gelder, M.G. (1976). Hormonal changes and mood in the early puerperium. *Brit. J. Psychiat.* **128**, 379-83.

Oppenheim, G. (1962). Psychological aspects of Pregnancy and Childbirth. Lecture to the RMPA quoted by Pitt (1973).

Paul, M.I., Cramer, H. and Bunney, W.E. (1971). Urinary adenosine 3' 5' Monophosphate in the switch from Depression to Mania. *Science* **171**, 300-303.

Paffenbarger, R.S. (1964). Epidemiological aspects of para partum mental illness. *Brit. J. Prev. Soc. Med.* **18**, 189-195.

Pitkin, R.M. and Gebhart, M.P. (1977). Serum calcium concentration in human pregnancy *Am. J. Obstet and Gynaecol.* **127**, 775-778.

Pitt, B. (1968). Atypical depression following childbirth. *Brit. J. Psychiat.* **114**, 1225-1235.

Pitt, B. (1973). Maternity blues. *Brit. J. Psychiat.* **122**, 431-435.

Reid, R.L. and Yen, S.S.C. (1981). The pre-menstrual syndrome. *Am. J. Obstet. Gynaecol.* **139**, 85-104.

Riley, D.M. (1979). A study of serum calcium in relation to puerperal psychiatric illness. *In Emotion and Reproduction* (Eds L. Carenza and L. Zichella), pp.829-835. Academic Press, London and New York.

Robin, A.M. (1962). Psychological changes associated with childbirth. *Psychiat. Quarterly* **36**, 129-150.

Robinson, D.S., Davis, J.M., Nies, A., Ravario, C.L. and Sylvester, D. (1971). Relation of sex and ageing to Monoamine Oxidase brain, plasma, and platelets. *Archs. Gen. Psychiat.* **24**, 536-539.

Robson, K.M. and Kumar, R. (1980). Delayed onset of maternal affection after childbirth. *Brit. J. Psychiat.* **136**, 347-353.

Savage, G.H. (1975). Observations on the insanity of pregnancy and childbirth. *Guys Hosp. Rep.* **20**, 83.

Sachar, E.J., Hellman, L., Roftwanz, H.P. and Halpern, E.S., (1973). Disrupted 24 hour patterns of cortisol secretion in psychotic depression. *Archs. Gen. Psychiat.* **28**, 19-24.

Scadding, J.G. (1967). Diagnosis, the clinician and the computer. *Lancet* ii, 877-882.

Schildkraut, J. (1965). The catecholamine hypothesis of affective disorder. *Am. J. Psychiat.* **112**, 509-522.

Schottsdead, W.W. and Wolff, H.G. (1955). Variation in fluid and electrolyte excretion in association with vascular headache of the migraine type. *Archs. Neurol. Psychiat.* **73**, 158.

Sinanen E., Keating A.M.B., Beckett, P.G.S. and Clayton Love, W. (1975). Urinary Cyclic AMP in endogenous and neurotic depression. *Brit. J. Psychiat.* **126**, 49-55.

Snaith, R.P., Ahmed, S.N., Mehta, S. and Hamilton, M. (1971). Assessment of the severity of primary depression illness. *Psychol. Med.* **1**, 143.

Sheikh, G.N. (1971). Weight changes after delivery. *Am. J. Obstet, ad Gynaecol.* **iii**, 244-258.

Starkman, M.N., Schiteingart, D. and Schork, M.A. (1981). Depressed mood and other psychiatric manifestations of Cushings Syndrome. Relationship to hormone levels. *Psychosomatic Medicine* **43**, 3-17.

Stein, G.S., Milton, F., Bebbington, P., Wood, K. and Coppen, A. (1976). Relationship between mood disturbance and free plasma tryptophan in post partum women. *Brit. Med. J.* **2**, 457.

Stein, G.S., Morton, J. and Keating, P. (1978). Peripartum heart failure. *Lancet*, 1214.

Stein, G.S. (1979). An enquiry into the nature and aeitology of the maternity blues syndrome. M. Phil. Thesis. London University.

Stein, G.S. (1980). The pattern of mental change and body weight change in the first post partum week. *J. Psychosom Res.* **24**, 165-171.

Stein. G.S., Ebeling, J. and Desagea, U. (1980b). Vasopressin and mood in the first post partum week. Abstract XI International Congress of psychoneuro-endocrinology. Florence 1980.

Stein, G.S. (1981b) Headaches in the first post partum week and their relationship to migraine. *Headache* **21**, 201-205.

Stein, G.S., Marsh, A. and Morton, J. (1981). Mood, weight and urinary electrolytes in the first post partum week. *J. Psychosom. Res.* **25**, 395-408.

Steiner, M. Psychobiology of mental disorders associated with childbearing. *Acta Psychiatr. Scand.* **60**, 449-464.

Stengel, E., Zeitlyn, B. and Rayner, E.H. (1958). Post operative psychosis. *J. Ment. Sci.* **104**, 389-402.

Thune, G.S. (1968). Sleep and wakefulness in normal human adults. *Brit. Med. J.* **2**, 269-272.

Treadaway, C.R., Kane, F.J., Ali Jarrehi-Zadeh and Lipton, M.A. (1969). A psychoendocrine study of pregnancy and the puerperium. *Am. J. Psychiat,* **136**, 1380-83.

Victoroff, V.M. (1952). Dynamics and management of parapartum neuropathic reactions. *Dis. Nerv. Syst.* **10**, 291-298.

Weeks, D., Freeman, C.L.L. and Kendell, R.E. (1980). Enduring cognitive defects following E.C.T. treatment in depression. *Brit. J. Psychiat.* **137**, 26-37.

Wing, J., Cooper J. and Sartorius, N. (1974). *The Measurement and Classification of Psychiatric Symptoms.* Cambridge University Press, Cambridge.

Wing, J.K. Bebbington, P. and Robins, L.N., (1981) What is a case? *The Problem of definition in Community Surveys.* Grant Macintyre, London.

Yalom, I., Lunde, D., Moos. R. and Hamburg, D. (1968). Post partum blues syndrome, *Archs. Gen. Psychiat.* **18**, 16-27.

Zuckerman, M. and Lubin, B. (1965). Manual for the multiple affect adjective check list. *Education and Industrial Testing Science, San Diego.*

6

Early Maternal Attachment

Kay Mordecai Robson and Elisabeth Powell

Introduction

There have been numerous attempts recently to investigate the development of mother–infant relationships. Several issues have been raised. For instance, do the mother's initial feelings and behaviour towards her neonate have any long-term consequences for their future relationship? Do events in the early postnatal period (such as mother–infant separation) affect the nature of the relationship and is there evidence for a "sensitive period" in the first few hours and days after delivery, when the human mother is optimally primed to "bond" with her newborn?

This chapter reviews the empirical and theoretical work on the development of attachment between mothers and their newborn infants; a process which has also been called "bonding". Much of the impetus for this research derived from animal studies in which a sensitive period for maternal "bonding" was found in species of ungulates in the period immediately after birth (e.g. Collias, 1956; Hersher et al., 1963).

The review will cover:

(1) The concept of attachment and problems of measurement.
(2) The theoretical background to studies which investigate early mother–infant attachment.
(3) A review of the studies which have investigated early maternal attachment and behaviour.
(4) An integration of the research findings and their implications for future research and practice.

This present review focuses on empirical research which has been conducted with mothers in Western societies. The study of maternal behaviour in animals and the work of psychoanalysts and anthropologists have stimulated many ideas

155

and hypotheses about maternal attachment, but these are beyond the scope of this chapter. Comparisons between animal species unrelated by descent and occupying dissimilar ecological niches have limited scientific use (Lockard, 1971). However, relevant animal studies have been briefly alluded to where the insights can be tested in human mothers. Psychoanalytic concepts, although usually based on a small number of clinical cases, have made fruitful contributions to the research which will be presented. For example, the increasing use of obstetrical procedures and the associated passivity of the mother was considered likely to have an adverse effect on the mother–infant relationship (Deutsch, 1944; Winnicott, 1958, 1960). Similarly, the anthropological research (e.g. Mead, 1935, 1950, 1954; Whiting, 1963; Hubert, 1974) has also shed light on the variety of practices surrounding the birth process and motherhood and has emphasized the importance of cultural values and beliefs with regard to maternal behaviour. The society in which a woman lives in can crucially influence her role as a mother (e.g. Chodorow, 1978; Kitzinger, 1978; Oakley, 1980).

The Concept of Attachment and Problems of Measurement

Definitions of Maternal Attachment

Much of the research on maternal attachment has been influenced by the work on attachment between the infant and mother. In this work close proximity has frequently been used as one of the most important indices of attachment (e.g. Bowlby, 1969; Ainsworth, 1973). Similarly, many researchers focusing on the mother–infant relationship have used proximity as a key indicator of maternal attachment (e.g. Kennell *et al.*, 1975). Ainsworth (1973) wrote:

> An attachment is an affectional tie that one person forms to another specific person, binding them together in space and enduring over time. Attachment is discriminating and specific ... and we usually think of attachment as implying affection or love.

Ainsworth's definition therefore rests on three criteria for attachment: firstly, an ability to recognize the object of attachment; secondly, a preference for the attachment figure; and finally, some response to the removal of the object of attachment (Ainsworth, 1973).

The distinction between "attachment" and "attachment behaviours" is stressed by Ainsworth. "Attachment" refers to the bond, tie or the enduring relationship between individuals; whereas "attachment behaviours" are those behaviours through which such a bond is first formed and which later serve to mediate the relationship (Ainsworth *et al.*, 1978). Attachment need not necessarily be the same as overt attachment behaviour, although the "... hallmark of attachment is behaviour that promotes proximity to or contact with the specific figure or figures to which the person is attached." (Ainsworth, 1973).

Klaus and his colleagues have given a similar definition: "An attachment can be defined as an enduring and unique emotional relationship between two people which is specific and endures through time." (Kennell *el al.*, 1975, 1979).

Behaviours like fondling, kissing, cuddling and prolonged gazing are said to be indicators of attachment. Kennell and his colleagues have suggested that optimal attachment behaviour is expressed when the mother shows interest, attentiveness, commitment and protectiveness towards her infant. Conversely, "disinterest, neglect, indiscriminate attention, abandonment, failure to protect, nurture or interact" are examples of a failure to attach. Klaus and Kennell have tended to concentrate on the measurement of such maternal behaviours as fondling, and have recorded the amount of time devoted to each behaviour. They, like many other workers in this field (e.g. Hales *et al.*, 1977; De Chateau and Wiberg, 1977a, b; Carlsson *et al.*, 1978, 1979), have limited their observations to the mothers behaviour and made no attempt to look at sequences of behaviour where the contributions and responsiveness of each individual can be assessed.

Bakeman and Brown (1977) suggested the notion of a dialogue to describe the mother–infant relationship. They viewed the mother–infant interaction as a conversation between two individuals (see also Trevarthen, 1979). Within this conversation "good" interaction involved some degree of balance between the activities of the partners, with both active concurrently for a proportion of the time. They suggest that the "good" mother should be responsive to the infant and should continue to respond until the infant is satisfied.

Similarly, using a detailed analysis of filmed observations of five mother–infant pairs, Brazelton *et al.* (1975) reported a rhythmic, cyclic quality about the mother–infant relationship, and an attention—non attention behavioural cycle, with the mother's pattern usually synchronized to the baby. It was argued that the interdependency of rhythm was at the root of maternal "attachment", and was evident when the pair were sympathetic to each other's needs. When a rhythmic quality was present, the observer senses that a "positive" interaction was taking place; when the balance was not equalized, the interaction had a "negative" quality.

Maternal attachment has also been defined as the ". . . extent to which a mother feels that her infant occupies an essential position in her life." (Robson and Moss, 1970). In the early stages of life, maternal attachment is said to be reflected in feelings of love or warmth, a sense of possession, devotion, protectiveness and concern for the infant's well-being, a positive anticipation of prolonged contact, and a need for pleasure in continuing transactions. These researchers interviewed mothers postnatally and asked them about their feelings towards their infants after birth and in the ensuing weeks.

Caretakers of infants (not just mothers), typically behave differently when interacting with babies as opposed to adults (Stern, 1977). For instance, their voices become high-pitched, are often slower, and "baby-talk" words are used.

They gaze a lot at the infants; the faces they make are often exaggerated, as are all movements. Stern noted that it is a highly unusual and very ineffective caretaker who behaves towards an infant as he/she would towards an adult. Through filmed observations of social interactions with mothers and their infants, Stern concluded that the "free play" situation provided the optimal setting for the evaluation of mothering, because it was during "free play" that the child had the most opportunity for learning and participating in social communications.

Schaffer's (1977a) definition of maternal attachment stressed the quality of the mother and infant's relationship and the mother's "heightened sensitivity to the child", based on "mother-love". He cautioned that love for an infant leads to an intensification of all emotions—negative as well as positive—an opinion which has been ignored by most of the researchers in the area and therefore not put to the test.

Similarly, Hinde and Simpson (1975), working with Rhesus monkeys, have emphasized that it is the quality of the mother–infant relationship that indicated most about maternal attachment. Inferences regarding the quality and meaning of the mother's actions must be made in order to assess attachment. It is not sufficient to limit the observations to counting behavioural acts. For instance, direct eye contact has been widely used as an index of maternal attachment, but may have a variety of meanings. Direct eye contact can express aggression as well as affection. Hinde and Simpson paid special attention to maternal warmth, maternal rejection, maternal control, and the synchronization of the interaction between mother and infant. They argued, however, that the usefulness of these measures can only be assessed by their predictive power in longitudinal studies.

"Attachment" has often been equated with "good" mothering, and it is "good" mothering which has usually been assessed in empirical research.

Labelling maternal behaviour as "good" or "sensitive" implies that we know what measures reflect "good" or "bad" mothering, and that in some way these measures are interrelated. To date, there have been few studies which show that behaviours such as fondling, kissing, attentiveness, protectiveness, and prolonged gazing are indeed indicators of good mothering (although it would appear likely), nor that they are interrelated. Dunn and Richards (1977) showed that different styles of mothering behaviour were associated with different infant and delivery factors (e.g. a longer labour was associated with increased feeding problems in the first postnatal days), but there were no intercorrelations amongst the behaviours generally described as indicating maternal affection (e.g. touching the infant was not correlated with other affectionate behaviours such as smiling, talking affectionately, and looking at the baby).

It has been asserted (Dunn and Richards, 1977) that beyond being fairly confident that a few aspects of parental behaviour are damaging to children (e.g. violence), there are still no widely accepted grounds for evaluating maternal behaviour in terms of outcomes in the child. Some recent research does, however, indicate stable relationships between maternal style and the quality of the infant's reaction in a strange situation (Blehar *et al.*, 1977; Sroufe *et al.*, 1978; Waters *et al.*, 1979). For example, mothers who were more responsive to their infants and who encouraged interaction in the first few months were more likely to have their one-year-old infants described as securely attached to them.

As well as the difficulty of assessing what "good" mothering is, it also seems apparent that what might be "good" mothering for one infant–mother dyad, might be wrong for another, and even for one particular dyad at different times (Winnicott, 1960).

Techniques used to Evaluate Maternal Attachment

It is very difficult to find agreement about ways of measuring "attachment" because there are fundamental differences of opinion about this concept.

Self-rating Scales

Some researchers have relied on self-administered rating scales (e.g. Broussard and Hartner, 1971; Parker *et al.*, 1979). In Broussard and Hartner's Neonatal Perception Inventory, the mother's perceptions of her infant are compared with her perceptions of the "average baby", on such factors as amount of crying, and trouble with feeding and sleeping. It is argued that maternal perceptions, either negative or positive, may be related to the degree of satisfaction which the mother is experiencing in her relationship with the infant.

In general, rating scales have the advantage of being speedy, so that the collection of a large sample is relatively easy. However, they do have disadvantages. The mothers may construe the questions differently and their response set (e.g. the tendency to always answer positively) can distort the results. The mothers may also tend to give responses which are perceived as being socially acceptable.

Interviews

In other studies (Robson and Moss, 1970; Robson and Kumar, 1980), mothers have been interviewed about their caretaking behaviours and feelings towards their babies. Although more time-consuming than self-rating scales, interviews allow the mother to expand on her perceptions of the infant. A skilled interviewer can also reduce the ambiguity of questions and answers can be probed for clarification. However, the skill and personality of the interviewer and the importance the subject attaches to the research may crucially influence the quality of the data collected. Mothers may distort their responses, either because of "social desirability" or because they simply do not remember or are unaware of their mothering behaviour.

Observations

Observations of behaviour have been widely used to investigate maternal behaviour, and attachment. Direct observations can be made either through a one-way mirror, or by an observer who is in the same room (e.g. Bakeman and Brown, 1977) such observations may sometimes show how differences in behaviour can occur. For instance, many studies have described parity differences in maternal behaviour and in general, multiparous mothers are usually more efficient and appear to have more harmonious relationships with their newborn infants (see pp.166). However, through extensive observations of mother–infant interaction in baboons, Ransom and Rowell (1972) noted that multiparous females have significantly longer nipples, which enable their infants to suckle more easily and therefore experience fewer disruptions whilst feeding. From their observations, Ransom and Rowell concluded that differences in nipple length can lead to variations in the quality of maternal care and in the development of the mother—infant relationship.

Time lapse photography, (e.g. Klaus *et al.*, 1970) cine-filming and videotaping (e.g. Brazelton *et al.*, 1975; Stern, 1977; Carlsson *et al.*, 1978) have the advantage that coding can be carried out at a later time, and fine analyses of behaviour can be made. It is also much easier to assess sequential interaction and the relative contributions of both partners.

All observational techniques do have certain disadvantages. It is necessary to select data from the large mass of available information and such decisions are open to bias. For example the observer's preconceptions about "good" mothering may cause him to ignore crucial features of the mother–infant interaction. Although both the quantity of individual behaviours (e.g. Kennell *et al.*, 1975) and sequences of behaviour (e.g. Bakeman and Brown, 1977) can be observed in the research situation, in practice they have rarely been combined.

Many studies which use observational methods employ "one-off", small time-samples of interaction as a data base. The variability of mother–infant interactions over time is usually ignored. For instance, Levy (1958) (cited in Macfarlane, 1977) looked at mothers' greeting responses when their babies were brought to them the first two or three times after birth. He noted great variations in their greetings at different times and maternal behaviour seemed to be dependent on what the baby was doing. Macfarlane suggested that "one-off" observations of mother's behaviour could be "grossly misleading about her actual feelings". Chappell and Sander (1979) recommended that the same mother–infant pair must be observed several times before any conclusion about their relationship can be made.

With direct observations, the presence of an observer may also be disconcerting to the mother, and even the presence of a one-way mirror does not completely overcome this difficulty. Filming and videotaping are not particularly naturalistic. Some mothers might be more concerned that they are filmed with the "right" (i.e. the most flattering side of their face) to the camera, rather than interacting with their babies. The camera lens covers a limited area, and may, therefore, exclude important details. Analysis of filming is usually extremely time-consuming and microanalytic techniques can invariably be carried out on a small sample only, from which it is difficult to generalize.

Finally, all methods of assessing maternal behaviours and feelings are beset with the problem that mothers may also have an idea of what the observer thinks "good" mothering involves. For instance, any mother who has read about the "bonding" research, may spend a great deal of time *"en face"* with her infant while she is being observed.

Many definitions of maternal attachment have been used and within these definitions three main elements can be identified. These are that the mother has a strong affection for her baby; that the affection will endure over time and that she has an awareness of her baby's needs and will respond appropriately.

The majority of researchers have relied upon behavioural indices of attachment and although a variety of behaviours have been considered important, almost all have included measures of mother–infant proximity and eye contact. So-called "attachment behaviours" do not, of course, necessarily reflect the strength of maternal "attachment" (Freud, 1943). For example, a mother who has little affection for her child may display excessive caring behaviour. Some research has concentrated simply on the quantity of different maternal behaviours observed (e.g. Klaus *et al.*, 1975; de Chateau and Wiberg, 1977). Others have tried to assess the quality of the mother–infant relationship (e.g. Hinde and Simpson, 1975) and yet others have placed emphasis on sequences of mother-infant interaction, accepting the participation and contributions of both mother and infant to the interactional sequence (e.g. Brazelton *et al.*, 1975; Stern, 1977; Bakeman and Brown, 1977). Most researchers using observational techniques have, however, tended to ignore the mother's reported feelings and perceptions of her infant.

Ideally, more than one technique should be employed to compensate for the weaknesses of any one method of investigation. Like Schaffer (1977b), we feel that the best way of trying to assess the mother–infant relationship is to treat the interaction in dyadic terms. Even the earliest interactions are two-way affairs, because the infant is already capable of organized spontaneous behaviour (see pp.169).

The Theoretical Background to Research on Early Maternal Attachment

The human infant has to be cared for over many years and as in all mammals, the mother is the main source of this nurturance in early life. There are two extreme views of the mother's function. Firstly, it has been argued that the role of the caretaker is circumscribed in influencing the development of children. In this view, apart from providing food, shelter and physical protection, the main contribution of the parent is to provide a stable context in which the young can develop (Harper, 1970). The converse view, which appears to have had more influence on the research into early maternal attachments, has been that the mother shapes the child's early experiences to such an extent that the infant's relationship with the mother forms a "prototype" for the subsequent social relationships in which the child may engage (Bowlby, 1969). The earliest attempts by the infant to manipulate the environment and to develop competence, are directed towards the mother and so her reactions are a major influence on the infant's development (Turner, 1980).

Bowlby and Ainsworth

Bowlby (1969) and Ainsworth (1969) assume that attachment behaviour has a biological function of its own which is independent of other functions, such as taking in nourishment. To Bowlby, human attachment behaviour has a biological base, and is only understood within the context of evolutionary adaptedness. Mothers are genetically programmed to respond appropriately (e.g. to provide physical closeness) to the human infant's five built-in signals and responses (crying, smiling, sucking, following and clinging). If culturally learned responses and events (such as separation of the mother and infant) interfere with the biological process of attachment formation, then the consequences for the infant could be serious and long-lasting (Bowlby, 1958, 1969; Ainsworth, 1969). Bowlby and Ainsworth therefore emphasized the importance of the infant's signals in eliciting and maintaining maternal proximity. They hypothesized that the biological function of the infant's attachment and attachment behaviours was to ensure maternal protection.

Richards (1970) however, disagreed with Bowlby's proposal that there are five stable infant behaviour systems that are particularly effective in bringing about proximity of mother and child, and ultimately mutual attachment:

> During feeding, his sucking certainly patterns the mother's behaviour but so do his facial movements, sneezes, burps, defaecations, and particularly his changes in state. In fact, almost any change in infant behaviour may be used by the mother to pattern her behaviour. This is rather unlike the very restricted and specific signals that are typical of the releasing system described in animal species.

Sociobiological Ideas

Sociobiologists have suggested that the mother obtains equal benefit from her attachment to the infant, by increasing the likelihood of the infant's survival which, in turn, perpetuates her genes in subsequent generations. This idea is termed "inclusive fitness" (Hamilton, 1964). Porter and Laney (1980) tried to integrate Bowlby's ideas on attachment within the framework of sociobiology.

They argued that both infant and mother benefit in an evolutionary sense from becoming attached to each other. Specific attachment behaviours have evolved because they increase the inclusive fitness not only of the infant, but also the caretaker who responds to the baby's signals. The "... love of parent for child is an evolutionary strategem insuring that parents will invest in the child in a manner that maximises each parent's fitness" (Barash, 1980).

The "Sensitive" Period

"Bonding" theory has been rooted in ethological and evolutionary ideas. Richards (1979) has suggested that, in effect, Bowlby's notion of attachment in infants has been transposed to the mother; has been given a new name "bonding" and has been shifted to a much earlier phase in development. The implications of Bowlby's theory are that there is a "critical period" for infant–mother attachment to develop. The child and biological mother (or mother surrogate) must not be separated, as all separations, even for a few days, are inevitably damaging and if they are for longer periods, they can do irreversible damage. Although Bowlby has modified his views regarding maternal separation, the concept of a "critical period" has influenced much research on maternal attachment (Dunn, 1979).

Similarly, researchers on early maternal attachment have also been influenced by the animal literature. Studies with several species of ungulates have suggested the existence of a "critical" period immediately after birth for the expression of appropriate maternal behaviours, and for the development of maternal attachment to the infant.

> Immediately after birth (and for some females shortly before giving birth), the motivation of the dam to 'mother' a young animal is strong. This maternal drive fades rapidly within a few hours after parturition, however, if the maternal-filial bond is not cemented within that time, it can be established only with difficulty at a later time (Hersher *et al.*, 1963)

The term "sensitive period" has been preferred by Poindron and Le Neindre (1980) to that of a "critical" period. They found in ewes that there was a period of high sensitivity to a neonate (any neonate) in the period immediately after birth, although selective responsiveness to the ewe's own lamb took several hours to develop.

The regulation of maternal behaviour in rats has been found to undergo a shift of control in the period after birth. The onset of maternal behaviour in the rat is determined by hormonal secretions, and the postpartum maintenance of this behaviour depends chiefly on stimulation from the young.

> The importance of the female rat's first contact with the newborn pups after parturition can now be understood in the context of her cycle of maternal behaviour: she depends on this contact for establishing a relationship which enables her to make the transition from prepartum hormonal to post-partum non-hormonal regulation of her maternal behaviour. (Rosenblatt, 1975)

Klaus and Kennell (1978) have proposed that separation between mother and infant in the first three days after birth has a profound effect on the mother because she is denied contact with her baby during a period when she is particularly sensitive to the neonate. They have suggested that an increased amount of contact (for details see p.174) between the mother and her baby at any time during the first three postpartum days appears to result in improved mothering. Klaus and Kennell distinguish between the concept of an early "sensitive period" and imprinting. They argue that imprinting usually refers to reaction in the infant and cannot take place after a certain period. Nor do Klaus and Kennell feel that the early period should be called a "critical" period, as there is no doubt that mothers can form attachments to their infants after the first three days. They argue that the increased contact between mother and infant somehow sets in motion a sequence of innate behaviours, which they describe as a "maternal sensitive period". Klaus and Kennell hypothesized that during this time a . . .

> . . . cascade of reciprocal interactions begins between mother and baby . . . locks them together and mediates the further development of attachment . . . this period is the optimal, but not the only one during which an attachment can develop.

Freedman (1974) and Macfarlane (1974), while still basing their arguments on an evolutionary point of view, suggested that there may be an advantage in a more gradual development of maternal attachment. Should the baby die in the immediate perinatal period, then the mother is not so attached that she cannot continue to function in a way that will maximize her reproductive potential, and should the mother die, the baby can develop a relationship with another caretaker.

Although these seemingly opposing explanations are based on evolutionary evidence for the development of maternal attachment, it is clear that they place quite different importance on the first few days. Whether or not Klaus and Kennell postulate a sensitive or a critical period, they still give a crucial role to early events. Experiences in the early postnatal period are seen as having a formative influence on mother–infant relationships, whereas Macfarlane and Freedman discount the crucial nature of the few days after parturition.

A "critical period" model has been considered by many researchers as being too simple (e.g. Sameroff, 1975; Schaffer, 1977). Both mother and child mature and develop different needs. It is difficult to predict the child's later development from earlier events, as the child, caretaker and environment are constantly changidng. A "transactional" model has been proposed to account for the complexity of development (Sameroff, 1975). The model implies that there is mutual modification between the parent and child at all stages of growth. The fact that a child is separated from his mother early in life will, therefore, not necessarily predict anything about the eventual outcome. Many other factors, such as socio-economic status, will also contribute to the child's development (Sameroff and Chandler, 1975).

Review of the Studies which have Investigated Early Maternal Attachment and Behaviour

For the sake of clarity, we consider separately five factors which may affect early maternal attachment:

(a) The mother's background.

(b) Pregnancy and birth.

(c) The newborn infant.

(d) The mother's reported feelings towards her infant in the early postnatal days.

(e) Early contact between mother and infant and its possible long-term effects.

All the research included in the review is subject to the methodological difficulties mentioned earlier.

The Mother's Background

Many factors in the mother's background can influence how she will relate to her infant. The effects of cultural factors and social class have been clearly demonstrated (Kagan and Tulkin, 1971; Tulkin and Kagan, 1972; Hubert, 1974; Klaus *et al.*, 1975; Dunn, 1979). For example, the cultural backgrounds of newly delivered mothers seemed to affect how they greeted their babies (Klaus *et al.*, 1975). Guatemalan mothers appeared to be more subdued and were less likely to have face-to-face contact with their newborns than were Californian mothers. Social class factors have also been associated with a mother's choice of feeding method. More middle-class women than working-class mothers choose to breast-feed their babies (Hubert, 1974).

There are several factors in the mother's background that may affect how she relates to her infant in the early postnatal period. Here we shall consider the mother's own experiences of being parented; her personality and her previous experience with young infants. A fourth factor, her emotional state, will be considered elsewhere in this volume by Margison (Chapter 7) and Stein (Chapter 5).

The Mother's own Experiences of her Parents

Several studies have investigated the effects of a woman's childhood experiences on her own subsequent mothering behaviour. For instance, Frommer and O'Shea (1973) reported that mothers, who had experienced disrupted childhoods, such as separation from either parent before 11 years of age, were more likely to report disturbances in their 2–13 month old infants, and they experienced more problems in managing them. Similarly, women whose family of origin had been disrupted by parental separation, divorce or death before the age of 16 years, showed reduced levels of interaction with their 20-week-old infants when compared to mothers without a disrupted background (Hall *et al.*,

1980). Uddenberg (1974) has also suggested that difficulties in adapting to motherhood may be associated with a woman's current relationship with her own mother.

The Mother's Personality

Although psychoanalysts have placed great importance on the mother's personality and emotional health for determining mother–infant relationships in the early days, there has been little empirical work testing this. Breen (1975) gave pregnant women a projective test (Franck and Rosen, 1948) which purported to measure traits of masculinity/femininity. She found that those who scored within the "feminine" range on the test were more likely to encounter problems of adjustment with their infant in the postpartum period. Breen interpreted these results as indicating that successful adaptation to motherhood requires a certain amount of assertiveness and self-confidence and other traits culturally rated as "masculine" (see Seiden, 1976, 1978).

In contrast, Robson and Kumar (1980) found that women who scored "masculine" on the Franck test were significantly more likely to report initial feelings of detachment towards their newborn babies. It was suggested (Robson, 1981) that women who are more "masculine" (more active) are likely to need more time before accepting their offspring (i.e. need to work at developing a relationship) rather than passively accepting what is given.

These two studies appear to be contradictory in that high "masculinity" was found to be associated with both better maternal adjustment postnatally (Breen, 1975) and feelings of detachment from the neonate (Robson and Kumar, 1980). However, the findings in the later study do not necessarily contradict Breen's results, as Robson and Kumar found no association between initial maternal reactions to the neonate and subsequent maternal postnatal depression, breast-feeding problems and aggression towards the baby.

The Mother's Previous Experience with Young Infants

In general, multiparous women seem to be more efficient in managing their babies than primiparae and are less likely to be influenced by outside disturbances. Thoman *et al.* (1970) found that although primiparae were more attentive to their infants, they had more difficulty in quietening them. Thoman *et al.*, (1972) reported that infants of multiparae sucked more during breast-feeding and consumed more during bottle feeding, even though primiparae spent more time feeding their infants and tried to stimulate them more to suck. These latter findings were confirmed by Brown, *et al.*, (1975). Multiparae were also found to respond more quickly to their babies' crying and were subsequently more likely to feed them (Bernal, 1972).

Newton (1955) reported that multiparous women were more likely than primiparae to express joy and satisfaction about caring for their babies during their hospital stay. When mothers were separated from their prematurely born babies, a greater decrease in self-confidence was found in primiparae than in multiparous women (Seashore *et al.*, 1973).

However, a primiparous mother's previous experience in caring for young infants can override differences due to parity. Both multiparous and primiparous mothers experienced in caring for young infants, were significantly more likely to report feelings of affection for their newly delivered babies than were primiparae without such experience (Robson and Kumar, 1980).

Studies of the consequences of the mother's own childhood experiences have relied on retrospective accounts, which are coloured by current factors and emotional state. They have also tended to ignore the influence of the respondent's age and social class (Crook and Eliott, 1980). It is therefore not possible to make definitive comments about the impact of maternal childhood experiences on subsequent mother–infant relationships. Similarly, there are too few studies assessing the influence of maternal personality on the development of attachment to make any conclusions. The data relating to parity differences and previous experience in childcare do however seem convincing. Using a range of methods and investigating the influence of prior experience on maternal care-taking, satisfaction and self-confidence, researchers have consistently found that more experienced mothers have fewer problems.

Factors during Pregnancy and Birth

Several workers have claimed to find a relationship between stress during pregnancy and subsequent mothering and the neonate's state (e.g. Ferreira, 1960; Sontag, 1966; Cohen, 1966a, b). However, none of these studies have convincingly demonstrated an association. Copans (1974) pointed out that, in general, most studies have failed to control for postnatal variables that may have confounded the results. They have used postnatal interviews to retrospectively assess prenatal anxiety. Variables such as parity, length of labour and obstetric medications, which may covary with anxiety, have rarely been controlled. Finally, the evaluation of the newborn's behaviour was often done by the same person who interviewed the mother.

Clinical reports (e.g. Bibring *et al.*, 1961) have suggested that the timing and the manner in which a mother is prepared to accept her foetus as a "separate" person during pregnancy may have a bearing upon the ways in which she will relate with her baby after its birth. During the course of a prospective study, it was found that women who perceived their foetus as a person by the third trimester, were more likely to feel immediate affection for their newborn babies (Robson and Kumar, 1980 see also Leifer, 1980). The increasing use of routine ultrasound scans during pregnancy may increase the woman's perceptions of her unborn baby as a "separate" person (Reading, 1980).

A wide range of obstetric procedures have been associated with infant and maternal condition at birth, which, in turn, may influence mother–infant interactions. Richards (1975b, 1978), for example, has suggested that although no randomized trial of induction and acceleration of labour has been carried out in Britain, these procedures may be associated with a raised incidence of Caesarian sections (Bonnar, 1975), forceps deliveries (Tipton and Lewis, 1975), higher incidence of preterm babies (Blacow *et al.*, 1975) and resulting separations of mother and infants (Richards, 1974). Dunn (1976) warned that because increased inductions of labour might lead to a higher maternal drug intake, more forceps deliveries and to a greater incidence of maternal separation from the child, this, in turn, could lead to adverse effects on the mother–child relationships (see also Bardon, 1973; Richards, 1974; Kitzinger, 1975; Robinson, 1976; Dunn, 1976 and Oakley, 1977).

More painful and difficult childbirth experiences have been linked with early maternal detachment, as has amniotomy and the amount of maternal analgesic used during delivery (Newton and Newton, 1962; Robson and Kumar, 1980). Caesarian sections have also been considered to adversely affect the initial mother–infant relationship (Tryphonopoulou and Doxiades, 1972).

Maternal drug intake can influence the neonate's state at birth. For instance, pain-relieving drugs administered to the mother during labour seemed to make the baby more difficult to console and increased its irritability (Aleksandrowicz, 1973); they reduced the infant's alertness (Borgstadt and Rosen, 1968); increased the likelihood of the newborn's eyes being closed (Brown *et al.*, 1975) changed sucking patterns and decreased sucking efficiency in the neonate (Brazelton, 1961; Kron *et al.*, 1966; Richards, 1974). However, in a recent study where maternal and infant drug intake was carefully monitored, no differences were found in the infant's behaviour at birth, but in the ensuing weeks those babies who had absorbed high pethidine doses were more likely to be irritable, more variable in mood, more difficult to console when upset and less likely to smile and less attentive to other people (Rosenblatt *et al.*, 1979).

It has been argued that the place of birth influences the mother's earliest interactions with her baby. Mothers delivered at home were said to be in a state of ecstasy immediately after birth and showed intense interest in the infant, especially in the first 15–20 minutes. Hospital-delivered women were more subdued in their initial greetings to the baby (Klaus *et al.*, 1975). Although it seems likely that women would be more subdued in a strange hospital environment, it is also probable that women who choose to have their babies at home differ from other women quite markedly. In the UK and USA they have invariably had to make a considerable effort to have a home delivery and their doctors must have considered them in the lowest risk group for birth complications.

Several factors therefore seem to be both directly and indirectly implicated in influencing the mother's earliest interactions with her infant. For example, the mother's perception of her foetus as a separate person is a possible indicator and perhaps precursor of subsequent attachment. Also, some obstetric procedures can affect the state of the mother and baby at birth and may therefore, colour the nature of the earliest interactions. There is a possibility, however, that women with certain personality characteristics may be predisposed to receive particular obstetric care. The early mother–infant relationship could be associated more with the differing maternal personality rather than the obstetric procedures themselves. For instance, the differing coping strategies women use throughout pregnancy, labour and delivery could well influence their experiences during childbirth and the early postnatal period (Cohen and Lazarus, 1973; Vaillant, 1977).

The Infant at Birth

Human infants look helpless and their large foreheads, full cheeks and large, dark eyes are usually very attractive to adults (Brooks and Hockberg, 1960; Fullard and Relling *et al.*, 1976; Sternglanz 1977). Lorenz (1944) suggested that these physical features could serve as innate releasers for infant caretaking behaviour. Any child who does not conform to the stereotyped image of "babyness" may cause initial pain and distress to the parents (Stern, 1977). For example, mothers often show an emotional reaction to a premature baby which is similar to the reaction evoked by a deformed newborn (Bentovim, 1972; Stratton, 1977).

The sex of the child may affect the way the mother initially responds to the baby. Mothers vocalized more to their male infants and spent more time stimulating them (Brown *et al.*, 1975; De Chateau and Wiberg, 1977a). The newborn's sex is the characteristic most commented upon in the immediate postnatal period (personal communication, Woollet and White, 1981). There are also sex differences in neonatal behaviour (e.g. Moss, 1967; Berger, 1972). For example, males tend to sleep less and cry more (Korner, 1969).

The newborn infant's state varies after birth and shows marked individual variations which appear to be closely related to the amount of maternal medication received during labour and delivery (Alexandrowicz, 1973; see p.168 for details). If only small doses of medication have been given then the infant is usually alert in the hour or so after birth. In 20 infants observed without intervention for 10 hours, the average length of this period of wakefulness was 2.2 hours. There was, however, a significantly longer period of arousal and wakefulness in those infants whose mothers had received no drugs (Emde *et al.*, 1975).

Neonates are very competent at using perceptual skills for social interaction (Stone *et al.*, 1973; Hunt, 1979). Neonates can recognize the smell of their own mother's breast pads at five days of age (Macfarlane, 1975a). By three days of age, neonates will suck selectively on a non-nutritive nipple to produce their own mother's voice, rather than that of another woman (De Casper and Fifer, 1980). Condon and Sander (1974) found that there was a close synchrony between the motor patterns of 16 neonates and the speech of an adult speaker. Slightly older neonates (between 12 and 21 days old) were able to imitate both the facial and manual gestures of an adult model, implying that the neonate can in some way adapt his own behaviour to that of others (Meltzoff and Moore, 1977).

It is apparent that much of the newborn's behaviour helps to ensure the close proximity of the mother for caretaking, e.g. crying, fussing and other signs of agitation. Other infant behaviours help to ensure social exchanges, e.g. eye contact, imitation and visual following (Thoman *et al.*, 1972). The importance of eye contact has been emphasized by Robson (1967). Congenitally blind infants were described by Fraiberg (1974) and Als *et al.* (1980), who both noted that the absence of eye contact was found to be a major problem which disrupted the mother's responsiveness towards the baby from birth onwards.

The mother's reported feelings towards her infant in the early postnatal days

Several investigators (e.g. Robson and Moss, 1970; Broussard and Hartner, 1971; Robson and Kumar, 1980) have asked mothers about their early feelings towards their neonates. They have tried to find associations between the mother's initial reactions and such variables as maternal personality, pregnancy, labour and delivery experiences and infant characteristics.

Newton and Newton (1962) obtained data from medical students' observations of 552 mothers' initial reactions to their newborn babies. It was not clear, however, which maternal criteria were being evaluated in their assessment. The analysis of the results is also questionable, as 60 of the mothers' reactions were considered unclassifiable; and these, along with 263 of the remaining mothers, who "smiled a little" were also excluded. The analysis of data only involved 229 subjects (41%). Newton and Newton compared the 157 women who seemed "greatly pleased" with the 65 who seemed indifferent and the 7 who seemed disgusted with their babies. They reported that women who seemed indifferent or disgusted were more likely to express negative attitudes towards breast-feeding and tended to have had more difficult childbirth experiences and were less cooperative with their attendants.

Three months after giving birth, 54 primiparous women were asked about their first feeling for their babies (Robson and Moss, 1970). Thirty four percent of the mothers said that the first contact elicited no feeling at all. Seven percent experienced dislike and the remaining 59% described affection (seven expressing intense love). Of the 41% of mothers with initial neutral or negative feelings for their babies, nine ("late attachers") expressed no love for their babies by nine weeks postnatally. The majority of these nine women had not wanted their babies. In contrast, the seven women who had initially described intense love for their babies ("early attachers") had had strong desires to be pregnant. When the mothers were asked the time at which they had first felt positive feelings and love for their infants, the third week of the infant's life was most frequently mentioned. By the end of the third month, most mothers said they felt strongly attached to their babies.

The authors concluded that the release of human maternal feelings was closely related to the infant's capacity to exhibit behaviours which typified adult forms of social communication. In particular, the mothers took great pleasure in the infant "seeing" them, and felt that eye contact, smiling and visual fixation elicited positive feelings in them (Robson, 1967; Robson and Moss, 1970). However, the evidence presented relating to the women who were "atypically" attached (i.e. either "late" or "early" attachers) do not support these interpretations. Most of the factors described as leading to "atypical" attachment pertain to characteristics of the mother herself, such as desire to have a baby and not to any inadequacies in the infant's social communications.

Robson and Kumar (1980) asked 104 women, on the seventh postpartum day, about their feelings for their babies when they first held them. Forty percent were rated as having felt mainly indifferent about their newborn babies. The numbers of women expressing indifference diminished rapidly over the first week. Of the 43 women who had reported detachment from their babies after birth, 31 spontaneously mentioned the time when they first experienced some liking for their babies. Four women said they had first felt affection towards the end of the first postpartum day and 20 mentioned experiencing a spontaneous feeling of affection during the second and third postpartum days. The remaining seven women said it took four days or longer before they felt any affection whatsoever.

Robson and Kumar tested factors such as individual differences between the mothers (e.g. occupational status and childhood separation from parents); prospective data collected during their pregnancies (e.g. antenatal depression, perception of the foetus as a person) during labour and delivery (e.g. obstetric medication and delivery complications) and on the characteristics of the baby (e.g. Apgar score, weight) to see whether any were associated with initial indifference for neonates.

They found that eight variables were significantly associated with initial indifference: separation from own father before the age of 11 years; a masculine score on a projective test (Franck and Rosen, 1948); no prior experiences of looking after babies; higher negative self-reports about being pregnant; not perceiving the foetus as a person at 36 weeks antenatally and, finally, having had an amniotomy and receiving more than 175 mg of pethidine and/or recalling that pain in labour was severe and worse than expected.

Log linear and discriminant function analyses showed that three variables (amniotomy, painful labour and pethidine dosage) were intercorrelated and were most predictive of the mother's initial feelings for her baby:

If a woman did not have an amniotomy, nor reported excessive pain, nor received more than 125 mgs. of pethidine, she had a *90%* chance of expressing *predominantly positive* or mixed feelings about her baby. If, however, she had:

(a) had an amniotomy *and*

(b) reported that pain in labour was severe and worse than expected *or*

(c) had had more than 125 mgs. of pethidine

then she had a *74%* chance of expressing *indifference* for her neonate. (Robson and Kumar, 1980)

Robson and Kumar suggested that the association of amniotomy with pain and pethidine dosage may imply some sort of physiological or hormonal basis. It was very tentatively proposed that there may be an hormonal "readiness" to mother in humans and that artificially rupturing the membranes somehow interferes with complex mechanisms. There may be different processes regulating the onset and maintenance of human maternal behaviour (Robson, 1981), as has been demonstrated in rats (Rosenblatt, 1975) and also sheep (Poindron and Le Neindre, 1980). In both these species, hormones appear to play a crucial role in the initiation of maternal responses, but infant characteristics and behaviour appear to maintain maternal responsiveness. It may also be useful in humans to differentiate between the mother's immediate postpartum reaction to the baby and subsequent maternal attachment (Robson, 1981).

Carek and Capelli (1981) reported a study of 49 primiparous women who were videotaped after delivery and rated on various indices including the mother's emotional and physical state. Forty one percent of the women appeared to be preoccupied and anxious when first presented with their babies. Carek and Capelli found that being in pain was associated with concern over the child's physical state and negative comments about the child. An expression of happiness with the sex of the child was significantly correlated with the appearance of being generally happy and joyful, with having a name for the child and general expressions of a sense of achievement.

In another study, Packer and Rosenblatt (1979) made direct observations of hospital deliveries. They pointed out that the circumstances were unfavourable for mother–infant interaction. For instance, the two periods when contact between the mother and baby was most likely were immediately after the cord was clamped, and after the infant was cleaned up. During the periods of contact the baby was often crying. Packer and Rosenblatt assessed the mother's behaviour in terms of the amount of holding and the quality of contact with the baby. The criteria for these assessments were not described. Even though the delivery room conditions appeared to be so unfavourable, Packer and Rosenblatt assessed 62% of mother–infant reaction as "good"; 31% as "indifferent" and 7% as "negative".

The difficulties of making predictions from the mother's immediate behaviour and reported feelings towards her neonate

Dunn and Richards (1977) have cautioned against making predictions from the first few days:

The rapid increase in co-ordination and adaptation shown in the interaction measures over the first 10 days suggests it would be mistaken to make wide generalisation about the relationships between mother and baby on the basis of information gathered on a single day early in the postnatal period.

It is difficult, however, to make generalizations from Dunn and Richard's subjects, who were medically "normal" and "socially secure", but Broussard and Hartner's research (1971) would again seem to confirm the difficulties of making predictions from the first postnatal days. They found that primiparae's negative perception of their infants (as measured on the Neonatal Perception Inventory) on the first or second postpartum day did not associate with any reported problems (such as crying, sleeping, feeding) in their month-old babies. This suggested to Broussard and Hartner that the earlier perceptions of the babies were based on fantasy, perhaps reflecting the women's own feelings of worth or their identification with other people in their lives. The socio-economic status of their subjects was not, however, mentioned, in the paper, so it is impossible to assess how far their results can be generalized. The mothers' perceptions of their month-old babies did associate with behavioural problems when the child reached 4½ years of age. Broussard and Hartner concluded that the processes for successful mother–child interaction had been established by one month after delivery. However, the usefulness of the Neonatal Perception Inventory as a predictive tool has recently been questioned (Palisin, 1980). In a replication study (n = 50), no association was found between the mothers' perceptions of their infants at one month and the subsequent development of behavioural problems at 4½ years.

Kempe and Kempe (1978) tried to develop screening tests for women who might encounter problems in looking after their children. They interviewed mothers during pregnancy about their feelings towards pregnancy and towards the unborn child. They later observed the mothers' reactions in the labour and delivery rooms and recorded how they greeted the baby and finally they used global ratings to observe the families during the first six weeks postpartum and from these assessed the mother–child relationship. Kempe and Kempe (1978) found that the most useful information for the prediction of unsuccessful parenting was that from the labour wards and delivery rooms. They noted whether either parent did not touch, hold or examine the baby, or did not talk in an affectionate tone, or spoke disparagingly or seemed disappointed over the baby's gender. They suggested that such observation should become a routine part of all obstetrical and postnatal care because the information gathered could significantly improve a child's chance of "escaping physical injury ..." (see p.182 for further discussion of this research).

For most women, initial detachment from their newborn infants dissipated within a few days (Robson and Moss, 1970; Robson and Kumar, 1980). At three months postnatally there was a significant association between initial detachment and negative scores on an "attitude to baby scale", but no associations between any other factors such as breast-feeding problems and later aggressive feelings towards the baby (Robson and Kumar, 1980). Again, the majority of women in both of these studies came mainly from the higher social classes and Robson and Kumar wrote that: "Similar investigations in relatively disadvantaged mothers may therefore reveal more accurately whether or not early reactions of maternal indifference are of any lasting significance."

All the foregoing studies have obvious methodological flaws. No study has used more than one technique for assessing maternal feelings: retrospective interviews (Robson and Moss, 1970; Robson and Kumar, 1980); rating scales (Broussard and Hartner, 1970); videotaped observations (Carek and Capelli, 1979) and direct observations (Packer and Rosenblatt, 1979). The majority of subjects have also belonged to the higher social classes, thus reducing the extent to which the findings can be generalized.

However, given the obvious limitations, it is significant that in four of these studies, using different methods in differing settings and samples, approximately 40% of primiparous women appear to be initially detached or have negative feelings for their babies in the immediate postnatal period.

Early contact between mother and infant and its possible long-term effects

Several researchers have tried to evaluate the influence of early mother–infant contact on later mothering behaviour. One group (e.g. Klaus and Kennell) manipulated the amounts of contact which mothers had with their newborn infants, either in the period immediately after delivery, or during the hospital stay. Most of these studies randomly allocated the mothers to early contact conditions, and used "blind" raters to assess maternal behaviour. A second group (e.g. Leifer *et al.*, 1972) has used the opportunity provided by infants being admitted to special care units, and therefore separated from their mothers, in order to evaluate the effects of separation between mother and infant after birth.

Early Contact Studies

Klaus *et al.* (1972) randomly allocated 28 young, black, low socio-economic status women to either an early contact condition or to a control condition of routine hospital care. The experimental group had contact with their naked infants for one hour immediately after delivery, and had five hours a day extra contact on each of the three days after delivery. The control mothers had a glimpse of their infants at birth and then saw them every four hours for 20–25 minutes feeding while they were hospitalized. It is not clear from the papers exactly what "contact" entails. The babies were given to the mothers, but whether they held the babies continually for the "extra contact" hours is not stated. Initially, there were no apparent differences between the groups, except in the treatments they received. One month later, the early contact mothers were found to be more reluctant to leave their babies with another person. When the mothers were observed, the early contact mothers fondled their infants more and engaged in more eye contact with them (Klaus and Kennell, 1972).

One year after the birth, while the babies were being examined, the early contact mothers were observed to spend more time near the babies assisting the physician examining them, and soothing the infants when they cried (Kennell *et al.*, 1974). At two years of age, five mothers and infants in each group were randomly selected for follow-up (Ringler *et al.*, 1975). Early contact mothers used significantly more questions, adjectives, words per proposition, fewer commands and content words than did control mothers. When the children were five years old, 9 extra contact and 10 control children were evaluated for their speech and language comprehension. No significant differences were found between the mean scores of the two groups of children on any of the tests. However, an association was found between the children's speech at 2 years of age, and language comprehension at 5 years, but only in the children whose mothers experienced extra contact (Ringler *et al.*, 1978).

Klaus and Kennell claimed that this series of studies demonstrated that 16 hours of extra contact within the first three days of life could affect maternal behaviour for one year and possibly longer, and, they argued, offered support for the existence of a maternal sensitive period after birth. However, their study, the first of its kind, has met with criticism and scepticism (e.g. Richards, 1975a; Haith and Campos, 1977). The extent to which the findings of these studies can be generalized has been questioned because of the small size and possible bias of the lower-class sample (Carlsson *et al.*, 1979). It has been suggested that the women must have known that they were being treated differently, and that preferential treatment may have influenced the outcome rather than extra contact (Bronfenbrenner, 1979). The strengths of the Klaus and Kennell studies are several, however: there was random allocation of subjects to conditions; the raters of the observational and interview data were ignorant of the subjects' experimental status; and a relatively long-term follow-up of the children has been undertaken.

In an attempt to clarify the timing of the "sensitive period", 60 primiparous women were studied in Guatemala (Hales *et al.*, 1977). The mothers were randomly assigned to three groups, which were comparable for maternal age and for the sex of the infant. The mothers in the early contact group were given their babies while on the delivery table and were taken, with the infant, to a private room where they lay in skin-contact with the naked infant for 45 minutes. The delayed contact mothers received an identical type of skin contact with their infants, but it was delayed for 12 hours after delivery. The control mothers had a glance at the baby at birth, then contact at approximately 12 hours when the wrapped babies were given to the mothers. All babies in the study from then on remained with their mothers during the day, and all were breast-fed during the two-day hospital stay.

Observations were made at 36 hours by a "blind" rater. Maternal and infant behaviours were recorded, such as the baby crying and sleeping and whether the mother was holding, looking at, talking to, fondling, kissing the baby, etc. or preoccupied by other people present in the room. The time of first physical contact did appear to affect maternal behaviour: the early contact mothers showed more affectionate behaviour particularly *"en face"* regard, than did the controls, with the delayed contact mothers showing an intermediate amount. The time of contact did not affect either maternal proximity to the infant, or caretaking behaviours. Hales *et al.* (1977) argued that these differences in affectionate behaviour underline the importance of physical contact between the mother and her infant during the first twelve hours after birth at least.

Although Klaus and Kennell hypothesized "that during this early sensitive period a series of reciprocal interactions begins between the mother and infant which bind them together and insures the further development of attachment", there is little evidence of any "series of reciprocal interactions" other than *"en face"* interactions, in the Klaus and Kennell series of studies or in Hales *et al.* (1977).

De Chateau and Wiberg (1977a, b) have attempted to assess the importance of skin-to-skin contact between the mother and baby during the first hour after delivery. In a middle-class Swedish sample (n = 62), randomly assigned primiparae were given 15 minutes of extra skin-to-skin contact with their infants immediately after birth, and 20 primiparae and 20 multiparae were given routine care which involved only brief contact with the baby at birth. At 36 hours postpartum, the extra contact primiparae held their infants more often, held them in an "encompassing" manner and looked at them *"en face"* more than did the mothers who had not had such contact, whether primiparae or multiparae. The usual differences between primiparous and multiparous breast-feeding behaviour seemed to be eliminated by the extra skin contact, and suckling contact after birth.

The primiparous mothers and their infants were followed up at both three months and at one year after the infant's birth. The extra contact mothers spent more time looking *"en face"* and kissing, and their infants laughed and smiled more frequently. The mothers in the control group spent more time cleaning their infants, who cried significantly more often. The effects of extra contact during the first hour of the infant's life were more pronounced for boys and for their mothers. Mothers and their sons in the extra contact group smiled at each other more often than did mothers and sons in the control group. No such differences were found for girls. Interview data revealed that extra contact mothers said they had adapted to their babies more easily, whereas control mothers were more likely to say that they found adaptation to their infants "as expected".

When the infants and mothers were seen one year after the birth, a similar pattern of behaviour and interactions was observed. The extra contact mothers held their infants in closer body contact and for a longer part of the observation period than did control mothers. Touching and caressing, not related to caretaking, were more frequent amongst extra contact mothers. A greater warmth in what the extra contact mothers said to their infants was noted.

There was a marked difference in the duration of breast-feeding in the groups: extra contact mothers breast-fed for 175 days (mean duration), whilst the control mothers fed for 108 days (mean duration), but there was a wide range in each group (extra-contact: 21–365 days; control: 10–240 days).

De Chateau concludes that:

> In our view, the relatively short period of "extra contact" during the first hour following delivery is hardly sufficient by itself to explain the differences in maternal and infant behaviour later on. Mothers and infants might have an opportunity during this early contact to exchange signals that may be important to the establishment of mother-infant synchrony. Consequently, the development of the mother-infant relationship may proceed more smoothly.

In another Scandinavian study, 62 primiparous women were given either limited contact with their infants after birth (i.e. five minutes holding and then the baby placed in a crib at the side of the bed); or extended contact in which the mother kept the naked baby in the bed for one hour immediately after delivery (Carlsson *et al.*, 1978). The baby was placed in a nursing position at the mother's breast. Two feeding sessions at two and at four days were observed. There were no differences between the groups in length of time spent feeding or in the amount of infant sucking. However, mothers who had extended contact showed more contact behaviours (e.g. rubbing and petting the infant) and fewer non-contact behaviours (e.g. the mother talking to someone other than the infant) than did the mothers who had limited contact at birth.

Carlsson *et al.* (1978) noted how the findings from this Swedish study appeared to confirm Klaus and Kennell's finding that events taking place after birth influence subsequent maternal behaviour. However, in their follow-up study six weeks after delivery, there were no apparent differences between the two groups of women (Carlsson *et al.*, 1979).

In a recent study involving 30 mother–infant pairs Svejda *et al.* (1980) ensured that the participating mothers were not aware of their inclusion in a study investigating the effects of early contact. Only one subject mother at a time was present in the hospital unit, and all other mothers sharing a room with the study mother were treated in the same way. Mothers were randomly assigned to either 10 hours of extra contact over the first 36 hours postpartum (including 15 minutes skin contact at birth), or to routine care.

Mothers were videotaped at 36 hours with their infants for 10 minutes free play and then for 15 minutes breastfeeding. Blind raters then scored the videotapes. No significant differences were found for any of the behaviours scored. Only when the data were analysed by sex, within contact groups, were significant differences found: early contact mothers talked more to females than to males; routine care mothers touched females more and spent more time "*en face"* with their male infants. The failure to replicate the earlier findings relating to early maternal attachment and the effects of early contact between the mother and infant, indicates a need for still more research in this area to try and identify the factors which determine differences in maternal attachment.

A different approach has been used to study the effects of early maternal contact by O'Connor *et al.* (1980). In this study, 143 mothers were randomly assigned to rooming-in care for the duration of the hospital stay and 158 women were randomly assigned to routine care, in which the infant was kept, apart from feeding times, in the hospital nursery. The average amount of contact that mothers in each group experienced with their infants over the first 48 hours was 11.44 hours for the rooming-in group and 2.15 hours contact for the control group.

At an average age of 17 months (range 12–21 months), the children were investigated for their experience of "parenting inadequacies", which may be regarded as reflecting the extreme negative end of the attachment continuum. Parental inadequacies were said to have occurred if the child's growth was adversely affected; if more than one admission to hospital had been required to remedy the inadequacy; if investigation by the Protective Services organization confirmed child maltreatment; if abnormal development resulted; if the parents surrendered caretaking of the child; or if the child was physically abused by the parent.

In the rooming-in group, two children were found to have experienced parenting inadequacies, but in the control group, 10 children had had one or more of these experiences. Although the number of affected children was small (12 in total), and there was a wide range in the number of parenting inadequacies that each child experienced (range one to six), the difference between the groups suggests that rooming-in improved the mother–infant relationship, and in some way enhanced parenting. This study used a double blind methodology, randomly assigned mothers to contact conditions and used outcome measures which were related to the concept of attachment.

Greenberg (1973) has shown that mothers who have roomed-in with their infants for the duration of the hospital stay rated themselves as being more confident and competent in caring for their infants when compared to mothers who had not roomed-in.

Separation Studies

Other workers have investigated mothers of infants who were separated after birth by the infant's admission to special care units. In one of these studies, Whiten (1977) describes 20 such mothers and infants. Although short-term difficulties were experienced by many mothers, Whiten attempted to identify "development effects", i.e. the long-term effects of early separation in the mother–child relationship. Ten infants, separated from their mothers for 2–14 days after birth due to admission to special care units for minor medical reasons (e.g. mild jaundice), formed the experimental group. A matched control groups was used, of mothers and infants not separated from their infants. In a limited analysis of several videotaped observations over the first few months (limited in both the data chosen for analysis and the behavioural categories used to analyse the data), Whiten found that at one month the only differences between the separated and "normal contact" groups were found in the "purely social group of behaviours". Normal contact mothers smiled and vocalized more with their infants. Mutual looking was seven times more frequent in the normal contact group. Whiten suggests that this is probably one of the first reciprocal communications in which the infant engages. Normal contact infants cried half as much as separated infants and contact mothers responded to a significantly higher proportion of cries.

Despite the findings of some early behavioural differences between the two groups, Whiten concludes that it is unlikely that any of the observed differences have important long-term consequences for the mother–child relationship. By four months there were no apparent differences between the two groups.

In another study involving separated mothers and premature infants, no long-term differences were reported between a "contact" group and a separated group (n = 42) (Leifer *et al.*, 1972; Leiderman and Seashore, 1975). However, the distinction between the amounts of contact that the two groups experienced was not great. For instance, the "contact" mothers could only handle their babies through the portholes of the incubator, and saw their babies on average every six days. Although there were no measurable maternal–infant differences, two of the separated mothers relinquished custody of their infants, and there were five marital breakdowns, compared to only one in the non-separated group, in the year after the infant's birth. The mothers of premature infants appeared less "committed" and had less confidence, when compared to the mothers of normal, full-term infants, but these differences disappeared one month after discharge.

Leiderman (1979) argues that if there is a sensitive phase after birth, it must last at least until three months, which was the maximum length of time his separated infants were in the unit, without any apparent long-term harmful effects. Even after a two to three month separation, the mothers in the separated groups did establish social bonds with their infants and these bonds or attachments could not be differentiated from those formed by mothers in the "contact" group. It was noted that the socio-economic standard of the family, the play behaviour of the infant and the gender of the infant became more important factors in differentiating maternal and infant behaviours, than did the initial experience of separation (Leiderman, 1979). These comments confirm Sameroff's findings (1975), that socio-economic status appears to have a much stronger influence on the course of development than any aspects of perinatal history. Environmental disadvantage will tend to exacerbate any adverse perinatal conditions, whereas more advantaged rearing will diminish the impact of such initial experiences.

Several of these studies do seem to show measurable differences in maternal behaviour in the first few postnatal days (e.g. increased *"en face"* eye contact, closer proximity and more successful breastfeeding) in mothers who had extra contact with their newborn infants. Although many of these differences constitute only a small part of maternal behaviour, they have been demonstrated in a range of social classes, in different countries and within different hospital settings, and this suggests that there may be some short-term benefits accruing to the mother from early contact with the infant.

However, the complexity of the experience being investigated is enormous and it is certainly not clear whether it is simply "contact" *per se* which is being manipulated or the many other confounding variables. For instance, the timing and length of early contact has varied markedly, from 15 minutes within the first postnatal hour (De Chateau *et al.*, 1977a) to the rooming-in study where mothers had at least five hours contact each day (O'Connor *et al.*, 1980). The quality of contact has also varied between studies. In some baby and mother are both naked (e.g. De Chateau *et al.*, 1977a) and in others, one or both are clothed.

It is rarely made clear whether or not other people are present while the mother and infant have extra contact. When the father is present, for example, the mother may have a reduced opportunity for holding the infant (personal communication, White and Woollet, 1981). Mothers may also be influenced by hospital routines and may assume that there is a "right" way to behave with their babies. If they are allowed to see their babies only at intervals they may think that this is the expected pattern which they should continue when they go home (Richards, 1975a). Another factor that may have been confounded with "early contact" is the mother's self-confidence (Richards, 1975a). The more contact and responsibility mothers have with their neonates the sooner they will become confident of their ability to look after them. This factor could explain the absence of any parity differences beyond the first 36 hours in the De Chateau and Wiberg study (1977a).

It is, of course, extremely hazardous to think in terms of a simple one-to-one causal relationship:

> ... interpretation of the effect of a particular variable should not be made in isolation. Separation may be damaging in the case of the premature infant, but this may be the effect of separation on an emotionally disturbed mother who is presented with an unattractive baby in surroundings of intense medical activity. (Stratton, 1977)

As can be seen, therefore, the apparent short-term effects of early contact may not be solely attributable to extra contact. The long-term effects are even more equivocal. Although Ringler *et al.* (1975) reported differences in the children of extra-contact and routine contact mothers at five years, it should be emphasized that even by one year after the birth, there were many more outcome measures which were not significant than were significant. It should also be noted that with the number of variables assessed in the studies, the probability of getting at least one significant result at the 0.05 level by chance alone are extremely high.

Discussion of the Concept of a Sensitive Period

Discussion

Human mothers in a hospital environment (Klaus *et al.*, 1970) seemed to function in a highly stereotyped manner when first making contact with their offspring. The women behaved in an orderly and predictable fashion; first touching the infant's extremities with their fingertips and then caressing the trunk with their palms. Klaus *et al.* (1970) suggested that the regularity of their behaviour might be a behaviour pattern specific to human mothers which could facilitate "bonding" between the mother and her neonate.

After observing women from various cultures and in differing environments, Klaus *et al.* (1975) found that interaction with the newborn did not always follow the same pattern. For instance, women delivering in their own homes picked up their babies immediately; stroked the babies' faces with their fingertips and started breast-feeding within minutes. Klaus *et al.* (1975) suggested that the more familiar settings of home deliveries probably elicited the most natural behaviour, but it should be remembered that Western women who have their babies at home probably differ significantly from women who deliver in hospitals (see earlier comments, p.168).

Macfarlane (1975b), in a preliminary analysis (of 14 videotapes) of the initial contact between mothers and their babies, suggested that his data did in part confirm that mothers ". . . tend to go through an orderly and predictable pattern of behaviour" (Klaus *et al.*, 1975). Macfarlane wrote, however, that in many cases, the behaviour recorded was only a very small part of the total behaviour patterns. The mothers verbalized, imitated their babies and put their own interpretation on the child's behaviour. Maternal behaviour also seemed to be influenced by the type of delivery; amount of medication used; whether the father was present or not; how well the mother knew her medical attendants; and how much contact was encouraged by the staff (Packer and Rosenblatt, 1979; White and Woollett, personal communication, 1981).

The empirical research on the "sensitive period" is difficult to assess, because there are many other important influences which affect maternal behaviour and feelings towards neonates such as the mother's own childhood experiences, her parity, obstetric experiences and, perhaps most importantly, the neonate's role in eliciting and maintaining maternal–infant interaction. Although several researchers have interpreted their findings on early contact as facilitating the development of reciprocal interactions between mother and infant, the absence of any data on the baby's contribution to these interactions is striking. The absence of any information about the mother's physical state and her feelings towards her infant must also limit the extent to which observed behaviours in the "early contact" studies can be interpreted. After delivery many women say they are disinterested in their babies. They may also be exhausted, in pain, drugged and emotionally distressed. Similarly, Schaffer (1977a) has made the point that a temporary separation after delivery may not necessarily influence subsequent attachment.

So the notion that a mother's attachment may be seriously affected by a temporary separation immediately after her baby's birth remains without support.

And this is just as well, for what hope would there otherwise be for adoptive parents and their children? If mothering was completely dependent in some simple way on hormonal changes that occur only in conjunction with childbirth, adopting would need to be discontinued, since it would be producing a lot of affectionless and empty relationships.

Although in the "early contact" studies no evidence is presented relating to the rhythmic, cyclic quality of early mother–infant interaction (cf. Brazelton *et al.*, 1975; Brown *et al.*, 1975; Stern, 1977), it seems likely, however, that the earlier the mother becomes aware of her infant's communicative signals, the sooner and the more smoothly a synchronous interaction will develop. Obviously, different mother–infant dyads will develop different modes of communication and empathy.

It has already been show that there is no unitary index of maternal attachment. So-called maternal "attachment behaviours" such as "*en face*" regard, holding the baby, length of breast-feeding, do not necessarily mean that the mother is "attached".

The studies of mothers' feelings about their newborn infants (e.g. Robson and Moss, 1970) all point to a gradual increase in the strength of such feelings over the first few weeks postnatally. Temporal changes in maternal attachment have not been commented on in the "early contact" observational studies. Obviously, the two approaches need to be integrated if a fuller understanding of the development of maternal attachment is to be reached. It may be useful to differentiate between early maternal feelings and the development of "attachment" to see, as has been suggested (Robson, 1981), whether there are different mechanisms and processes regulating the onset and maintenance of human mothering.

From the present studies, however, it does appear that allowing mothers to have more contact with their neonates may have short-term influences. The long-term associations are not clear and attempts to assess infants likely to be "at risk" on the basis of mothers' and fathers' reactions in the labour ward must be regarded with caution (e.g. Kempe and Kempe, 1978).

Initial feelings of maternal indifference dissipated quickly for most women (Robson and Kumar, 1980). It was suggested that the preparation given to mothers in the antenatal classess may have helped them understand that their initial feelings would not last. Given the consensus from several studies that approximately 40% of primiparae experience indifference for their neonates, it would seem appropriate to forewarn women routinely about the possibilities of feeling detached from their infant after childbirth.

Similarly, information about the baby's communicative skills and perceptual abilities, if passed on to the mother, could alert her to the interactive potentials of the neonate. This feedback may well facilitate the development of synchronous interactions (Widmayer and Field, 1980).

It could be that the methods used for assessing maternal attachment are just not sensitive enough to pick up long-term sequelae. However, present knowledge about the impact of the first few postnatal days on mother–infant interaction is extremely ambiguous. It is, therefore, important that the studies do not acquire pessimistic connotations (i.e. a separation has occurred, therefore "trouble" can be expected). Such implications, if taken to extreme, could adversely affect the helping professions and, of course, the mothers themselves (Herbert *et al.*, in press).

However, even if no long-term effects of immediate postnatal experiences can be discerned, anything which can make the quality of life better for women at such an important time in their lives is surely worthwhile. Even a year after childbirth women remember those first moments after birth quite vividly (Robson and Kumar, 1980). If unnecessary aspects of current obstetric practice and hospital routines make this time less satisfying for the woman and her baby, then this in itself should be enough to bring about change. If what happens to a mother in labour and after delivery can affect her initial feelings for her baby and subsequent behaviour (even for a short time), then the medical indications for obstetric interventions and hospital routines need to be carefully re-evaluated.

Future Research

The are still no generally agreed criteria for assessing "good" or "bad" mothering and the methodological problems of studying mother–infant interactions are formidable. Individual research studies have tended to focus on a single aspect of maternal experience (e.g. the mother's feelings or observed behaviours). Most researchers have also concentrated on "positive behaviours" and emotions when evaluating "good" outcome and have ignored the possibility that love, an important component of maternal attachment, may involve both intense positive *and* negative emotions (Schaffer, 1977a).

Future research on maternal attachment should use a range of methods to get at different perspectives on maternal attachment. There may be a lack of agreement in the findings from observational and interview data, but at least if the two are combined within a particular study, then the possibility of integration exists and it may be possible to check reliability and validity. Different methods may give us access to different aspects of the same experience. It may also be of value to concentrate further on studies of special groups of women, whose situations suggest that adaptation to mothering may be more difficult, e.g. very young, single mothers; those with known psychiatric disturbances (see Chapter 7) and those whose babies need to be separated for medical reasons. One of us (EP) is currently undertaking such a project in a group of mothers with premature and very ill babies, using a wide range of measures of maternal attachment.

References

Ainsworth, M.S. (1969). Object relations, dependency and attachment: A theoretic review of the infant-mother relationship. *Child Development* 4, 4, 969-1025.

Ainsworth, MS. (1973). The development of infant-mother attachment *In Review of Child Developmental Research* (B.M. Caldwell and H.N. Riccuiti, eds). University of Chicago Press, Chicago.

Ainsworth, M.D., Blehar, M.C., Waters, M.C. and Wall, S. (1978). *Patterns of attachment: assessed in the strange situation and at home.* Lawrence Erlbaum, Hillside N.J.

Aleksandrowicz, M.K. (1973). Neonatal behavioral patterns and their relation to obstetrical medication. Unpublished doctoral dissertation, University of Kansas.

Als, H., Tronick, E. and Brazelton, T.B. (1980) Affective reciprocity and the development of autonomy. *J. of Amer. Acad. of Child Psychiat.* 20, No. 1.

Bakeman, R. and Brown, J.V. (1977). Behavioral dialogues: An approach to the assessment of mother-infant interaction. *Child Development* 48, 195-203.

Barash, O. (1980). *Sociobiology: The Whisperings Within.* Souvenir Press, London.

Bardon, D. (1973). Psychological implications for provision of childbirth. *The Lancet,* ii, 7828, 555-558.

Bentovim, A. (1972). Handicapped preschool children and their families. *Bristish Medical Journal* 3, 579-581, 634-637.

Berger, M. (1972). Early experience and other environmental factors: An overview. I. Studies with humans *In Handbook of Abnormal Psychology.* (ed. H.J. Eysenck) 2nd Ed., pp.604-624. Pitman, London.

Bernal, J. (1972). Crying during the first 10 days of life and maternal responses. *Dev. Med. Child. Neurol.* 14, 362.

Bibring, G.L., Dwyer, T.F., Huntington, D.S. and Valenstein, A.F. (1961). A study of psychological processes in pregnancy of the earliest mother-child relationship I. Some propositions and comments. *The Psychoanalytic Study of the Child* 16, 9-27.

Blacow, M., Smith, M.N., Graham, M. and Wilson, R.G. (1975). Induction of labour. *The Lancet* i, 217.

Blehar, M.C., Lieberman, A.F. and Ainsworth, M.D.S. (1977). Early face-to-face interaction and its relation to later mother-infant attachment. *Child Develop.* 48, 182-94.

Bonnar, J. (1975) Induction and acceleration of labour in modern obstetric practice. Paper presented at a Study Group on Problems in Obstetrics organised by the Medical Information Unit of the Spastics Society. Tunbridge Wells, April.

Borgstadt, A.D. and Rosen, M.C. (1968). Medication during labour correlated with behavior and EEG of the newborn. *American J. of the Disturbed Child* 115.

Bowlby, J. (1958). The nature of the child's tie to his mother. *International J. Psychoanalysis* 39, 350-373.

Bowlby, J.D. (1969). *Attachment and Loss Vol. 1. Attachment.* Basic Books, New York.

Brazelton, J.B. (1961). Psychophysiological reaction in the neonate II. The effects of maternal medication on the neonate and his behaviour. *Journal of Pediatrics* 58, 508-512.

Brazelton, T.B., Koslowski, B. and Main, M. (1975). The origins of reciprocity: The early mother-infant interaction *In The Effect of the Infant on its Caregiver* (eds M. Lewis and L.A. Rosenblum), pp.49-76. Wiley, New York.

Breen, D. (1975). *The Birth of a First Child.* Tavistock, London.

Bronfenbrenner, U. (1979). *The Ecology of Human Development.* Harvard University Press, Cambridge Mass.

Brooks, V. and Hockberg, J. (1960). A psychophysical study of "cuteness". *Perceptual and Motor Skills* II, 205

Broussard, E.R. and Hartner, M.S.S. (1971). Further considerations regarding maternal perception of the first born *In Exceptional infant 2. Studies in abnormality.* (ed. J. Hellmuth) pp. 432-449. Butterworths, London.

Brown, N.J.V., Bakeman, R., Snyder, P.A., Fredrickson, W.T., Morgan, S.T. and Helper, R. (1975). Interactions of black inner-city mothers with their newborn infants. *Child Development* **46**, 677-686.

Carek, D.J. and Capelli, J.A. (1981). Mothers reactions to their newborn infants. *J. Am. Acad. Child Psychiat.* **20**, No. 1.

Carlsson, S.G., Fagerberg, H., Horneman, G., Larsson, K., Rodholm, M., Schaller, J., Danielsson, S. and Gundewall, C. (1978). Effects of amount of contact between mother and child on the mother's nursing behaviour. *Devel. Psychobiol.* **11**, 2, 143-151.

Carlsson, S.G., Fagenberg, H., Horneman, G., Hwang, C.P., Larsson, K., Rodholm, M., Schaller, J., Danielsson, B. and Gundewall, C. (1979). Effects of various amounts of contact between mother and child on the mother's nursing behavior: A follow-up study. *Infant Behav. Develop.* **2**, 209-214.

Chappell, P. and Sander, L.W. (1979). Mutual Regulation of the neonatal-maternal interactive process: Context for the origins of communication. *In Before Speech: The Beginning of Interpersonal Communication* (ed. M. Bullowa). Cambridge University Press, Cambridge.

Chodorow, N. (1978). *The Reproduction of Mothering: psychoanalysis and the sociology of gender.* University of California Press, London.

Cohen, F. and Lazarus, R.S. (1973). Active coping processes, coping disposition and recovery from surgery. *Psychosom. Med.* **35**, 5.

Cohen, R.L. (1966a). Pregnancy stress and maternal perceptions of infant endowment. *J. Ment. Subnorm.* **12**, 18-23.

Cohen, R.L. (1966b). Some maladaptive syndromes of pregnancy and the puerperium. *Obstet. Gynae.* **27**, 562.

Collias, N.E. (1956). The analysis of socialization in sheep and goats. *Ecology* **37**, 228-239.

Condon, W.S. and Sander, L. (1974). Neonate movement is synchronized with adult speech: Interactional participation and language acquisition. *Science* **183**, 99-101.

Copans, S.A. (1974). Human prenatal effects: Methodological problems and some suggested solutions. *Merrill-Palmer Quarterly* **20**, 1, 43-52.

Crook, T. and Eliot, J. (1980). Parental death during childhood and adult depression: A critical review of the literature. *Psychol. Bull.* **87**, 252-258.

De Casper, A.J. and Fifer, W.P. (1980). Of human bonding: Newborns prefer their mothers' voices. *Science* **208**, 6th June.

De Chateau, P. (1977). The importance of the neonatal period for the development of synchrony in the mother-infant dyad — a review. *Birth and the Family Journal* **4:1**, 10-23.

De Chateau, P. and Wiberg, B. (1977a). Long-term effect on mother-infant behaviour of extra contact during the first hour postpartum. I. *Acta Paediat. Scand.* **66**, 137-143.

De Chateau, P. and Wiberg, B. (1977b). Long-term effect on mother-infant behaviour of extra contact during the first hour postpartum. II. A follow-up at 3 months. *Acta. Paediat. Scand.* **66**, 145-151.

Deutsch, H. (1944). *The Psychology of Women* (Vol. 1 and 2). Grune and Stratton, New York.

Dunn, J. (1979). Understanding human development: Limitations and possibilities in an ethological approach *In Human Ethology.* (ed. Von Cranach, Foppa, Lenenies and Ploog) pp.623-662. Cambridge University Press, Cambridge.

Dunn, J.F. and Richards, M.P.M. (1977). Observations on the developing relationship between mother and baby in the newborn *In Studies in Parent-Infant Interaction* (ed.

H.R. Schaffer). Academic Press, London and New York.

Dunn, P.M. (1976). Obstetric delivery today. For better or worse? *The Lancet*, **i**, 790-793.

Emde, R.N., Swedberg, J. and Suzuki, B. (1975). Human wakefulness and biological rhythms after birth. *Archives of General Psychiat.* **32**, 780-783.

Ferreira, A.J. (1960). The pregnant mothers emotional attitude and its reflection upon the newborn. *Amer. J. Orthopsych.* **30**, 553-561.

Fraiberg, S. (1974). Blind infants and their mothers *In The Effect of the Infant on its Caregiver* (eds M. Lewis and L. Rosenblum) pp.215-233. Wiley, New York.

Franck, K. and Rosen, E. (1948). Projective test of masculinity-feminity. *J. Consult, Psychol.* **13**, 247-256.

Freedman, D.G. (1974). *Human Infancy: An Evolutionary Perspective.* Lawrence Erlbaum Associates, N.J.

Freud, S. (1943). *A General Introduction to Psychoanalysis.* Garden City Publishing Co., New York (First German Edition, 1917).

Frommer, E.A. and O'Shea, G. (1973). Antenatal identification of women liable to have problems in managing their infants. *Brit. J. Psychiat.* **123**, 149-156.

Fullard, W. and Relling, A.M. (1976). An investigation of Lorenz's babyness. *Child Develop.* **47**, 1191-1193.

Greenberg, M. (1973). First mothers rooming-in with their newborns: Its impact on the mother. *Amer. J. Orthopsychiat.* **43**, 5. 783-788.

Haith, M.M. and Campos, J.J. (1977). Human infancy. *Ann. Rev. Psychol.*, **28**, 251-293.

Hales, D.J. Lozoff, B., Sosa, R. and Kennell, J.H. (1977). Defining the limits of the maternal sensitive period. *Dev. Med. Child Neurol.* **19**, 4, 454-561.

Hall, F., Pawlby, S.J. and Wolkind, S. (1980). Early life experiences and later mothering behaviour: A study of mothers and their 20 week old babies. *In The First Year of Life: Psychological and Medical Implications of Early Experience* (eds D. Schaffer and J. Dunn). John Wiley, Chichester.

Hamilton, W. (1964). The genetical evaluation of social behavior. II. *J. Theoret. Biol.* **7**, 17-52.

Harper, L.V. (1970). Ontogenetic and phylogenetic functions of the parent-offspring relationship in mammals. *Advances in the Study of Behavior* **3**, 75-117.

Herbert, M. Sluckin, W. and Sluckin, A. (in press). Mother-to-infant bonding. *J. Child Psychol. Psychiat.*

Hersher, L., Richmond, J.B. and Moore, A.U. (1963) Maternal behaviour in sheep and goats. *In Maternal Behavior in Mammals* (ed. H.L. Rheingold), pp.203-232. Wiley, Chichester.

Hinde, R.A. and Simpson, M.J.A. (1975). Qualities of mother-infant relationships in monkeys. *In CIBA Foundation Symposium 33*, pp.39-67. Assoc. Scientific Publishers, Oxford.

Hubert, J. (1974). Belief and reality: social factors in pregnancy and childbirth. In Richards M.P.M. (ed.) *The integration of a child into a Social World.* Cambridge University Press, Cambridge.

Hunt, J. McV (1979). Psychological development: Early experience. *Ann. Rev. Psychol.* **30**, 103-143.

Kagan, J. and Tulkin, S.R. (1971). Social class differences in child rearing during the first year *In The Origins of Human Social Relations* (ed. H.R. Schaffer). Academic Press, London and New York.

Kempe, R.S. and Kempe, C.H. (1978). *Child Abuse.* Fontana, London.

Kennell, J.H., Jerauld, R., Wolfe, H., Chesler, D., Kreger, N.C., McAlpine, W., Steffa, M. and Klaus, M.H. (1974). Maternal behaviour one year after early and extended postpartum contact. *J. Develop, Med. Child Neurol.* **16**, 172-179.

Kennell, J.H., Trause, M.A. and Klaus, M.H. (1975). Evidence for a sensitive period in the human mother In CIBA Foundation Symposium 33: *Parent-Infant Interaction*, pp.87-101. Assoc. Scientific Publishers, Oxford.

Kennell, J.H., Voos, D.K. and Klaus, M.H. (1979) Parent-infant bonding. *In Handbook of Infant Development* (ed J. Osofsky), Wiley, Chichester.

Kitzinger, S. (1975). *Some Mothers' Experiences of Induced Labour*. National Childbirth Trust, London.

Kitzinger, S. (1978). *Women as Mothers*. Fontana, London.

Klaus, M.H. and Jerauld, R. (1972). Maternal attachment—Importance of the first post-partum days. *New Eng. J. of Medicine* **286**, 460-463.

Klaus, M.H. and Kennell, J.H. (1980). An early maternal sensitive period? A theoretical analysis *In Intensive Care in the Newborn. II* (ed. D. Stern). Masson Pub., USA.

Klaus, M.H., Kennel, J.H., Plumps, N. and Zuehlke, S. (1970). Human maternal be-haviour at the first contact with her young. *Pediatrica* **46**, 187-192.

Klaus, M.H., Trouse, M.A. and Kennell, J.H. (1975). Does human maternal behaviour after delivery show a characteristic pattern? In CIBA Foundation Symposium 33: *Parent-Infant Interaction, pp.69-85. Assoc. Scientific Publishers, Oxford.*

Korner, A.F. (1969). Neonatal startles, smiles, erections and reflex sucks as related to state, sex and individuality. *Child Dev.* **40**, 1039-1053.

Kron, R., Stein, M. and Goddard, K.E. (1966). Newborn sucking behaviour affected by obstetric sedation. *Pediatrics* **37**, 1012-1016.

Leiderman, P.H. and Seashore, M.J. (1975). Mother-infant separation: Some delayed consequences *In* CIBA Foundation Symposium 33: *Parent-Infant Interaction*. Elsevier-Excerpta Medica, North Holland.

Leiderman, P.H. (1979). Human mother to infant social bonding: Is there a sensitive phase? Unpublished manuscript.

Leifer, G.D., Leiderman, P.H., Barnett, C.R. and Williams, J.A. (1972). Effects of mother-infant separation on maternal attachment behaviour. *Child Dev.* **43**, 1203-1218.

Leifer, M., (1980). *Psychological Effects of Motherhood*. Praeger, New York.

Levy, D.M. (1958). *Behaviour Analysis*. Thomas, Springfield.

Lockard, R.B. (1971). Reflections on the fall of comparative psychology. Is there a message for us all? *Amer. Psychol.* **26**, 168-179.

Lorenz, (1943). Die Angeborenen Formen Moglicher Erfahrumg. *Z. fur Tierpsych.* **5**.

Macfarlane, A. (1974). If a smile is so important . . . *New Scientist* **62**, 164-166.

Macfarlane, A. (1975a). Olfaction in the development of social preferences in the human neonate *In* CIBA Foundation Symposium 33: *Parent-Infant Interaction*, pp.103-117. Assoc. Scientific Publishers, Oxford.

Macfarlane, A. (1975b). The first hours and the smile *In Child Alive* (ed. R. Lewin). Temple Smith, London.

Macfarlane, A. (1977). *The Psychology of Childbirth*. Fontana, London.

Mead, M. (1935). *Sex and Temperament in Three Primitive Societies*. William Morrow, New York.

Mead, M. (1950). *Male and Female*. Victor Gollanz, London.

Mead, M. (1954). Some theoretical considerations on the problem of mother-child separa-tion. *Amer. J. Orthopsychiat.* **24**, 471-483.

Meltzoff, A.N. and Moore, M.K. (1977). Imitation of social and manual gestures by human neonates. *Science* **198**, 75-78.

Moss, H.A. (1967). Sex, age and state as determinants of mother-infant interaction. *Merrill-Palmer Quart.* **13**, 19-36.

Newton, N. (1955). *Maternal emotions: A study of women's feelings towards menstruation, pregnancy, childbirth, breast feeding, infant care and other aspects of their feminity.* Psychosom. Med., Mono. Paul Hocber, Harper & Bros., New York.

Newton, N. and Newton, M. (1962). Mothers' reactions to their newborn babies. *J.A.M.A.* **181**, 206-210.

Oakley, A. (1977). Cross-cultural practices *In Benefits and Hazards of the New Obstetrics.* (eds Chard and Richards). S.I.M.P., London.

Oakley, A. (1980). *Women Confined.* Martin Robertson, Oxford.

O'Connor, S., Vietze, P.M., Sherrod, K.B., Sandler, H.M. and Altemeier, W.A. (1980). Reduced incidence of parenting inadequacy following rooming-in. *Pediatrics* **66**, 176-182.

Packer, M. and Rosenblatt, D. (1979). Issues in the study of social behaviour in the first week of life *In The First Year of Life* (eds D. Schaffer and J. Dunn). Wiley, Chichester.

Palisin, H. (1980). The Neonatal Perception Inventory: failure to replicate. *Child Develop.* **51**, 3, 737-742.

Parker, G., Tupling, H. and Brown, L.B. (1979). A parental bonding instrument. *Brit. J. Med. Psychol.* **52**, 1-10.

Poindron, P. and Le Neindre, P. (1980). Endocrine and sensory regulation of maternal behaviour in the ewe. *Advances in the Study of Behaviour,* Vol. II. Academic Press, New York and London.

Porter, R.H. and Laney, M.D. (1980). Attachment theory and the concept of inclusive fitness. *Merrill-Palmer Quart.* **26**, 1.

Ransom, R. and Rowell, T. (1972). Early social development of feral baboons. *In Primate Socialization* (ed. F. Poirier). Random House, New York.

Reading, A.E. (1980). Psychological affects on a mother of real time ultrasound. Paper presented at the conference of the Division of Clinical Psychology of the British Psychological Society, September, 1980.

Richards, M.P.M. (1970). Social interaction in the first weeks of human life. Paper presented at Netherlands Interdisciplinary Society for Biological Psychiatry.

Richards, M.P.M. (1974). The one-day-old deprived child. *New Scientist,* 28th March.

Richards, M. (1975a). Early separation. *Child Alive* (ed. R. Lewin). Temple Smith, London.

Richards, M.P.M. (1975b). Innovation in medical practice: Obstetricians and the induction of labour in Britain. *Soc. Science Med.* **9**, 595.

Richards, M.P.M. (1978). A place of safety? An examination of the risks of hospital delivery. *In The Place of Birth* (eds S. Kitzinger and J.A. Davis) pp. 66-84. Oxford University Press, London.

Richards, M.P.M. (1979). Effects on development of medical intervention and the separation of newborns from their parents *In The First Year of Life* (eds D. Shaffer and J. Dunn). Wiley, Chichester.

Ringler, N. Kennell, J.H. Jarvella, R., Navojosky, B.J. and Klaus, M.H. (1975). Mother-to-child speech at 2 years: Effects of early postnatal contact. *J. of Pediatrics* **86**, 141-144.

Ringler, N., Trause, M.A., Klaus, M. and Kennell, J. (1978). The effects of extra postpartum contact and maternal speech patterns on children's I.Q, Speech and Language Comprehension at Five. *Child Devel.* **51**, 775-779.

Robinson, J. (1976). How hospitals alienate mothers. *Mind Out,* March.

Robson, K.M. (1981). A study of mothers' emotional reactions to their newborn babies. Unpublished Ph.D. thesis, London University.

Robson, K.M. and Kumar, R. (1980). Delayed onset of maternal affection after childbirth. *Brit. J. Psychiat.* **136**, 347-353.

Robson, K.S. (1967). The role of eye to eye contact in maternal-infant attachment. *J. Child Psychol. Psychiat.* **8**, 13-25.

Robson, K.S. and Moss, H.A. (1970). Patterns and determinants of maternal attachment. *J. of Pediatrics* **77**, 976-985.

Rosenblatt, D., Redshaw, M., Packer, M. and Leiberman B. (1979). Drugs, birth and infant behaviour. *New Scientist* 15 Feb., 487-489.

Rosenblatt, J.S. (1975). Prepartum and postpartum regulation of maternal behaviour in the rat *In CIBA Foundation Symposium 33*, pp.17-37. Assoc. Scientific Publishers, Oxford.

Sameroff, A.J. (1975). Early influences on development: Fact or Fancy. *Merrill-Palmer Quart.* **21**, 4.

Sameroff, A.J. and Chandler, M.J. (1975). Reproductive risk and the continuum of care-taking casualty *In Review of Child Development Research Vol. 4* (eds F.D. Harawitz, M. Hetherington, S. Scarr-Salapatek and G. Siegel) pp. 187-244. University of Chicago Press, Chicago.

Schaffer, H.R. (1977a). *Mothering: The Developing Child.* Fontana, London.

Schaffer, H.R. (ed.) (1977b). *Studies in Mother-Infant Interaction.* Academic Press, London and New York.

Seashore, M.J., Leifer, A.D., Barnett, R. and Leiderman, P.H. (1973). The effects of denial of early mother-infant interaction on maternal self-confidence. *J. of Personality & Social Psychology* **26**, 3, 369-378.

Seiden, A.M. (1976). The maternal sense of mastery in primary care obstetrics. *Primary Care* **3**, 717-726.

Seiden, A.M. (1978). The sense of mastery in the childbirth experience *In The Woman Patient* (eds Notman and Nadelson). Plenum Press, New York.

Sontag, L.W. (1966). Implications of fetal behaviour and environment for adult personalities. *Ann. N.Y. Acad. Sci.* **134**, 782-786.

Sroufe, L.A. and Waters, E. (1977). Attachment as an organizational construct. *Child Develop.* **48**, 1184-1199.

Stern, D. (1977). *The First Relationship: Infant and Mother.* Fontana, London.

Sternglanz, S.H., Gray, J.L. and Murakami, M. (1977). Adult preferences for infantile facial features: An ethological approach. *Animal Behaviour* **25**, 108-115.

Stone, J., Smith, H. and Murphy, L. (1973). *The Competent Infant.* Basic Books, New York.

Stratton, P.M. (1977). Criteria for assessing the influence of obstetric circumstances on later development *In Benefits and Hazards of the New Obstetrics* (eds T. Chard and M. Richards). Heinemann Medical Books, London.

Svejda, M.J., Campos. J.J. and Emde, R.N. (1980). Mother-infant "bonding" failure to generalise. *Child Develop.* **51**, 6, 1009-1013.

Thoman, E.B., Turner, A.M., Leiderman, P.H. and Barnett, C.R. (1970). Neonate mother interaction: Effects of parity on feeding behaviour. *Child Dev.* **41**, 1103.

Thoman, E.B., Liederman, H.P. and Olson, J.P. (1972). Neonate-mother interaction during breast-feeding. *Devel. Psychology.* **6**, 110-118.

Tipton, R.H. and Lewis, B.V. (1975). Induction of labour and perinatal mortality. *Brit. Med. J.* **1**, 391.

Trevarthen, C. (1979). Communication and co-operation in early infancy *In Before Speech: The Beginning of Interpersonal Communication.* (ed. M. Bullowa). Cambridge University Press, Cambridge.

Tryphonopoulou, Y. and Doxiadis, N. (1972). The effect of elective Caesarian section on the initial stage of mother-infant relationship *In Psychosomatic Medicine in Obstetrics and Gynaecology* (ed. N. Morris), pp.314-317. Kasger, Basel.

Tulkin, S.R. and Kagan, J. (1972). Mother-child interaction in the first year of life. *Child Develop.* **43**, 31-41.

Turner, J. (1980). *Made for Life: Coping, Competence and Cognition.* Methuen, London.

Uddenberg, N. (1974). Reproductive adaptation in mother and daughter. *Acta Psychiat.*

Scand. Suppl. 254.

Vaillant, G.E. (1977). *Adaptation to Life*. Little, Brown & Co., Boston.

Vaughn, B., Egeland, B., Sroufe, L.A. and Waters, E. (1979). Individual differences in infant-mother attachment at twelve and eighteen months: Stability and change in famililes under stress. *Child Develop.* **50**, 971-975.

Waters, E., Wippman, J. and Sroufe, L.A. (1979). Attachment, positive effect and competence in the peer group: Two studies in construct validation. *Child Develop.* **50**, 821-829.

Whiten, A. (1977). Assessing the effects of perinatal events in the success of the mother-infant relationship *In Studies in Mother-Infant Interaction* (ed. H. Schaffer). Academic Press, London and New York.

Whiting, B.B. (1963) (ed.). *Six Cultures: Studies of Child Rearing*. Wiley, Chichester.

Widmayer, S.M. and Field, T.M. (1980). Effects of Brazelton Demonstrations on early interactions of preterm infants and their teenage mothers *Infant Behaviour and Development* **3**, 79-89.

Winnicott, D.W. (1958). Through paediatrics to Psychoanalysis *In Primary Maternal Preoccupations*, pp.300-305. Hogarth Press, London.

Winnicott, D.W. (1960). The theory of the parent-infant relationship. *Int. J. of Psychoanalysis* **41**, 585-595.

7

The Pathology of the Mother–Child Relationship

F. Margison

Introduction

The previous chapter has discussed in detail the research evidence concerning the early relationship between mother and baby. This chapter is concerned with the pathology of that relationship. The first section deals with the assessment of the mother–baby relationship, the second with the psychopathology of bonding, the mother–baby relationship in psychiatric disorder and a brief overview of aetiological features. The second section also includes a section on prevention and treatment with a summary of the available means to protect the safety of the baby under British law.

Assessing the Mother–Baby Relationship

Assessment Methods used in Research

Hinde (1978) has distinguished between social behaviour and social relations in the assessment of interpersonal relationships. Relationships may be described in terms of a series of interactions at the behavioural level. Interactions can be described by their content and less reliably by their quality. To characterize a relationship, however, we need to describe not only the content and quality but also how the interactions are patterned in time.

A number of research strategies for studying mother–baby relationships are described in the Proceedings of the Loch Lomond symposium on Mother–Infant interaction (Schaffer, 1977) and many of the methods attempt sophisticated behavioural analyses of the patterns, as well as the content, of mother–infant interactions as suggested by Hinde. Such detailed assessments of mother–baby interaction have not, however, been used widely in mother and baby psychiatric units or with mentally ill mothers. The clinical research which is reviewed here typically relies upon less sophisticated and precise measures.

Lytton (1973) in a general overview of research into parent–child interactions distinguished three approaches: ethological, interview and experimental. Most of the clinical work on abnormalities in the mother–baby relationship cannot be fitted into any of these approaches. Typically, unstructured observations and data from a variety of sources are synthesized into global ratings such as "able to cope with baby at home." Problems of reliability and validity arise whenever clinical judgements are made and this review describes some of the ways in which information is gathered and evaluated. Six types of assessment are distinguished by Cox (1975):

(a) Interviews with individual parents.
(b) Conjoint family interviews.
(c) Observation of structured interactions
(d) Unstructured observation at home.
(e) Use of a diary kept by the parents.
(f) Questionnaire techniques.

The least reliable techniques (a), (b) and (d) are the ones which are most often used.

Interview Techniques

Peterson and Mehl (1978) studied 46 families in an attempt to determine which of a number of variables best predicted maternal attachment. Although the authors describe some observational data, most of their data were coded from individual and conjoint interviews carried out between the sixth and eighth month of pregnancy, one week after delivery and again one, two, four and six months later. Three raters coded the interviews from recorded tapes until 85% agreement was reached. Scores were derived for prenatal attitude, birth experience and attachment and these were analysed with other information about birth experience and sociodemographic data using a stepwise multiple regression analysis.

The attachment score was derived from a semi-structured interview eliciting information from the mother about feelings of closeness, feeling the baby was hers, caretaking behaviour, confidence in her ability to care for the baby, feelings about caring for the infant in the middle of the night and behaviour in comforting the child. Discrepancies in the mother's account and differences from behaviour observed by the interviewer were noted. The most important variable predicting maternal attachment was neonatal separation.

This study attempts to produce a measure of attachment but the content of the interview is not clearly linked with the derived attachment score. Also some of the criteria for good attachment are unclear, for example, "she sought and maintained close contact with the infant a high percentage of the available time," "she felt reasonably happy and satisfied with the infant and with motherhood, expressing more positive feelings than negative in general."

Observations of Mother–Infant Interactions

Roberts and Forehand (1978) have described six "observation technologies" for assessing parent–child interactions, namely descriptive-narrative, event recording, three types of interval sampling and sequential event recording. The sequential event recording method was found to be most advantageous in terms of four assessment criteria: precise description of the parent–child interaction; target selection (of abnormal behaviours); identification of an intervention strategy and evaluation of that strategy. Although this work applied to older children it is likely that sequential event recording can also be applied to the detailed assessment of mother–baby interaction when the aim is to try and alter an abnormal mother–baby relationship by means of a specific intervention.

An interesting variant of the observational technique was used by Massie (1978) and his co-workers, they obtained unstructured "home movies" of mother–baby interactions taken for reasons which had nothing to do with the research. He compared the interactions recorded in *pre-existing* films between mother and baby in a group of children later diagnosed as mentally ill ("prepsychotic") and for a control group whose home movies were produced in response to an advertisement requesting help in "a study of child development." Groups were matched for numbers of first and second-born children.

Three judges were trained for approximately five hours to use a five-point scale ranging from maternal or infant aversion to intense responsiveness and clinging. They were asked to rate four areas of interaction which were present on most of the films, i.e. feeding, holding, eye contact and touching. Inter-rater correlations of between 0.39 and 0.54 were produced for these apparently crude measures of attachment. This study found that mothers of prepsychotic children exhibited less eye gaze and touching. There are considerable difficulties in evaluating this method of assessment. The measure of attachment assumes an interval scale which is probably inappropriate, and also describes "clinging" behaviour (which has much in common with the concept of *insecure* attachment) as high attachment. Nevertheless, Massie was able to produce moderate levels of inter-rater agreement with minimal training on a simple scale of attachment using unstructured film material.

Diary Techniques

These have not been used widely in the assessment of mother–baby interaction, but Reavley and Gilbert (1976) described the use of diaries kept by parents undergoing treatment because they were thought to be at risk of causing non-accidental injury. The parents kept a diary of interactions with the child and were told to rate how much pleasure and enjoyment they experienced. The diary was then used to monitor progress in coping with situations the parents found to be stressful, such as changing the child's soiled nappy.

Questionnaire Techniques

Questionnaires have not been widely used in the direct assessment of the mother–baby relationship, but they have been used in the form of a screening device in the antenatal period, to detect mothers at high risk of having problems in managing their infants (Frommer and O'Shea, 1973). Frommer and O'Shea's questionnaire was designed to test the assumption that early childhood separation from the expectant mother's own mother might predispose to later difficulties. The women were then interviewed postnatally and were given a semistructured interview exploring the mother's feelings towards the child and an assessment of the mother's actual coping (details not given). The mother was interviewed on four occasions postnatally (2–3 months, 6–7 months, 9–10 months and about 13 months.)

Women who had been separated in childhood from their own mothers were found to have babies with major sleeping problems and the authors considered that such problems reflected mothers' difficulties in managing their infants. The separated group, however, were also more often rated as depressed and an alternative explanation for the difficulties experienced by the mother could be her depression.

Clinical Assessment

The methods of assessment described above are not generally suitable for clinical purposes. Clinical assessment needs to take into account the mother's life history and any psychiatric disturbance in the past, the environment and family situation, and the mother's relationship to the child. The following schema is useful in the clinical assessment of the mother–baby relationship. This information is gathered over the course of several days by the whole team and especially by the nursing staff in constant contact with mother and baby.

(a) *Previous medical history*, including psychiatric history and history of previous pregnancies.

(b) *Relationships to other important figures*, including parents, boyfriends, spouse, other children and friends. Changes affecting other attachment figures of the mother are important, for example by bereavement.

(c) *History of this pregnancy and delivery*, including the mother's response to being pregnant, her antenatal health, details of the delivery, whether the delivery was painful, whether she held the baby; separations and fears about the baby's health.

(d) *Early response to the baby*, including success in feeding, adopting a routine, the presence, if any, of feelings of warmth and acceptance towards the baby.

(e) *Changes in attachment*. The work on potential child abuse by Reavley and Gilbert (1976) assesses changes in attachment using a behavioural analysis. Abnormal responses are divided into two categories; inappropriate actions (for example violence, or shouting at the baby) and maladaptive emotional responses (for example, anxiety, disgust or rage). "Triggering" situations for feeling of rejection or violence are determined. For example, triggering stimuli to feelings of rejection may include the baby crying or soiling his nappy. Other factors modifying the mother's response are recorded (for example, the presence of others).

Fahlberg (1981) has described a series of simple check-lists of attachment which can easily be adapted for clinical use. There are four observation checklists for different age groups (birth to one year, one to five years, school-children and adolescents). Separate items are given for parents and children. The checklist is not designed to give an overall score but can be used in two ways: first, as a way of structuring observations in the clinical situation, particularly when staff are inexperienced, and second, as a measure of change during a treatment programme.

Both of the techniques described have in common the importance of observation of the mother–baby interaction and the importance of dividing attachment and its abnormalities into components which can be evaluated separately.

(f) *Assessment of the baby*. The role of the baby in causing difficulties in the relationship is dealt with in more detail later. During the assessment, attention should be paid to the baby's responsiveness. Some babies cry frequently, are difficult to feed and are relatively unresponsive to attention. Babies are sometimes "difficult" as a result of the mother's abnormal handling, and it is always helpful to get independent accounts from relatives or the health visitor.

(g) *Observation of the mother and baby together*. Eye contact, feeding, playing and handling can be assessed by direct observation. Mothers who have difficulty in relating to their babies often hold the baby stiffly at arms length like a doll. They avoid eye contact and may ignore the baby's social signals interpreting smiles or gurgling as "wind" rather than as social interactions.

(h) *Mother's psychopathology and attitudes toward baby*. The mother's feelings for the baby should be evaluated by direct discussion with the mother, although it is possible for her to cover up abnormal feelings.

Some of the mother's feelings may have a phobic or obsessional component. The mother may describe intense anxiety and distress associated with particular aspects of caring for the baby. Some mothers describe intense revulsion or disgust when changing the baby. The mother may avoid skin contact with the baby, for example only holding the baby against clothing or a towel and avoiding direct physical contact and may describe specific feelings of revulsion rather than a general rejection of the baby. The feelings of revulsion may be associated with marked somatic anxiety.

It is important to determine whether the baby is involved in any delusions. These are described in more detail later and they commonly include grandiose ideas that the baby has a special purpose (e.g. is the new Messiah), beliefs that the baby is physically ill or dying and bizarre delusions that the baby is changing shape, colour or size, or delusions that the baby is changing into an animal or the Devil. Mothers rarely describe the baby in the role of an active persecutor (Bärtschi Rochaix, 1937) even in the presence of extensive persecutory delusions.

In the context of experiencing a general loss of feelings, the mother may describe a lack of feelings for the baby. This often occurs in depression and should be differentiated from active rejection or hostility to the baby. The significance of psychopathology to the mother–baby relationship is described later.

(i) *Longitudinal information.* The above schema for recording information about the mother–baby relationship is largely dependent on cross-sectional accounts with the exception of the assessment of attachment. It is useful to develop a system to record clinical information longitudinally so that changes can be detected over time.

The Mother and Baby Psychiatric Unit at University Hospital of South Manchester has developed a system which uses narrative recordings from any member of the nursing staff who is on duty. The nurses record a narrative account of the mother's behaviour and record any statements about the baby twice daily under the following headings:

(1) Statements about the baby.
(2) Response to baby (including any affection or rejection shown).
(3) Practical competence.
(4) Incidents (this is interpreted broadly and includes episodes where the baby was at risk, or any other observation the nurse considers significant).

This technique is useful when there is a likelihood that relatively untrained nurses may work on a ward as relief staff. Frequently, there are changes in the pattern of responses *before* clear evidence of rejection or hostility occurs.

Case Example

A 28-year-old mother of a three-month old boy admitted with depression.

Day 1 The mother appeared increasingly preoccupied with the baby's health, frequently asking the nurses to contact the paediatrician. She asked the nurses to feed the baby on three occasions which was unusual for her. *Day 2* A student nurse recorded that the mother had commented about her painful delivery and that she would never have a baby again. She appeared to be affectionate towards the baby but was noted to be playing less with him. *Day 3* She expressed concern about the baby's health, left him crying for long periods, and left the ward to go to the shops without telling the nurses. She still seemed practically competent. *Day 4* She announced "out of the blue" that she could not cope with the baby and wanted someone else to care for him. She asked to see an Adoption Agnecy. *Day 5* She expressed infanticidal ideas.

It was clear in retrospect that numerous clues had been given to her aversive feelings and that definite changes in all areas of her behaviour had been recorded. The significance of each individual change was not possible to assess but a clear *pattern* emerged from the detailed observations made by the nurses.

The nurses' accounts separate the mother's statements from her observed behaviour and from her practical care of the baby. It is possible to conceptualize a hierarchy of relationship difficulties according to the extent the difficulties are present in different aspects of the mother and baby interaction.

Stage 1. No relationship problem noted.

Stage 2. Isolated areas of difficulty noted, for example, expressing abnormal ideas, or deficits in practical competence alone.

Stage 3. Miscellaneous problems—no evidence of overt rejection or hostility but difficulties noted in several areas. For example, the mother lacks practical competence, is inconsistent in her handling and is socially unresponsive.

Stage 4. There is evidence of overt rejection and/or hostility to the baby.

These stages are used only as a framework to assess changes in the mother's relationship. Some single abnormalities, such as a statement that the baby had to die to save the world would, of course, be seen as indicating high risk to the babies in the absence of any other abnormality. Despite the limitations, however, a retrospective review of each incident where a child has been put at risk on the unit has shown that episodes of rejection are often preceded by abnormalities in other areas first, the significance of which are likely to be overlooked unless systematically recorded and reviewed.

The advantage of a simple narrative recording system is that it can be used by staff who are new to the unit, the more experienced nursing staff being able to detect underlying changes in the relationship by reviewing the whole record of the mother–baby interaction.

When a mother and baby are admitted to the Manchester Mother and Baby Psychiatric Unit it is usually possible to assess the relationship in considerable detail within two weeks. The nurses make regular observations of the mother's interactions as described above. A psychiatric history and assessment of psychopathology, a social and family assessment by the psychiatric social worker and, sometimes, a psychological assessment are also made soon after admission. Further assessment of the mother's practical capacity is possible in the occupational therapy department and when necessary the mother may live with the baby for a one or two week assessment period in a flat in the occupational therapy department. The nursery nurses are closely involved in the general nursing assessment, but they are also able to give an independent view about the ease with which the baby can be managed. A paediatric assessment of the baby including its level of development is also made. At the end of the two week assessment the staff are able to provide a report and treatment plan.

The Psychopathology of Bonding

Rejection

In *The concept of the rejecting mother*, Anna Freud (Freud, 1970) described rejection from the point of view of the older child. She distinguished a number of different types of rejection including rejection by unwillingness, by abnormality of the mother, by separation, by inconsistency and what she called "rejection in spite of devotion."

The concept of rejection from the child's viewpoint described by Anna Freud differs considerably from the rejection felt by the rejecting mother herself. Delay in the onset of maternal affection has been described in detail in the previous chapter. Rejection differs from this in several ways. Negative thoughts about the child are present, there is often a wish that the child had never been born or could be changed in some fundamental way (for example by being of the opposite sex) and in some instances the mother may totally deny that the child is hers or even that she has given birth at all.

Some authors have taken an extremely wide view of rejection based on psychodynamic theories. Brew and Seidenberg (1950) in a review of 83 postpartum psychoses admitted to the Syracuse Psychopathic Hospital between 1933 and 1946 stated that "in both the schizophrenic and manic-depressive postpartum reactions, one point in common was the rejection of the new-born infant. This manifested itself in many ways—by actual expression or by *symbolization*" (my italics)

The instances of actual violence were high in this series; three mothers attempted infanticide by strangulation and another tried to throw the child out of the window. However, the other patients showed a wide variety of symptoms which were interpreted as rejection—delusions, hallucinations, amnesia and over-solicitude to the baby. The delusions were commonly in the form of fears that the baby was dead, disfigured or dying. Some patients disavowed their husbands or re-enacted parturition. One patient with schizophrenia was reported to have said "I didn't have a baby but a balloon and it burst." Some patients had fears that they were poisoning their children. This broad view of rejection has been influential since Zilboorg (1931) attributed postpartum psychiatric illness to maternal rejection of the child.

Few authors give sufficient details of the psychopathology of their patients to enable one to delineate a group where overt rejection is apparent from the larger group where the rejection is symbolic. Anderson (1933) compared 50 patients with postpartum psychotic illnesses which began within six weeks of childbirth with 50 control patients with non-puerperal psychoses. He noted that nine of his 50 postpartum psychotic patients showed aversion to the child, although no details were given. Tetlow (1955) gave a much more pessimistic view of the frequency of abnormal relationships in a study of 67 consecutive admissions to

Warwick Central Hospital for psychotic illnesses with onset in the six months after delivery. She stated that the mothers showed "... no constructive effort (on their part) to overcome the normal difficulties of motherhood." In women with affective psychoses (60% of the total) "... there was in every case an abnormal emotional relationship to the child, expressing itself as perverted hatred, indifference or phobia that the child would be injured or killed or even a denial that the child was theirs." Tetlow described fears of the child falling downstairs or troubling dreams of the baby dying of starvation or being murdered. One mother described a feeling that the baby was not hers and another the idea that she had "no mother instinct." Less detail is given of the mothers with schizophrenia, but Tetlow described these mothers as tending "to deny the existence of the child."

In an unselected series of obstetric admissions in Sweden (Jacobson *et al.*, 1965) the frequency of various psychiatric symptoms in the postnatal period was determined by questionnaire. Twenty-eight of 404 mothers (7%) were rated as having a fear of hurting their child but no mention is made of rejection as such. Seager (1960) in a descriptive study of 40 postpartum mental illnesses gave incidental details of one patient killing her twins, two wishing to harm their children and one complaining of having lost love for her child. At follow up between six months and five years later the two mothers who had wished harm to the babies and the mother who felt no love had normal relationship with their children, although six mothers who had previously had normal relationships now blamed their children for their illnesses and were antagonistic to them.

Another retrospective clinical study which gives incidental data about the mother-child relationship and rejection is that of Ostwald and Regan (1957). They studied 54 patients admitted to the Payne Whitney Clinic of the New York Hospital between 1937 and 1955 with psychiatric disorders in the 90 days postpartum. They divided their patients into three groups; disorganized, depressed and paranoid. Hallucinations and delusions were common in the disorganized group, the content "frequently" involving injury to, or destruction of, the infant as well as themes of sex and impending punishment. In addition they attempted to measure masculine and feminine personality attributes and in the process of doing this recorded a number of items said to reflect "maternal" characteristics. Combining the three groups, only 21 patients (39%) had wanted the pregnancy and only five patients (9%) were reported to display maternal warmth. The criteria for maternal warmth were, however, not stated. More descriptive information derived from psychotherapy interviews with these patients stated that the patients often felt proud of the appearance or behaviour of their offspring but were aware of a sense of remoteness; feelings of love or warmth were absent and hostility present in 19 patients (35%).

The relationship of feelings of rejection to the pregnancy being wanted originally is unclear, but Matejcek *et al.* (1978) in a controlled study of 220 nine-year-old children of mothers refused termination of those pregnancies showed that the majority of mothers became more accepting with time, although the unwanted children were more often maladjusted.

Zemlick and Watson (1953) in a study of 15 primiparous patients attempted to relate maternal attitudes of acceptance and rejection during and after pregnancy. They used a large number of predictor variables assessed during pregnancy, at parturition and postpartum which included obstetric data, complex measures of physical symptoms and emotional symptoms, a projective test derived from the Thematic Apperception Test, a Pregnancy Attitude Scale devised locally and validated separately on a group of 266 pregnant patients and a psychosomatic inventory. The criterion variables are described elsewhere (Boggs, 1951) and consisted of detailed observational measures using a time sampling technique during feeding. The assessment produced scores of the mother's verbalization, the baby's sucking time, a measure of persistence of sucking and a composite score. The wide range of measures used makes it difficult for the authors to come to clear conclusions, but they note a significant increase in acceptance postpartum. Another interesting finding was that prenatal attitudes of rejection were *inversely* related to some postpartum criteria of adjustment. The authors suggest that "overprotection" may be a covert manifestation of rejection. An alternative explanation would be that expressed attitudes do not necessarily correspond to observed rejecting behaviour and vice versa. This would support the view expressed earlier that different aspects of the mother–baby relationship need to be assessed simultaneously in the clinical setting.

Non-accidental Injury (NAI)

This is one of the clearest examples of breakdown of the normal mother–baby relationship (Helfer and Kempe, 1974). NAI has been studied in great detail (e.g. Carver; 1978; Scott, 1977; DHSS, 1975) and will not be fully reviewed here. Some authors imply that NAI and bonding failure are inextricably bound. This is probably an overstatement but the research on NAI may throw light on other mother–baby relationship problems.

Workers at Park Hospital, Oxford, (Lynch et al., 1976, Lynch and Roberts, 1977) have listed a number of predictors of NAI which seem to be related to difficulties in the mother–baby relationship. The major significance of this work lies in the possibility of detecting difficulties early and arranging appropriate intervention to prevent NAI. Lynch and Roberts (1977) compared 50 children referred because of actual or potential child abuse. A control group was derived from the next live child born after the index child in the same hospital. A separate check was made to be certain that the control children were not thought to be at risk of NAI. Information about the children was derived from the case notes—using paediatric, obstetric and nursing records, and also any available social work notes.

The following significant predictors of NAI were found:

(a) Mother's age—more mothers of an index child had had their first babies before 20 years of age.

(b) "Emotional disturbance" (derived from information recorded in the psychiatric illness section of the notes but not otherwise verified.) This had been attributed to 23 mothers of abused children compared to seven mothers of controls.

(c) Referral to social worker. Twenty-nine mothers of index children compared to three control mothers had been referred to the hospital social worker.

(d) Admission to special care baby unit. The infants had more often been admitted to the special care baby unit.

(e) Adverse comments about mothering. A systematic search for any comment indicating concern about mothering showed that concern was expressed about the mothers of 22 abused babies and three controls.

Overall, 35 of 50 abused children had two or more of these five predictors. Only five of the control group had more than one adverse factor.

Lynch (1976) assessed 25 consecutive abused children with one or more siblings to clarify the factors which put a particular sibling at risk. The factors which occurred significantly more commonly in the life histories of the abused group were:

(a) Abnormal pregnancy (defined as any complication requiring investigation and/or admission to hospital, mothers who concealed the pregnancy, mothers refusing antenatal care or where an abortion had been refused).

(b) Abnormal labour (defined as prolonged labour over 24 hours, premature labour, and all operative deliveries apart from "easy forceps").

(c) Any separation after delivery.

(d) Any separation in the first six months.

(e) Illness in the child in the first year of life.

(f) Illness in the mother in the first year of the child's life.

"Failure to Thrive without Organic Cause"

This refers to a syndrome in which the infant does not grow, gain weight or develop normally in the early months of life and yet shows leaps in development and weight gain with routine hospital care. An association has been noted between "failure to thrive" and early separation (Ambuel and Harris, 1963; Shaheen *et al.*, 1968, Evans *et al.*, 1972). Failure to thrive can be seen as a physical consequence of emotional deprivation.

Infanticide

In British law the killing of a child under the age of 12 months by its mother under circumstances which would otherwise amount to murder may be classed as infanticide and dealt with as manslaughter providing that "the balance of her mind was disturbed by reason of her not having fully recovered from the effect of giving birth to the child or by reason of the effect of lactation consequent upon the birth of the child . . ." (Infanticide Act, 1938.)

This has a great effect on the sentence received because murder receives a mandatory sentence of life imprisonment but in the Criminal Law Revision Committee's review of sentencing from 1969 to 1974 the majority of women found guilty or pleading guilty to infanticide received non-custodial sentences.

The Infanticide Act, 1938, formalized an increasingly merciful reponse to mothers who had killed their babies (Bluglass, 1978). A number of authors have provided evidence of coexisting psychiatric disturbance at the time of infanticide which supports the need for special provision in these cases. In British law it is not necessary to prove that the mother's mental condition was the cause of her actions, it is sufficient simply to demonstrate that there was mental disturbance.

Many mothers who have committed infanticide also commit suicide (Gibson, 1975). Gibson and Klein (1961) in a study of 113 mothers who had killed their children found that 62% also committed suicide. West (1965) concluded on the basis of his series (whose psychopathology he assessed retrospectively from relatives) that those mothers who killed their child and committed suicide usually showed significant evidence of depression.

Clinical reviews of infanticide (Hopwood, 1927; Morton, 1944; Batt, 1948) draw attention to the preponderance of psychiatric symptoms and apparent psychiatric disorder. D'orban (1979) reviewed a series of 89 women who had killed their children. He divided the women into six groups; battering mothers 36, mentally ill mothers 24, neonaticide 11, retaliatory killing 9, unwanted children 8, mercy killing 1. The categories were not clearly differentiated nor were they mutually exclusive. The number of mothers in the mentally ill category may be an underestimate because mothers in other categories may also have been mentally ill. Of the whole series, 50 (56%) had psychiatric symptoms such as depression, irritability, exhaustion and apathy. The main diagnoses in the mentally ill group were psychosis, "acute reactive depression associated with a suicide attempt" and "personality disorder with sufficient depressive symptoms to warrant admission."

Gregger and Hoffmeyer (1969) discussed the relationship between schizophrenia and the patient killing her child, but they quote only a small number of patients and were unable to draw any overall conclusions about the risk to children of schizophrenic mothers. The psychopathology of infanticide was also discussed by Harder (1967). He gave case histories of eleven mothers following the killing of their children in the first year of life but outside the newborn period. He considered that they were all depressed.

The psychopathology of murderous impulses was discussed by Chapman (1959) in a clinical account of 20 mothers who had obsessional fears of infanticide. He described fear of mutilating the child by stabbing or decapitation and a linked fear of becoming insane. Many of these mothers avoided the presence of knives or scissors. Many mothers had elaborate and distressing fantasies of standing over the bleeding body of the child, headlines in the newspaper and being taken away to a psychiatric hospital. Many mothers feared being left alone with the child. The author described most of these mothers as being passive with a fear of expressing anger towards parents.

Homicidal wishes towards the child may represent hostility to a hated spouse which the child represents. This was described in a clinical account of seven cases by Stern (1948). He called this constellation of feelings "The Medea Complex." Typically, a mother would feel intense hatred towards a child who resembled its father. The hatred of the child's father could not be expressed because of desertion or fear of retribution.

Few of the accounts of infanticide and murderous impulses make clear how the risk to a particular child can be assessed in advance. Clinical guidelines which may be helpful are:

(1) The mother's previous history of violence to this child or others. Even minor acts of aggression in the setting of homicidal thoughts reflect a major change from their presence in imagination only.

(2) Mothers who have true obsessional phenomena, where impulses are recognized as foreign to the personality and strongly resisted, probably represent a lesser degree of risk than mothers with other forms of aggressive impulses.

Historically, the supposed presence of hostility played a large part in the management of puerperal mental illness. MacDonald (1899) suggested that the child be removed as his "presence may be obnoxious to the mother." He further noted that if the illness "turns to depression she may lose interest in all about her, especially her child towards whom she may exhibit a marked dislike or even hatred." Savage (1875) compared allowing a mother contact with her baby during a puerperal mental illness to exposing the child "to the danger of a mad nurse." These quotations make clear the complexity of the interrelationship of hostility, rejection and potential violence in the puerperium. As discussed earlier, the policy of separating the mother from her baby continued until the 1950s.

The Mother–Baby Relationship during Various Forms of Psychiatric Disorder

There has been very little systematic work on evaluation of the mother–baby relationship during psychiatric illnesses. In the section on "rejection" a number of incidental findings about the mother–baby relationship were reported. In this section other information about the qualities of the mother–baby relationship will be summarized.

Psychosis

Gamer *et al.* (1976) studied aspects of the social and cognitive development of the children of 15 psychotic mothers not all with onset in the puerperium. The mother's diagnoses were schizophrenia (three), schizoaffective (six), psychotic depression (five), and borderline (one), and the children were aged between one and eleven months (mean four months.) The children of psychotic mothers differed from controls on a measure of "object permanence" which is of theoretical interest in that it may reflect the capacity of the child to form stable attachments. Other data were given about the children's response to their mothers. Two children showed a lack of positive interactions with their mothers but responded to their fathers preferentially. One subject although being described as "good with the baby" was "somewhat coercive" and two other mothers were described as not appearing "to enjoy her child." There were also frequent comments about abnormal handling of the child by these mothers.

Sobel (1961) studied eight infants of schizophrenic mothers comparing four reared by their natural parents with four reared by foster parents. Three of the four infants reared by their natural parents showed evidence of "depression" although the criteria were not made explicit. Sobel describes the natural mothers as showing little pleasure themselves when interacting with their infants and engaging in little active play. A review of children at risk of schizophrenia described schizophrenic mothers as responding vocally but showing less touching and playing less with their infants than other mothers (Garmezy, 1974).

Overall, little detailed work has been done on the mother–baby relationship during the mother's psychiatric disorder. Practical competence is often relatively intact, at least at the crude level at which it has been measured but social activities such as play and touching were more frequently disrupted.

Neurosis

Uddenberg (1974) commented that puerperally disturbed mothers showed abnormal relationships to their children "characterised by a combination of rejection, anxiety and overprotection. Feelings of guilt towards the child and of inadequacy in the mothering role were also common." Uddenberg studied 95 nulliparous pregnant women randomly selected from women attending the antenatal clinic at Lund, in Southern Sweden. One source of information was from a semistructured interview administered four months after delivery. During this interview the mothers described their situation and their experience of the maternal role. Uddenberg assessed the degree of handicap based on this information, a checklist of symptoms and observations during the interview.

Uddenberg and Englesson (1978) followed up 69 of the original sample of 95 women using a similar semistructured interview and also information derived by a psychologist observing and talking to the children in a play session. The psychologist was not aware of the mothers' psychiatric status. A summary score of the mother's positive or negative attitude to the child was based on six three-point scales assessing parental qualities of being punishing, rewarding, restricting, helping, rejecting and comforting. Sixteen mothers had been categorized as "severely mentally handicapped" during the first paranatal period. ("Severe mental handicap" was taken to mean "the woman had experienced very painful mental symtoms and the emotional disturbance had resulted in definite deterioration of social and interpersonal functioning. The women in this group also had obvious signs of mental disturbance".) These 16 mothers were compared with the remaining 53.

Mothers who had been defined as "severely mentally handicapped" more often described their children in negative terms at follow up. They described their children significantly more often as "causing much trouble", "insisting on too much attention", or as "having temper tantrums". These mothers were also more likely to feel they could not influence their children and described losing their temper more often.

The overall opinion about the mother's general attitude to her child was that the attitude was negative for 16 mothers overall. Eight of these came from the "severely handicapped" group, significantly more than would have been expected by chance. Children whose mothers had been severely mentally handicapped described their mothers in a more negative way overall. In particular these children described their mothers as "not comforting" or "strongly restrictive."

Although the criteria were not explicit, most of the severely mentally handicapped group had neurotic disorders. The follow-up study showed many to have chronic or recurrent symptoms. The study assessed maternal function and attitudes in some detail gathering information in the postnatal period and four years subsequently. The main drawback to the study is that the investigator assessing maternal function and attitudes also assessed the degree of psychiatric disturbance. Moreover one of the criteria for "severe mental handicap" was disruption of interpersonal functioning which presumably included the maternal relationship. Despite these drawbacks this study is one of the very few attempting to follow up mentally ill mothers and report their maternal functioning.

Personal Observations

The aspects of psychopathology in the mother which most interfere with the mother–baby relationship may vary between different psychiatric states. The clinical observations recorded are derived from patients admitted to the Manchester Mother and Baby Psychiatric Unit (see later).

Mania and Acute Schizophrenia

Manic patients usually show a marked disorganization of practical care. The mother may relate very warmly to the baby but only for brief periods and then inconsistently. Grandiose ideas about the child having a "special purpose" (for example being "the infant Jesus", "born of the Devil with special powers to take over the world"), are common. Other common delusions include the belief that the baby can control the television or influence the mother's thoughts, and bizarre ideas about the child changing appearance or shape (for example, "He's turning into a cockroach").

Deliberate physical injury to the child is uncommon but many mothers need to be separated during the most severe phase of the illness because she may be acting in a disinhibited, disorganized way. For example, one woman in the Manchester Mother and Baby Unit crawled about the floor reliving the birth of her child. She then put roses in all the prams and roughly lifted the babies in and out of the prams.

Chronic Schizophrenia

This is one of the most difficult and disabling conditions which affects the mother–baby relationship. As described earlier the mother often describes a flatness and deadness of feeling and an inability to play with and respond to the baby. These mothers very frequently show gross deficits in the organization of a daily routine and practical competence. The overall prognosis, even with extensive help, for the small group of patients already suffering from chronic schizophrenia during pregnancy seems extremely poor, the baby often being placed in the care of the Local Authority eventually (Margison, 1981).

Depression

Mothers with depression frequently report a lack of feelings generally which may involve the baby. The mother may express concern about her lack of love for the baby, or anything else (anhedonia). "I feel no love for the baby like I should, I just feel nothing, no joy, not anything when the baby smiles at me." If the depressed mother is retarded or has poor concentration it may be difficult to maintain a daily routine; "I can never keep up, as soon as I've changed the baby he's woken up and I'm back to square one again. I feel like I just can't cope, I'm so slow and muddled in my thoughts."

The mother may show irritability or anger in the presence of the baby when she is unable to cope with an unexpected change in the daily routine. Abnormal ideas are common. These include guilt, fears about the baby's health, or regret about having harmed the baby. The mother commonly describes a feeling of being unable to cope which is disproportionate to her actual loss of competence. Less commonly she may have obsessional fears about killing or mutilating the baby.

Neurotic Illnesses other than Depression

Neurotic illnesses marked by an ambivalence to the baby with overt rejection and hostility or obsessional symptoms are described elsewhere.

Another common presentation is of a highly anxious mother with mild depressive symptoms and intense fears of not coping. These mothers have often had very high expectations of motherhood, have previously led a well-ordered lifestyle and find it extremely difficult to cope with the realities of the practical care of a young baby. Many of these mothers and babies get into a vicious circle of failed feeding, increased crying, increasing feelings of anxiety and panic about the baby. Many cope well with support outside hospital, and those who are admitted often settle very quickly and maintain a good relationship with the baby at follow-up.

The Mother's Abnormal Ideas about the Baby

As part of a pilot study about the mother–baby relationship based on case note information, all statements about the baby recorded in the medical and nursing notes for 245 admissions were examined. Each mother was assigned to one of six groups according to the predominant abnormal ideas she held, if any. The groups of abnormal ideas were:

(1) *Concern about the baby's physical health.* These included exaggerated forms of normal concerns held to a preoccupying degree, e.g. fear of cot death, concern about feeding, and also delusional beliefs about illness which were not open to reassurance. For example "The baby is all blue, he's withering away to a bare skeleton", "The baby has been poisoned by blow flies".

(2) *Delusions other than about the baby's health.*
   (a) Delusions referring to the child's "special purpose", e.g. "He's the new Jesus Christ", "He is the son of the Devil".
   (b) Delusions of special powers, e.g. "He can put thoughts into my head".
   (c) Delusions of bodily change, e.g. "He's developing a cockroach head", "He's changing into a vampire bat".

(3) *Ideas of rejection or hostility.* These were ideas beyond mild resentment or irritation. They involved intense hatred, resentment or rejection, e.g. "I wish he'd never been born, I hate him for ruining my life", "I feel like killing him, I'm not just saying that".

(4) *"No feeling".* This category as distinct from (3) involves no expression of negative feelings, but just a lack of feelings, e.g. "I feel empty like I'm drained of all love for her, and for everyone", "I just don't seem to be able to feel love like a mother should".

(5) *Ideas of not coping.* These involved intense ideas of inadequacy out of proportion to any actual impairment of competence, e.g. "I'm just not a fit mother, he won't take any food from me, he'd have starved if the nurses weren't here" "I'm just useless as a mother".

(6) *No abnormal ideas expressed.* Mothers who made brief comments about not coping or irritation which were not dominant could be included here.

The data recorded in Table 1 are tentative; they are derived from case notes and

Table 1. Abnormal ideas about child by diagnosis

	Puerperal psychosis	Non-psychotic depression
(1) Ideas of illness	26	12
(2) Other delusions	23	0
(3) Rejection or hostility	4	28
(4) "No feelings"	4	10
(5) Ideas of "not coping"	11	22
(6) No abnormal ideas	25	6
	—	—
	93	79

are subject to selection biases. The mothers have been allocated to the predominant category of disturbance but may have expressed ideas in other areas. However, some points are very striking even with the crude data available. Mothers with puerperal psychoses often expressed abnormal ideas about their children being ill and the babies were also the subject of other kinds of delusions. The psychotic mothers rarely expressed predominantly hostile ideas. Twenty-five of these 93 psychotic mothers expressed no recorded abnormal ideas about the child. The non-psychotic depressed mothers most frequently expressed ideas of rejection or "not coping."

The Causes of Disruption of the Mother–Baby Relationship

The Baby

The complex interaction between mother and baby in the early postpartum period has been described earlier (Robson and Powell, Chapter 6). A number of factors relating to the baby may be associated with abnormal "bonding". Richards and Bernal (1972) have shown that a group of persistently restless, sleepless, crying babies can be identified very soon after birth. Schaffer and Emerson (1968) have described a number of characteristics such as social orientation and assertiveness which are present within a few days of delivery. Scarr (1969) has shown that these characteristics may be heritable responses. Babies high on social orientation seem to be treated differently from babies low on social orientation. The mothers of babies showing high social orientation are more attentive.

Moss (1967) studied 30 normal children in the first three months of life. The boys in the sample were more irritable in the third week than the girls and their mothers spent more time responding to them. However, by the twelfth week the mothers of the irritable boys were finding them difficult to pacify and the girls were receiving more attention. This study draws attention to the complex interaction between the baby's irritability, the mother's initial response and how the response changes over time. Irritability of the baby may be important in predicting battering in that children who are battered tend to be more irritable, but it does not automatically follow that the irritability is an innate quality despite evidence that babies do tend to have some characteristics from birth for example assertiveness and social orientation as discussed earlier. Smith (1969) based on a clinical study of battering took the view that the irritability was probably a *result* of abnormal handling; "difficult, especially crying or clinging behaviour was encountered by the mothers and may have precipitated battering. After some time being in hospital, however, they (the children) were no more irritable than the controls."

Premature children are thought to be particularly at risk of rejection, failure to thrive and battering. Bicknell (1981) has described the reactions of the parents of children who are physically and/or mentally handicapped. Typically, the parents pass through phases similar to bereavement after the delivery period. The time required for the process of mourning and eventual adaptation varies. The process can be seen as mourning an idealized child (Solnit and Stark, 1961; Olshansky, 1962). The child clearly does not fulfil the parents' expectations but in addition may be deficient in producing behaviours which promote attachment, for example eye fixation. This lack may be exaggerated by medication which the baby is receiving for a coexisting state, for example, barbiturates to control epileptic fits.

Brazelton (1969) has found that many psychotropic drugs may pass into breast milk and thus alter the infant's habituation and orienting responses, as well as measures of "cuddliness" and smiling.

The Mother

The importance of psychiatric disorder in the mother has been discussed elsewhere. An important additional area of aetiological importance in mother–baby relationship problems is the mother's general capacity to form relationships. A mother who has unresolved difficulties about dependence may see the child as a threat to her own needs for dependence. Other possible personality factors include traits of impulsivity and a pattern of relationships characterized by instability and shallowness. Emotional deprivation in the mother's own upbringing is probably linked to the mother's capacity to form affectional bonds (Bowlby, 1977).

If the mother has previously related normally to another of her children the overall prognosis is better. However, the particular child may have a specific personal significance to the mother, for example, the child may be associated with a bereavement or a hated spouse or may be associated with painful recollections about the delivery.

> A young professional woman complained of a phobia for needles during a wanted pregnancy but was otherwise well. She had an extremely distressing delivery during which she was heavily sedated. On recovery from the birth she developed intense recurrent ideas that she had been deliberately tortured. She had not been able to hold the baby postnatally and her first experience with her baby was unfortunate. She had stated that she wanted to breast feed, but a baby, left in the ward without comment, was bottle fed. She was later told it was her baby, but was unable to accept the idea, saying the baby was "a monster", "too big", "that couldn't be a baby inside me." She became depressed and developed the conviction that the baby was not hers, and that another baby had been substituted to cover up her baby's death. These ideas came to light six months later when she described leaving the child at the top of the stairs hoping she would fall down. Intense feelings of disgust towards the baby were present and the mother avoided any skin contact with the child initially.

Although the main features of the illness were definitely affective, the central experience was that of her baby dying and another baby being substituted. This experience of the baby being a changeling is well recognized in folklore. These ideas of complete rejection were linked to an extremely distressing experience of delivery. At follow-up one year later, the depressive symptoms had improved, but there were still marked symptoms of phobic anxiety. She was able to hold the child and care for her physically, but the central belief that the child was not hers was unchanged.

Prevention and Treatment of Bonding Disorders

Prevention in the Non-psychiatric Setting

The importance of early separation in the causation of bonding disorders has been discussed earlier. Premature and sick babies are commonly treated separately from their mothers. As early as 1907 Budin commented on the rejection of premature infants. The policy on many special care baby units has changed to minimize the separation from the mother. Klaus and Kennell (1976) after reviewing the evidence about early separation recommended steps to minimize the risk of a later disorder of maternal bonding. The steps are summarized here:

(1) The mother should be allowed brief contact and the baby should be nursed in the same hospital if possible.
(2) If the baby has to be moved, the father should accompany the baby to the special care unit in the other hospital.
(3) The mother should be given a photograph of the baby.

(4) As soon as possible the parents should be encouraged to make physical contact with the baby. Eye contact should be established as soon as possible even if this means that the ultraviolet light (used to reduce bilirubin levels) has to be discontinued temporarily. This is in keeping with the findings of Robson (1967) about the important role of early eye contact in forming attachments.

(5) Even when the baby is severely ill pessimistic remarks should be avoided because these seem to delay attachment if the baby does survive. If the baby dies Klaus and Kennell see it as the responsibility of staff to help the parents with mourning.

(6) A particularly important step which Klaus and Kennell recommend is the keeping of a "contact diary" in which all contacts by the mother are recorded. The staff, therefore, record all telephone and personal contacts. If a mother telephones or visits less than three times in two weeks the baby is identified as being at high risk of non-accidental injury, failure to thrive or rejection. The use of this detection procedure is described by Fanaroff *et al.* (1972).

The suggestions discussed above apply particularly to sick babies, but the general principles could be applied in other situations, for example, during the mother's physical or mental illness.

The detection of mothers at high risk of NAI has been discussed earlier. It is possible to arrange postnatal care so that mothers thought to be at risk of rejection can be detected and referred for more detailed assessment, treatment and follow up (Roberts, 1980). This can be done by having a psychiatrist or psychiatric social worker in regular liaison with the obstetric unit. Mothers identified as "at risk" are referred to the liaison social worker or psychiatrist.

Prevention in a Psychiatric Setting

The use of a specialized mother and baby psychiatric unit is discussed elsewhere, but it is possible to maintain lesser degrees of contact in other psychiatric settings by bringing the baby to see the mother on the ward. Even when the mother has a severe psychiatric illness it is usually possible to maintain some degree of contact with the relatives present. The father, parents and parents-in-law are often keen to be involved in the mother's treatment.

The specialized mother and baby psychiatric unit is able to provide a comprehensive assessment of the mother–baby relationship. The mother is usually able to keep contact with the baby, helping to some extent in practical care even in the presence of a severe psychotic illness. The mother's capacity to help in the care of her child is often one of the few areas of relatively normal behaviour. Although these steps would seem appropriate in view of the evidence available about bonding disorders it must be emphasized that very little empirical evidence is available at present about the effects of psychiatric illnesses on maternal function.

Specific Interventions

After a period of assessment it should be possible to produce a treatment plan to deal with the observed areas of difficulty.

Practical Competence

The assessment of practical competence involves competence specifically with the baby and also general competence with housework. As discussed elsewhere, impairment of competence may be temporary as in most patients with puerperal psychosis when specific intervention may not be required, or may be prolonged as in many patients with chronic schizophrenia.

On a mother and baby psychiatric unit the nurses are able to care for the baby with the mother helping during all but the most severe phases of psychotic illnesses. The psychiatric or nursery nurse is therefore both giving practical instruction and acting as a role model. Other mothers on the unit may share these functions of giving practical help and acting as role models, particularly during group sessions (focusing on the practical problems of caring for the babies) which the nurses organize.

For the small group of mothers who have very severely impaired practical competence (for example, mothers with chronic schizophrenia) intensive help with rehabilitation may be needed, one aspect of which will be her ability to care for the baby. Many hospitals have temporary living accommodation attached to the psychiatric unit or occupational therapy departments for assessment and rehabilitation of domestic skills. It may be helpful for the mother to spend time with the baby in that setting before discharge.

For less severely ill patients at home, help with practical competence can be given by a community psychiatric nurse or health visitor, or alternatively the mother may be allowed to stay for a period in a local authority mother and baby home. Some local authorities have made use of "peripatetic house mothers" to provide a very high level of practical support in the mother's home after an assessment period in hospital, or as an alternative to admission.

A mentally handicapped mother whose previous child died of a chest infection and hypothermia at home was assessed for two weeks with her two-month-old baby on the Manchester Mother and Baby Unit in conjunction with the local authority social services. No evidence of psychiatric illness other than mental handicap was found and the assessment of her relationship with the baby showed no abnormality apart from marked impairment of practical skills. The local authority housing department rehoused the family and a peripatetic house mother attended daily to help with the practical care of the baby for a number of months after which close supervision was provided by a local authority social worker and the health visitor. Both mother and baby were well at one year follow-up.

Psychotherapy

Exploratory psychotherapy is particularly indicated when the baby triggers painful feelings which may be echoes of previous important relationships. For example, the birth of the baby may raise feelings which are associated with earlier unresolved sibling-rivalry. Supportive psychotherapy may help break a "vicious cycle" of increasing tension, feeding difficulty, sleeplessness and irritability. Personal support from nursing staff is an important part of the therapeutic milieu on a specialized mother and baby psychiatric unit as in other psychiatric settings. Family or marital therapy may be indicated when the birth of the baby activates an underlying family conflict. The baby may embody a family myth which recurs through generations, which may involve expectations of, say, the firstborn child of a generation having particular qualities, the child being rejected or made a scapegoat in the absence of these imagined qualities.

Behavioural Treatment Approach

The behavioural approach has been developed for use in families where there is evidence of rejection or NAI. A hierarchy of problem areas is constructed and the therapist uses a variety of behavioural techniques including desensitization and participant modelling. The therapist rehearses anxiety-inducing situations and models coping strategies (including appropriate ways of handling the child). As the mother's anxiety diminishes she attempts increasingly difficult tasks (Reavley and Gilbert, 1976; Reavley et al., 1978).

Reavley and Gilbert draw attention to a number of supplementary points:

(1) The mother can be taught "self-control" techniques similar to those used by Meichenbaum and Goodman (1971) with impulsive children. The mothers are taught a strategy of rehearsal with repeated self commentary (e.g. "I won't get angry with him"). The patients carry out repeated practice.

(2) The patients are encouraged to contribute by keeping detailed records of treatment in the form of a diary, and are also given feedback about progress by the therapist.

(3) The treatment ideally takes place in the patient's home, so that generalization is more likely to take place.

Behaviour therapy has been most often tried in mothers with personality disorders who have difficulties with impulse control or in mothers with phobic anxiety directed at the baby. However, such treatments can also be applied to some problems in the post-psychotic stage after a puerperal psychosis. The mother may feel she has lost confidence, she may be slow and may show marked anxiety when holding the baby. Techniques of anxiety control and participant modelling may be helpful.

The behavioural approach has the extra advantage of not "begging the question" of the nature of "bonding problems." The patient's problems with her baby are seen individually and the contingencies and triggers for each aspect of the problem can be kept separate. It is probably unhelpful to consider "bonding" as a unitary process following a single developmental sequence. Bonding problems are best seen as complex phenomena involving family, marital, intrapersonal and interpersonal levels. They are potentially open to a mixture of psychodynamic, interpersonal, cognitive and behavioural treatment approaches.

The Safety of the Child

The empirical findings referred to in the chapter on mother and baby units show that the risks to the baby can be kept low on such units with close observation and transfer of acutely disturbed patients to an adjacent ward. However, circumstances arise when legal steps need to be taken to ensure a child's safety because of the risk of injury or neglect from the child's mother. Legal aspects of child injury or neglect are discussed succinctly by Black and Hughes (1979). In the United Kingdom, if there is reason to believe that the child's "proper development is being avoidably impaired or neglected or he is being ill-treated", a Place of Safety Order application can be made to a magistrate under the powers of the Children and Young Persons Act, 1969. The application may be made to remove a child from home or to prevent a child being taken home from hospital and is usually made by the National Society for the Prevention of Cruelty to Children (NSPCC) or the Local Authority. The maximum duration is 28 days (although the Police also have power to keep a child in a place of safety for up to eight days without contacting a magistrate). The Place of Safety Order can be used in situations where the baby is likely to be put at immediate risk. It is usual where a child is considered to be at risk to call a case conference involving the social and health agencies involved (and often also the Police) to decide how to proceed further. Many local authorities keep registers of children thought to be at risk of abuse or neglect. The case conference is an opportunity to adopt a shared policy for coordinating the care of a family where a child is thought to be at risk. Liaison between different disciplines is essential to minimize the risk of abuse or neglect. The practical aspects of organizing a case conference are discussed by Carver (1978.) After a Place of Safety Order the case may be referred to the juvenile court for an Interim Care Order to be implemented. This lasts for 28 days but can be repeated until evidence for a Care Order is prepared. A Care Order gives parental rights to the local authority usually until the child is 18.

It is also possible to arrange for voluntary admission into care under Section 1 of the Children Act, 1948. When a child is in the care of the local authority under Section 1, it is possible for the authority to pass a Section 2 resolution to assume parental rights without going to a juvenile court unless the parents then object. A number of other provisions are also available in British Law to protect the rights of children at risk including Supervision Orders, Wardship and Guardianship. Further details of these procedures are available in Clarke Hall and Morrison's Law relating to Children and Young Persons (Jackson *et al.*, 1977.)

Case Examples

The following case examples have been selected as typical examples of patients with clear relationship difficulties with their babies from a series of patients admitted to the Manchester Mother and Baby Psychiatric Unit.

A Severe Bonding Problem

A 25-year-old married woman was admitted briefly to the mother and baby psychiatric unit for assessment of her relationship with her four-month-old son after an attempt to drown him. She described the pregnancy as unplanned and unwanted and had disliked the pregnancy and loss of freedom it entailed. The delivery was induced because of post-maturity. She had been heavily sedated and was not given the baby to hold until the following day. She described herself as uninvolved with the baby, a "spectator" and felt disgust when trying to breast-feed followed by a sense of failure when baby would not feed. She developed some depressive symptoms over the next four months and during this period put a towel over the baby's face and later tried to drown him in his bath. After the attempted drowning she recalled putting the baby in a towel on a chair and ringing the general practitioner in a daze. The doctor was able to save the life of the baby.

Her husband wanted to keep the child although the patient continued to say that she could not control her feelings of rejection and had impulses to kill the child if she were alone with him. A short period of assessment was arranged under very close supervision. The assessment revealed consistent evidence of total rejection. Most of her statements implied rejection or disgust. She often left the ward without arranging supervision for the baby. When accompanied she was physically able to care for the child but described feelings of revulsion and disgust when she had to tend him alone. She held the child at arms' length. There was minimal evidence of psychiatric disturbance other than the features described. She described herself as lacking feminine qualities.

After a brief assessment she and her husband agreed to have the baby adopted. This mother showed complete and consistent rejection of the baby. She may have been predisposed by a disturbed background of violence and an ambivalence about her sexual identity. The baby was unwanted and the abnormal delivery increased the chances of eventual rejection. After the initial assessment and the decision to have the child adopted, no specific treatment to increase the mother's attachment to the baby was attempted.

Spurious Rejection

Many of the presenting features in this example were similar to those in the above example but the assessment and outcome were entirely different. The mother was 32 years old and was admitted for assessment nine days postpartum. Her background had been very strict. She had mild obsessional traits and was sensitive to the opinion of others. The baby had been unplanned and she had considered abortion. Her pregnancy and delivery had been uneventful but had provoked feelings that she "should have been a man." She felt herself to be nasty and incapable of any loving relationship. On admission she was distressed at times but showed no evidence of psychiatric disorder. The nurses observed a marked discrepancy between her statements (for example, "I hate being a mother" "I feel nothing for babies, I hate them"), and her behaviour which was consistently warm, affectionate and practically competent. After a two week admission during which time she talked at length about her fears of being a mother and her fears of losing her identity, she acknowledged increasingly often that she felt warmth for the baby. After discharge she was followed up closely (a review case conference having been held with the social services department, health visitor and general practioners). Within two months at home she felt consistent warmth for the baby, had an improved relationship with her husband and had increasing self esteem.

These two examples have much in common at first sight; both women stating complete rejection for the initially unwanted baby. It was only by observation of discrepancies between the second mother's actions and her statements that it became apparent that this did not represent a true "bonding failure" at all.

Rejection of the Baby in a Setting of Depression

A 32-year-old mother who had previously had a successful professional career was admitted after a six month history of a depressive illness with preoccupying delusions of worthlessness. She expressed resentment about the baby for disrupting her previously settled life. For a few weeks she was separated from the baby because of her intense rejection. After considerable improvement during a three month admission she was eventually discharged home with the baby although anergic depressive symptoms continued. She described at this time a feeling of emptiness and deadness and a total lack of warmth towards her husband and baby. After a period of improvement, she relapsed soon after the child's first birthday with a recurrence of depressive symptoms, but she improved rapidly and returned home where she made further improvement, now seeing her son as an integral part of the family. Previously she had described her care of her son as "lacking spontaneity" or "unnatural" and this feeling continued even when her observed behaviour was normal. The depressive symptoms of deadness and the feeling that life had changed irretrievably for the worse with the birth of this child were the main features of this mother–child relationship. The treatment had been complex, including a long in-patient stay, a behavioural approach to her feelings of disgust for the baby and an individual psychotherapeutic approach focusing on her self-esteem, self-concept and her ability to take control of her life again. No attempt was made to explore any underlying conflicts about her role as a mother as attempts to do this produced increasing feelings of self blame.

A Further Case of Rejection during Depression

A 28-year-old woman had coped well with two previous children. During an unwanted and unplanned pregnancy she avoided antenatal care and made an ambivalent attempt to induce an abortion. She had a complicated premature labour during which she was sedated and was then separated postnatally for two weeks. Three months later she was admitted with depression including intense suicidal ideas. Her care of her child was not grossly abnormal at that time although she expressed regret about having become pregnant and intense guilt that she may have harmed the child through her actions during pregnancy. Over the next two weeks she felt the increasing conviction that the child was not hers in the context of a psychotic depressive illness. She developed auditory hallucinations with a judgmental quality and later became extremely perplexed and fearful. She made a slow recovery over the next year, and although there was still considerable guilt and mixed feelings about the child she was able to care for him competently and affectionately by the time of discharge. In subsequent follow up the content of many of the ideas expressed during the psychotic phase of the illness have become understandable in terms of her early experiences.

Severe bonding problem in the context of depressive, obsessional symptoms and phobic anxiety treated by a behavioural approach

A 27-year-old woman, had been married for a few years and had planned and wanted a baby. Despite some sickness during pregnancy she looked forward to the baby with high expectations of subsequent family life. The baby was born by Caesarean section and she was unable to see the child for about 12 hours. When she did see the baby she thought he looked too big to be newborn and wondered whether he was hers. She also said she recalled hearing under anaesthesic someone saying that the baby was dead. She failed to breast-feed on one occasion and then became frightened to feed the child in case she failed again. In the months postnatally she developed increasing obsessional symptoms focusing on the cleanliness of the baby and also her home. By seven months postpartum she had marked depressive and anxiety symptoms in addition and was admitted to hospital after shaking and smacking the baby and expressing infanticidal ideas.

During the next four years she was treated at various times as an in-patient, day-patient and out-patient for recurrent episodes of depression, tension, anxiety and obsessional symptoms. Throughout this period she felt almost complete rejection of the baby, which was later reinforced by the baby understandably failing to respond to her. Physical treatments included ECT, tricyclic and monoamine oxidase inhibitor antidepressants, and benzodiazepines. There were numerous attempts made at supportive and exploratory, individual and marital psychotherapy. There were several episodes of self-injury and during most of this period the child was cared for by relatives.

When the child was four, a behavioural treatment approach was initiated (Brierley, 1980) using some of the techniques described earlier. The aim was to use the therapy sessions to maximize pleasurable interactions with the child and later to generalize the pleasurable responses to situations outside the sessions, in the hope that this would increase the patient's self-esteem and feelings of competence and would later lead to a more positive affectionate relationship overall. Some of the sessions took place at home initially but her obsessional symptoms in that setting precluded further treatment there until that problem had been resolved in its own right. Some treatment sessions took the form of "outings" (i.e. taking the child out for the day.)

A hierarchy of increasingly difficult interactions was developed from looking at the baby directly, through smiling at him, touching him, dressing him, holding his hand, touching his face, touching faces together and finally kissing. The interactions were structured by the therapist in a number of ways to maintain a relaxed, pleasurable atmosphere, the therapist playing with the mother and child with the therapist taking a more active role when the patient's anxiety increased. A non-judgmental, light-hearted approach was taken by the therapist. Practical details in this form of therapy are very important. For example, the patient at one time lacked ideas for interacting with the child leading to further feelings of failure; one suggestion of telling nursery rhymes was initially unsuccessful until the mother learned some suitable nursery rhymes which allowed her to interact with the child.

Although the aims of therapy had been agreed with the husband and the patient it was necessary for the therapist to prevent competitive interaction from the husband for the baby's attention at times.

The case example illustrates a number of important themes running through this chapter.

(1) A psychiatric illness accentuated pre-existing obsessional traits to a disabling degree and these increased the relationship difficulties.

(2) The relationship between the multiple psychiatric symptoms of depression, tension, generalized and phobic anxiety and the resulting "bonding disorder" is complex and each component needed separate assessment and treatment. Although the results of treatment are tentative the successful resolution of the bonding problem has coincided with a marked reduction in her psychiatric symptoms.

(3) Adverse events around the time of delivery were important precipitants.

(4) After a long period of enforced separation the mother had to learn basic mothering "skills" such as playing with the child, and secondary problems such as the competitive interaction with her husband had to be resolved.

(5) Even after a long period of rejection treatment was effective. However, the needs of the child had to be considered as well. It is becoming customary to build in to treatment programmes a series of review dates at which the development of the child is an important consideration.

(6) This case example raises a major conceptual difficulty; when the mother eventually described herself as feeling "love" for the child, where did this love come from? One view would be that her psychiatric disorder had merely blocked her already present feelings and the behavioural approach was effective because it overcame a series of practical obstacles. A more contentious view would be that she had "learned" to love her child in some way. One component of the treatment may well have been the patient's opportunity to model herself on a therapist who related warmly both to the child and the patient in a setting where she could control her anxiety.

As yet there has been insufficient research to disentangle the effects of psychiatric illness, maternal attitudes and behaviour and the various aspects of treatment. An important prerequisite for future progress is to stop considering normal and abnormal bonding as two discrete categories and to consider separately the components of the bonding process and their relation to psychiatric disorders.

Achnowledgements

I am grateful to Sister Christine Keelan and the nursing staff of the Mother and Baby Psychiatric Unit, University Hospital of South Manchester for helpful discussions and their detailed clinical observations, and to Dr. Brockington who introduced the multidisciplinary assessment of mother–baby interactions. Eileen Brierley, Clinical Psychologist, Trafford and Judy Jackson, Clinical Psychologist, University Hospital of South Manchester have made valuable contributions to the section on behavioural treatment.

References

Aleksandrowicz, M.K. and Aleksandrowicz, D.R. (1974). Obstetric pain-relieving drugs predictors of infant behaviour variability. *Child Dev.* **45**, 935-45.

Ambuel, J. Harris, B. (1963). Failure to thrive: a study of failure to grow in height and weight *Ohio Med. J.* **59**, 997.

Anderson, E.W. (1933). A study of the sexual life in psychoses associated with childbirth. *J. Ment. Sci.* **79**, 137-49.

Baker, A.A. (1962). Puerperal Psychosis in Notes and comments *Br. Med. J.* **1**, 814.

Bärtschi-Rochaix, F. (1937). The position of the child in the delusional system of the mother. *Z. Neurol Psychiat.* **159**, 746.

Batt, J.C. (1948) Homicidal incidence in the depressive psychoses *J. Ment. Sci.* **94**, 782-92.

Bicknell, J. (1981). The psychopathology of mental handicap. Lecture to Department of Psychiatry, University of Manchester, 9 March 1981.

Black, J.A. and Hughes, F. (1979). Legal aspects of child injury or neglect *Br. Med. J.* **2**, 910-2.

Bluglass, R. (1978). Infanticide. *Bull of Royal Coll of Psychiatrists*, August 1978.

Boggs, J.W. (1951). An observational study of mother-infant relationships. Unpublished M.A. Thesis, Washington University 1951.

Bowlby, J. (1977). The making and breaking of affectional bonds: I, Aetiology and Psychopathology in the light of attachment theory. *Br. J. Psychiat.* **130**, 201-210.

Brazelton, T.B. (1969). The effect of prenatal drugs on the behaviour of the neonate. Paper presented to the American Psychol. Assoc., Miami Beach, 1969.

Brew, M. F. and Seidenberg, R. (1950) Psychotic reactions associated with pregnancy and childbirth. *J. Nerv. Ment. Dis.* **111**, 408-23.

Brierley, E. (1980). The treatment of bonding failure. Lecture to conference on puerperal. mental disorders, Manchester 1980.

Budin, P. (1907). *The Nursling.* Caxton, London.

Carver, V. (ed.) (1978). *Child Abuse: A study text.* Open University Press, Milton Keynes.

Chapman, A.H. (1959). Obsessions of infanticide *Arch Gen Psychiat* **1**, 28-31.

Cox, A. (1975). Assessment of parental behaviour *J. Child Psychol. Psychiat.* **16**, 255-9.

DHSS (1975). Non-Accidental injury to children. Proceedings of a conference held at the Department of Health and Social Security, 19 June 1974.

D'Orban, P.T. (1979). Women who kill their children *Br. J. Psychiat.* **134**, 560-71.

Evans, S. Reinhart, J. and Succop, R. (1972). A study of 45 children and their families *J. Am. Acad. of Child Psychiat.* **11**, 440-54.

Fahlberg, V. (1981). What is attachment? *Adoption and fostering* **103**, (i) 17-22. Reprinted from *Attachment and Separation* (1978). Michigan Social Services.

Fanaroff, A.A. Kennell, J.H. and Klaus, M.H. (1972). Follow up of low birth weight infants—the predictive pattern of maternal visiting patterns *Paediatrics* **49**, 288-90.

Freud, A. (1970). The concept of the rejecting mother. In *Parenthood: its psychology and psychopathology* (eds E.J. Reading and T. Benedek). Little Brown, New York.

Frommer, E.A. and O'Shea, G. (1973). Antenatal identification of mothers likely to have difficulty managing their infants. *Br. J. Psychiat.* **123**, 149-56.

Gamer, E. Gallant, D. and Grunebaum, M. (1976). Children of psychotic mothers: an evaluation of one year olds on a test of object permanence *Arch. Gen. Psych.* **33**, 311-7.

Gamer, E., Grunebaum, H., Cohler, B.J. and Gallant, D.H. (1977). Children at risk: performance of three year olds and their mentally ill and well mothers on an interaction test *Child Psychiat. Hum. Dev.* **8** (2), 102-14.

Garmezy, N. (1974). Children at risk: The search for antecedents of schizophrenia Part 1. Conceptual Models and Research Issues *Schizoph. Bull.* **8**, 14-90.

Gibson, E. and Klein, F. (1961). Murder: a Home Office Research Unit Report. HMSO, London.

Gibson, E. (1975). *Homicide in England and Wales. 1967-1971.* Home Office Research Study no 31. HMSO, London.

Gregger, J. and Hoffmeyer, O. (1969). Murder of several children by schizophrenic mothers. *Psychiatria Clinica* **2** (i), 14-24.

Harder, T. (1967). The psychopathology of infanticide *Acta. Psych., Scand* **13**, 196-244.

Helfer, R.E. and Kepe, C.H. (eds) (1974). *The Battered Child* 2nd Ed. University of Chicago Press, Chicago.

Hinde, R.A. (1978). Interpersonal relationships—in quest of a science. *Psychol. Med.* **8**, 373-86.

Hopwood, J.S. (1927) Child Murder and insanity. *J. Ment. Sci.* **73**, 95-108.

Hubert, J. (1974). Belief and reality: social factors in pregnancy and childbirth. *In The Integration of the Child into a Social World* (ed. M.P. Richards). Cambridge University Press, Cambridge.

Jackson, J., Booth, M. and Mains, B. (eds) (1977). *Clarke Hall and Morrisons's Law relating to children and young persons 9th Ed.* Butterworth, London.

Jacobson, L., Kaij, L. and Nilsson, A. (1965). Postpartum mental disorders in an unselected sample: Frequency of symptoms and predisposing factors Br. Med. J. **1**, 1640-3.

Kempe, H. (1962). The battered child syndrome *J. Ame. med. Assoc.* **181**, 17-22.

Klaus, M.H. and Kennell, J.H. (1976). Parent to infant attachment. *In Recent Advances in Paediatrics* (ed. D. Hull). Churchill, London.

Lynch, M.A. (1975). Ill health and child abuse. *Lancet* **ii**, 317.

Lynch, M.A. and Roberts, J. (1977). Predicting child abuse: signs of bonding failure in the maternity hospital *Br. Med. J.* **1**, 624-26.

Lynch, M.A. Roberts, J. and Gordon, M. (1976). Child abuse: early warning in the maternity hospital. *Dev. Med. Child Neurol.* **18**, 759-66.

Lytton, H. (1973). Three approaches to the study of parent-child interactions: ethological, interview and experimental. *J. Ch. Psychol. Psychiat.* **14**, 1-17.

MacDonald, C.F. (1899). "Puerperal insanity: a cursory view for the general practitioner"

Margison, F.R. (1981). Assessing the use of a psychiatric unit for mothers with their babies: Risks to the babies. M.Sc. Thesis, University of Manchester.

Massie, M.D. (1978) Blind ratings of mother-infant interaction in home movies of pre-psychiatric and nomal infants. *Am. J. Psychiat.* **135** (ii), 1371.

Matejcek, Z., Dytrych, Z. and Schuller, V. (1978). Children from unwanted pregnancies. *Acta Psych. Scand.* **57**, 67-90.

Meichenbaum, D. and Goodman, J. (1971). Training impulsive children to talk to themselves: a means of developing self control. *J. Abn. Psychol.* **77**, (i), 115-26.

Morton, J.H. (1934). Female homicides. *J. Ment. Sci.* **80**, 64-74.

Moss, H.A. (1967). Sex, age and state as determinants of mother-infant interaction. *Merrill Palmer Quart.* **13**, 19-36.

Olshansky, S. (1962). Chronic sorrow: a response to having a mentally defective child. *Social Casework* **43**, 190.

Ostwald, P.F. and Regan, P.F. (1957). Psychiatric disorders associated with childbirth. *J. Nerv. Ment. Dis.* **125** (2), 153-65.

Peterson, G.H. and Mehl, L.E. (1978). Some determinants of maternal attachment. *Am. J. Psychiat.* **135** (10), 1168-73.

Reavley, W. and Gilbert, (1976). The behavioural treatment approach to potential child abuse—two illustrative case reports. *Socialwork Today* **7** (6), 166-8.

Reavley, W., Gilbert and Carver, V. (1978). The behavioural approach to child abuse. *In Child Abuse: A study text* (ed. V. Carver). Open University Press, Milton Keynes.

Richards, M.P. and Bernal, J. (1972). An observational study of mother-infant interaction *In Ethological Studies of Child Behaviour* (ed. Blurton Jones). Cambridge University Press, Cambridge.

Roberts, J. (1980). The prediction and prevention of bonding failure. Lecture to Conference on Postpartum Mental Disorders University of Manchester.

Roberts, M.W. and Forehand, R. (1978). The assessment of maladaptive parent-child interaction by direct observation: an analysis of methods. *J. Abn. Child. Psychol.* **6** (2), 257-70.

Robson, K.S. (1967). The role of eye to eye contact in maternal-infant attachment. *J. Child Psychol. Psychiat.* **8**, 13-25.

Robson, K.M. and Kumar, R. (1970). Delayed onset of maternal affection after childbirth. *Br. J. Psychiat.* **136**, 347-53.

Savage, G. (1875). Observations on the insanity of pregnancy and childbirth. *Guy's Hospital Report* **20**, 83-117.

Scarr, S. (1966). Genetic factors in activity motivation *Child Dev.* **37**, 663-73.

Schaffer, H.R. (ed.) (1977). Studies in mother-infant interaction. Proceedings of the Loch Lomond Symposium, Ross Priory, University of Strathclyde, September 1975. Academic Press, London and New York.

Schaffer, H.R. and Emerson, P.E. (1968). Patterns of response to physical contact in early human development. *J. Child Psychol. Psychiat.* **5**, 1-13.

Scott, P.D. (1977). Non-accidental injury to children: memorandum of evidence to the Parliamentary Select Committee on violence in the family. *Br. J. Psychiat.* **131**, 366-80.

Seager, C.P. (1960). A control study of postpartum illness. *J. Ment. Sci.* 106, 214-230.

Shaheen, E., Alexander, D., Truskowsky, M. and Barbero, G. (1968). Failure to thrive: a retrospective profile. *Clinical Paed.* **7**, 225.

Smith, S.M. (1969). *The Battered Child Syndrome.* Butterworth, London.

Sobel, D.E. (1961) Children of schizophrenic patients: preliminary observation on early development. *Am J. Psychiat.* **118**, 512.

Solnit, A.J. and Stark, M.H. (1961). Mourning and the birth of a defective child. *Psychoanalytic Studies of the Child* **16**, 523.

Spitzer, R.L., Endicott, J. and Robins E. (1978). Research diagnostic criteria: rationale and reliability. *Arch. Gen. Psych.* **35**, 773-82.

Stern, E.S. (1948). The Medea complex: the mother's homicidal wishes to her child. *J. Ment. Sci.* **94**, 321.

Tetlow, C. (1955) Psychoses of childbearing. *J. Ment. Sci.* **101**, 629-39.

Uddenberg, N. (1974). Reproductive adaptation in mother and daughter. A study of personality development and adaptation to motherhood. *Acta. Psych. Scand.*, Suppl. 254.

Uddenberg, N. and Englesson, I. (1978). Prognosis of postpartum mental disturbance: A prospective study of primiporous women and their 4½ year old children. *Acta. Psych. Scand.* **58**, 201-12.

West, D.J. (1965) *Murder followed by Suicide.* Heinemann, London.

Zemlick, M.J. and Watson, R.I. (1953). Maternal attitudes of acceptance and rejection during and after pregnancy. *Am. J. Orthopsychiatry* **23**, 570-84.

Zilboorg, G. (1931). Depressive reactions related to parenthood. *Am. J. Psychiat.* **10**, 927.

8

Psychiatric Mother and Baby Units

F. Margison and I. F. Brockington

The Development of Mother and Baby Units

The admission of a child to a mental hospital with its mentally ill mother was pioneered in 1948 by Dr T.F. Main at the Cassel Hospital in Surrey, England.

At the time it was already established practice to allow mothers unrestricted visiting to paediatric wards, and in some hospitals to admit the mother with her sick child. As long ago as 1925 Sir James Spence had founded the Babies Hospital at Newcastle-upon-Tyne with the principal aim that the mothers would nurse their own babies. At the time Main began admitting children with their mothers, the dangers of separating a child from its mother were being spelled out by Spitz (1946), Bowlby (1953) and Robertson (1958). In this climate of opinion, Main (1958) pointed out that

> It seems odd that so much less attention is paid to the disruption in this same mother–child relationship when it is the mother who has to go into hospital.

As a student he had been influenced by Sir James Spence's views that separation was a danger not only to the child, but also to "the mother's confidence in her future capacities as a mother".

> Just as it seemed important to keep a man patient in touch with his job and to treat him for the difficulties he might meet there, so it seemed important that a mother should be kept in touch with her job, and the children who were part of it.

In 1948, therefore, when a patient asked for permission to bring in her toddler son, who had no one else to look after him, he agreed. Gradually the admission of mother and child became a commonplace event in the life of the hospital and by 1955 it had become a condition of admission that mothers should bring their babies and young children with them. At the time of his article in 1958, there were 18 toddlers or infants living "cheek by jowl" with the patients in a 100-bedded hospital. The problems presented by having toddlers around, e.g.

the need for quiet when babies were asleep, for laundry services and for furniture repairs, were gradually worked out by communal discussion involving patients and staff. For example, it was decided that mothers and children should have special mealtimes, that one of the common-rooms would be used as a play-room and that an hour of television time would be reserved for them. Each mother and child lived together in their own room with their own toys and possessions, the hospital "offering independence and providing support only where and when it is necessary". Under these conditions they had admitted up to three children with one mother and occasionally had to arrange classes for older children. Rarely (where the father was also ill) they admitted the whole family. Admission was preceded by a home visit by a senior nursing sister who assessed the need for admitting more than one child and anticipated the nursing problems involved. Initially many patients raised objections, especially in the winter when the children were driven indoors, but strong feelings gradually died down and few restrictions had to be imposed. Hostility of other patients to the children was not a major problem because

> the neurotic patient's difficulties lie mostly in relationships to other adults and rarely preclude the ordinary ambivalent altruistic responses that young children evoke in most people.

Only one patient was refused admission because of their presence—a man with homicidal impulses towards children.

Originally the intention was to treat neurotic women, and the child was admitted simply to make in-patient treatment possible. By 1954, however, they realized they had given themselves "an unusual opportunity for studying disturbances of mothering". As Dr Main points out, "Remarkably little has been written about mothering and its disturbances" and "psychiatry needs opportunities to study severe disturbances of the mother–child relationship".

The psychiatric practice at the Cassel Hospital was mainly concerned with neuroses. Chronic mental illness or severe disturbances leading to compulsory admission were not within its scope. The treatment was mainly by psychotherapy over long periods, and the average length of joint mother–child admission was over six months. From 1955 they started to admit patients with puerperal breakdowns, after consultation with Dr Gweneth Douglas who had worked in a maternity ward at the West Middlesex Hospital with newly delivered mothers who were having difficulty in accepting their babies. However, they only admitted puerperal depression and anxiety states, not patients with "gross confusional insanity or schizophrenia".

Dr Douglas reported her own experience of working with "psychotic mothers" in 1956. One of her premises was that "all cases had one feature in common—hostility to the baby".

> The patient's inability to bear this hostility causes her personality to break up and earlier infantile conflicts to be brought to life so that she becomes psychotic.

She had observed that the illness usually lasted several months and that there was a tendency to relapse as soon as the mother returned home and resumed her maternal duties. Douglas published a series of case reports which appeared to show that joint admission led to lasting cure, confirmed by two years follow-up. She had successfully treated six patients in all and the following is one of the examples she quotes:

> A pretty and intelligent young woman had always been pampered by her family. In childhood she had developed minor ailments without organic cause. She married a man much older than herself and became pregnant after three years. Towards the end she was worried whether she would be able to care for the baby adequately. She felt very inadequate when she got home but managed with much support from relatives until he was six months old, when she became tense and strained and expressed ideas that a film was being made about her and that other people were impersonating her and wearing her clothes. She was admitted to hospital and improved over the course of two weeks. At that time she could give no clear account of her state of mind on admission, and insisted on going home and taking full responsibility for her baby again. When seen in the out-patient clinic a week later she was again withdrawn and said, "Are you going to bury me? Is my baby dead?" She was readmitted and made a rapid superficial recovery. She was then given a course of ECT and deep insulin therapy lasting 3½ months. She left hospital against medical advice and tried once more to look after the child, this time succeeding for several weeks until she become as seriously disturbed as before and had to be readmitted. This time the baby was admitted too, and with psychotherapeutic treatment she gradually took over the care of the baby. She was discharged home after 3 months and remained well, caring for her child during the next 2 years."

Case reports like this are persuasive, though obviously they do not prove that joint admission is instrumental in promoting recovery.

Meanwhile at Banstead Hospital in Surrey, England, Baker *et al.* (1961) had been exploring the possibility of admitting "schizophrenic" mothers with their children. They believed that puerperal schizophrenia had a poor prognosis, and reasoned that it should have a good prognosis because it occurred under stress in mature socially adjusted women. It seemed possible that the poor prognosis was due to the practice of separating mother and infant. In the mid-1950s, therefore, they started studying the interaction between schizophrenic mothers and their children and concluded that they often had a normal emotional response to the babies and, while they might neglect them, rarely made an attempt to harm them. Only half these mothers, however, looked after their babies when they returned home. It was extremely difficult to assess their ability to care for the babies and to advise relatives on the wisdom of giving them this responsibility. For these reasons Baker and his colleagues opened a unit in 1959 capable of taking up to eight mothers, with babies up to one year of age.

They compared the first 20 patients admitted to this unit with a group of 20 treated by the same consultant without their babies. Duration of admission was shorter (11 weeks compared with 17), the relapse rate was less (three compared with 10 in the first six months after discharge) and, most impressively, all 20 returned home to take full care of their babies while seven of the comparison group were unable to do so. Treatment was with ECT and chlorpromazine and the patients admitted with their babies showed more recovery than the comparison group, although they were rather more severely ill on admission. This enterprising team "refused no patient because of the severity of her illness and accepted some patients with catatonic excitement". In addition to their other studies, they carried out a treatment trial which is reported elsewhere in Chapter 3 (p.55).

At the same time an American group at Massachusetts Mental Health Center were also beginning to admit babies with their mentally sick mothers. Their experience, including their nursing and administrative difficulties, is set out at length in a book entitled *Mentally Ill Mothers and Their Children* (Grunebaum *et al.*, 1975), although their first publications appeared 12 years earlier. They begin their account by quoting a custody case from England in 1606 in which a Dr Turner pleads with Lord Therle of Salisbury on behalf of a patient "as melancholick a creature as may bee without total loss of her wittes"). He says,

> Now if her belovedst chyld shold bee geven from her I am in great dowbt my Lord she wold with greef fall clene besydes her selff never to bee recovered by any arte.

As background they explain that the practice of separating psychotic mothers from their children is based on four assumptions: (1) that the psychosis is caused by the mother's inability to deal with her hostility to the child, and her recovery depends upon separating them; (2) the mother is a potential physical and psychological danger to the child; (3) the disturbed behaviour of other patients is also a danger; (4) the presence of young children on the ward would be extremely disruptive to the therapeutic milieu. They had, however, heard of the experience of Dr Main at Cassel Hospital and Dr Douglas at the West Middlesex Hospital in England, and were familiar with some unpublished work of James Haycock at the McLean Hospital, Belmont, Massachusetts involving the admission of the babies of several severely disturbed mothers. They did not regard their patients as suffering from an illness, but rather "as needing help in accomplishing certain tasks in living".

> Their first patient was "a 22-year-old woman who gave birth to a son the day before her college graduation in June 1959. This was a bitter disappointment to her because she wanted to continue her education in anthropology. In childhood she had come under strong pressure from her mother to achieve academic success, and grew up shy with no real friends. She married her husband on the understanding that they would both continue their studies. Her unplanned pregnancy meant that only the husband would be able to do so. During pregnancy, she became depressed and neglected her housework. Her husband took over, but in a critical spirit. After a difficult delivery her younger sister helped her, but the baby became ill and had to have surgery for pyloric stenosis. He recovered from the operation and became a charming, lively child, but his mother felt increasingly inadequate as a wife and mother and became seriously depressed with marked depersonalization ("My mind is full of sand"). She was admitted to hospital in September 1960, when her baby was 15 months old. Immediately the problem arose of who would look after the baby, and it was resolved after much debate by admitting him too, into a single room shared with his mother. They were in hospital for 4 months, during which time she had individual psychotherapy dealing with her anger towards her husband and her hatred of the baby,

motherhood and womanhood. At the same time she could observe the nurses and occupational therapists playing with him, and gradually she also played with him until they were all having 'a wonderful time together.' This also helped her in her relationship with her husband because she came to feel that the one thing she could do better than him was to be a mother and care for the baby.

Grunebaum and colleagues subsequently admitted 19 other mothers to their wards, and stimulated the interest of Dr Van der Walde who began a similar experiment in a large public mental hospital nearby; this was described in an article by Van der Walde and colleagues in 1968. Between autumn 1964 and spring 1966, nine joint admissions were made to a private room on a closed 45-bed female ward. They describe how the initial anxiety, ambivalence and resistance on the part of the administration, nursing staff, doctors, patients and relatives was replaced by a general increase in morale and even a receptiveness to other new ideas.

Another pioneering unit was established at Shenley Hospital near St. Albans, England in 1959 (Glaser, 1962). The theoretical background stressed the feelings of guilt experienced by mothers separated from their young children, even when this was due to unavoidable circumstances.

> If the separation is prolonged, there is a gradual slackening of longing and concern for the children, and this also precipitates guilt feelings, which may make a mother reluctant to resume the care of her young children.

They converted an empty ward into a specialized unit with 5–10 beds and a large playroom for the children. The mothers shared the facilities and group activities of the other patients. The first admission was a young mother with a seven-month-old baby, suffering from mild puerperal depression. By 1962, 20 mothers had been admitted for an average period of 3–4 months. Some of them were suffering from psychotic illness, exacerbations of which occasionally required transfer to another ward. When this happened the babies remained on the unit, in one case for as long as 6 weeks without the mother. However, Glaser (1962) gives her opinion that

> A mothers' and babies' unit, as described in this paper, can only cope with patients who have passed the acute stage of their illness and are willing and able to look after their children.

She suggests the creation of a combined obstetric and psychiatric unit for mothers who were mentally ill at the time of delivery, or who were at very high risk of an early puerperal breakdown.

Later papers (Bardon *et al.*, 1968; Bardon, 1977) describe experience of 193 and 633 admissions to this unit. By that time the facility had extended to 10 single rooms, a nursery, playroom and communal sitting room, looked after by two sisters and two assistant nurses working on opposing shifts. The majority of the patients were admitted with illnesses starting during pregnancy or the puerperium (i.e. within 12 months of childbirth) but others were admitted with long-standing personality disorders, neuroses or schizophrenia having no relationship to pregnancy, but in whom separation from their children would have been harmful. Although neither paper gives details of the ages of the babies, it is clear that they were prepared to admit children aged two years or over and to admit more than one child if necessary. The babies slept with their mothers, unless they were acutely disturbed in which case they slept in the nursery for a few nights. No actively infanticidal patient was admitted, but one instance of infanticide occurred. The average length of hospital admission for mothers becoming ill during pregnancy or the puerperium was about seven weeks. Two patients committed suicide during a relapse out of hospital, and one was found drowned in her bath, perhaps during a syncopal attack. Although, as they point out, they could not prove that their unit provided better treatment for puerperal psychosis than could be obtained elsewhere, it was certainly feasible to admit such mothers with their babies.

Another early unit was started in 1963 in Derby (Fowler and Brandon, 1965). This was again part of a larger ward with 2–5 joint admissions on a 20-bedded "villa". The interconnecting doors were sound-proofed to prevent the other patients being disturbed at night. They compared the length of stay of the first 33 patients admitted with that of women admitted without their babies and found it was shorter (44 days compared with 75).

Mitchell and Turton (1966) describe the admission of older children with their mothers to an adult psychiatric ward at Park Prewitt Hospital, in Hampshire. All categories of patient (schizophrenic, psychoneurotic) were admitted to a 25-bedded short-stay ward together with their children. The average number of children present at any one time was eight and the maximum 13. At least 17 of the first 50 mothers were admitted with more than one child. Eleven of the children were under the age of six months, four between six and twelve months, 16 between one and two years, seven between two and three years, 12 between three and four years and 17 between four and five years. The children rapidly fitted into the routine of the ward and enjoyed themselves; there was no evidence of their being even minimally upset by adult schizophrenic patients and no incidents of "schizophrenic aggression" occurred. Those children who were emotionally disturbed before admission (especially those cared for by inadequate and immature mothers) appeared to improve and became more easy to handle.

None of the above-mentioned pioneering ventures involved admission of children to a psychiatric day hospital. This was undertaken by Masson et al. (1977) in Lausanne. They describe the admission of 16 children, 14 with their mothers and two with their fathers, to a 20-patient Day Centre over the course of nine months in 1974–5. The parents were suffering from a variety of illnesses including psychoses and neurotic depression, and the children were mostly ill themselves, 10 with depression, one with extreme agitation, three with language retardation, two with striking "hyper-maturity" and two with physical illness; six of them had been battered by their parents. Ten of the children were over three years old, including two over six years old. Their message is the same—that joint admission was well tolerated by the children, the other patients and the staff.

A number of other articles have been published, describing joint admission programmes in Premontre in France (Racamier *et al.*, 1961), New York City (Schuurmans, 1966), Baltimore (Luepker, 1972), Auckland (Lindsay, 1975) and Jerusalem (Mester *et al.*, 1975). In 1978 Lindsay and Pollard published a follow-up study of 244 mothers admitted to their unit in New Zealand during a period of eight years (1965–72).

The conclusion of these pioneering studies is that joint admission can be achieved harmoniously without placing an impossible burden on the nursing staff, without an obviously increased risk of injury to the children, and without adverse effect on the mental health of the mothers, the children or the other patients. These conclusions apply to a variety of different settings—mixed wards with one or a few rooms given over to the mothers, day hospitals and purpose-built separate units—and a variety of diagnoses (schizophrenia and puerperal psychoses on the one hand, psychoneurotic disorders on the other). The fact that the children themselves are emotionally disturbed is no bar, and children of all ages up to six or even beyond have tolerated joint admission.

The remainder of this chapter will examine more closely the scope and value, and the special problems of such units, based on experience of the unit at the University Hospital of South Manchester (Withington Hospital) in England. This is a nine-bedded unit detached from, but close to, other psychiatric wards in a comprehensive psychiatric unit of about 240 beds, itself part of a District General Hospital with obstetric, paediatric and other services. The unit was opened in 1972 and has now admitted over 500 women and their babies up to 12 months old.

How Safe are Psychiatric Mother and Baby Units?

One of the risks of any hospital is cross-infection. Babies are particularly prone to gastrointestinal infections and on neonatal wards there is a policy of a division of labour, so that those preparing the feeds are not also changing the nappies and doing the laundry. This policy conflicts with one of the main aims of psychiatric mother and baby units—to preserve the mother's caretaking role so far as possible. The danger of gastrointestinal epidemics is therefore ever present. Margison found that 101 out of 245 babies had physical illnesses which required the attentions of a doctor. Of these, 27 were associated with injury (including non-accidental) 13 were congenital malformations, and nine others were disorders of early life not readily attributable to the environment on the ward (failure to thrive, lactose intolerance, transient jaundice). There were 75 instances of infections, as shown in Table 1.

It can be seen that upper respiratory infections were the most frequent, but

Table 1. Cases of Infection on the Manchester Unit.

	No. of incidents	Severe incidents
Gastroenteritis	23	11
Upper respiratory infection	24	4
Monilia	14	Nil
Salmonella carrier state	8	Nil
Urinary tract infection	3	Nil
Otitis media	2	Nil
Pyrexial skin infection	1	Nil

that gastrointestinal infections were more often severe. In all, 15 babies had to be transferred to paediatric care. All the babies recovered without sequelae. The figure of 15 severe infections out of 245 admissions is not negligible. However, it is hard to assess its significance without comparative data on the frequency of such infections at home when the baby is looked after by its mentally ill mother or other relatives.

In Manchester, gastrointestinal infection sometimes occurred in outbreaks, usually due to a rotovirus. Several babies would be affected, and perhaps one or two transferred to a neonatal ward for treatment. On these occasions we had the dilemma of deciding whether or not to close the unit. This would have been extremely disruptive to the psychiatric care of the mothers already in the unit. In these instances, therefore, our policy was to transfer the sick baby to a paediatric unit and to warn the consultant psychiatrists and general practitioners, seeking admission of a patient, of the risks to the baby (particularly to a very small baby). At the same time we consulted with the infectious diseases service and the paediatricians about the seriousness of the infection and the best means of dealing with it, and jointly took a decision whether or not to close the ward (so far, in all cases, not to close). We searched for the source and, if one of the mothers or her baby was a carrier, we raised this matter with the consultant in charge. Finally we arranged that all babies' feeds would be prepared centrally by one person not concerned with the general care of the babies. As a prophylactic measure it was routine to examine the stools of mothers and babies on admission to check for the presence of pathogens. Clearly the risk of infection must be one of the concerns of those running these units, and it is one reason for their being placed in close proximity to general hospitals with their laboratories and neonatal or paediatric units.

Mental illness is sometimes associated with violence. This violence may arise out of loss of control over emotion (as in mania), through despair (in depressive psychosis) and through delusional misinterpretation (in paranoid, schizophrenic and confusional illnesses); it is also a feature of personality disorder. All these kinds of mental disturbance are to be found on psychiatric mother and baby units, and one must be extremely concerned about the risks to babies of residing on wards which contain potentially aggressive persons.

The literature quoted so far has conveyed the impression that these units are safer than one might expect. There have, however, been two reported fatal incidents. Bardon (1977) reported one case of infanticide in 633 admissions, and Lindsay and Pollard (1978) one case of child murder by a 19-year-old unstable adolescent (not his mother) in a fit of rage because she was told drugs were not allowed on the ward. Bardon also reported 10 other incidents of violence by mother upon her own child "to a degree that caused concern".

Margison (1981) has examined the risks to the baby in study of 245 patients admitted to the Manchester unit over a five-year period. The sources of information were the hospital case notes (with their detailed nursing and medical reports), social reports, case conferences on non-accidental injury (NAI), cross infection data, hospital incident reports and regional statistical reports. There were 37 instances of possible NAI to a baby. The question arises in a retrospective study whether this was a low estimate. Cross-checking with the hospital incident records showed that eight of the 11 more severe incidents were documented in the incident reports and that no incidents were found which were not already recorded in the case notes. An additional source of information were the research records which were kept by nurses during one year of the study. All incidents recorded in these files were also found in the case records. It is, therefore, unlikely that any episodes of moderate or severe risk to the child were not reported in the case notes.

The 37 incidents included four episodes of throwing the baby on the cot, two of throwing him elsewhere, three of trying to suffocate him and the rest were more trivial incidents, e.g. shaking or slapping the baby. In addition, there were five other attacks which did not lead to injury because the patient was restrained, and one incident of the baby being dangled by the arm without injury. In all, 21 babies were involved, eleven of them only once and eight twice; one mother attacked her baby on four occasions, one serious assault preceded by three minor ones; another made six minor assaults none resulting in injury. In both of these cases of multiple attacks, the baby was eventually received into the care of the Local Authority.

Another way of looking at these assaults is by assessing their severity. The risk to the baby was minimal in 10 cases (e.g. slapping or shaking, rough handling, throwing him into the cot without violence); it was judged moderate in eight (throwing him into the cot violently, shaking or slapping violently, or attempting to smother him in the presence of nurses), and it was judged severe in three instances. In one incident a baby was thrown at least six feet across the room by a manic patient who thought he was invincible (fortunately in the direction of a nurse who caught him). In another, an attempt was made to kill a baby by suffocating him with a plastic bag. The third was the most serious: the mother had already made several attacks on members of staff and three on the baby and then managed suddenly to push him off her lap onto the floor in the presence of two nurses. This was the only baby to suffer injury (i.e. the only instance of actual harm in the 245 admissions); he sustained a parietal skull fracture from which he made an unevenful recovery.

The matter can also be viewed from the standpoint of maternal diagnosis. Only three of the 21 mothers who attacked their babies were suffering from puerperal psychosis (defined for the purpose of this study as an illness starting within four weeks of delivery); thus the puerperal psychotic patients had significantly less risk of harming their babies ($P = < 0.05$).

The results confirm that the babies are at risk, but that real injury is remarkably uncommon on these wards full of disturbed women. No doubt this is largely due to the vigilance of the nursing staff on this unit, maintained over a period of years at a high level. Rarely, however, a major incident occurs. Bearing in mind the skull fracture sustained by one of our babies and the two babies who have been killed on these units in the past 30 years, is the risk unacceptable? Unfortunately there are no data to make an informed judgement on this point. It is possible that other serious injuries have not been reported and a more extensive survey of serious injuries sustained on mother and baby units should be made. Secondly the risk of joint admission must be compared to the risks of leaving the baby at home, either in the care of its mentally ill and potentially aggressive mother or with others who may not be in a position to provide a high standard of care. Thirdly, Margison's data shows that the question has to be considered separately for puerperal psychotic women and those with other diagnoses. The former group are admitted at an earlier stage and their babies may be more vulnerable to gastrointestinal infections, but they are less likely to be harmed by their mothers. The risks of non-accidental injury are higher in mothers with depression, personality disorders or "bonding failure".

Is it possible to minimize the risk by setting up procedural rules for admission and care? Following the serious incident at Manchester it was decided that the unit could not care for mothers who *both* were psychotic *and* had already harmed their baby or attempted to harm him. It was believed that the unit could cope with non-psychotic mothers who had harmed their babies, and with mothers who had recovered from their psychosis even if they had acted dangerously during the psychosis, but the combination seemed to present too high a risk. Furthermore, after admission, certain mothers should never be left alone with their babies, (e.g. some with bonding disturbances, see Chapter 5); they should sleep apart from them, and should see them only in the presence of two nurses. As the clinical condition improves and the risk falls, protective cover is gradually withdrawn. Margison's data suggest a rider to these guidelines, namely that mothers who have attempted to harm their babies more than twice should not be allowed to care for them even under the intensive nursing supervision of these units until treated and cured of their psychiatric illnesses, but this rather drastic policy perhaps requires more backing in experience than is provided by the two patients in this category encountered in the five years under study.

How Expensive are these Units?

A psychiatric mother and baby unit is a pleasant place for doctors and nurses to work. Mothers with young children seem a particularly important group to treat and they often do extremely well, so these wards tend to have a high morale. However, there are considerable logistic problems. The Manchester Unit, for example, was intended as a regional unit meeting the needs of the North Western Region of the United Kingdom, with its four million inhabitants. Of these rather more than one million live a considerable distance away (in Lancaster, Blackpool, Preston, Blackburn, Burnley or Ormskirk) but the rest are concentrated within the conurbation of Manchester, Salford and surrounding towns (Stockport, Tameside, Trafford, Bolton, Bury, Oldham, Rochdale and Wigan), all within 30 miles. It was reasonable to expect that the specialist service would meet the needs of this large concentration of people, but in fact the admission statistics show that relatively few patients were admitted from North Manchester and the surrounding towns. Eighty-one percent of the parents come from seven areas near the unit (Manchester North, Central and South, Stockport, Salford, Tameside and Trafford) and only 10% from elsewhere in the Region (the remainder being admitted from outside the Region). Analysed by distance, 159 (65%) came from within 10 miles of the unit and a further 56 (23%) from 11–15 miles away, 24 (10%) from 16–20 miles away and only six patients from further afield. Furthermore, the average bed occupancy of the unit was not high. Built to house nine patients and their babies, it took three years (1972–5) to reach an average level of "half-full" (4.9 in 1975), and thereafter it climbed to a peak of 6.5 beds occupied (72%) in 1977. Even in that year it was full for only 35 days. In summary, on the average, only six beds were required for an effective catchment area of 2 million.

The unit requires regular staffing at the level of two nurses by day and one by night. In addition, nursery nurses are necessary (unless other nurses can be trained to do the job) to look after the babies of mothers temporarily unable to provide adequate care. The need for their help is shown by the fact that 143 of the 245 Manchester mothers required extensive supplementary care for their babies, 66 of them had to be separated from the infant at some stage and 62 (25%) showed prolonged incompetence, i.e. lasting at least eight weeks. At least one nursery nurse is required during the day. If the unit is placed within the confines of a psychiatric hospital, staffing problems are eased because at times of crisis additional nurses can be mobilized, and at slack periods, the unit can return these favours. This also enables the transfer of highly disturbed patients to intensive care, a resource which was required in 22 (9%) of the Manchester patients for at least a week. In order to provide the minimum level of three nurses and one nursery nurse per 24 hours, bearing in mind holidays, sick leave and study leave, an establishment of five day nurses, two night nurses and three nursery nurses is required, i.e. ten staff of all kinds for nine beds (1.1 nurses/patient). This is a very high ratio. In the same hospital a similar number of staff were required for a 24-bedded general psychiatric ward, whose bed occupancy was over 85%. The mothers and babies unit cared for 50 admissions per year, and the general ward 200 admissions. It is hard to avoid the conclusion that these units are at least three times as expensive per patient treated, but such preliminary figures make no allowance for the cost of providing alternative care for the babies, a few of whom may be ill in their own right.

How Useful are these Units?

The question of the positive value of these units is a complicated one, because the answer is different for each of several categories of patients treated. It seems appropriate, first, to deal with non-psychotic patients because these are the group who were historically the first to be admitted with their babies (by Main in 1948), and because their relationship problems with the baby often provide an obvious justification for joint admission. The theoretical background is clear, and has been stated by Main (1958) and Glaser (1962). Hospital admission is a treatment with its own side-effects, one of the most important being the atrophy of skills and the loss of confidence in one's ability to carry out a job and the tasks of daily living. A mother needs to remain, so far as possible, in touch with her normal role. If her mental distress is particularly associated with that role, even caused by abnormal or hostile feelings about motherhood and her baby it seems especially dangerous to take her out of the situation because she can hardly learn to live with it in the context of abstract discussion, and avoidance of the difficulties may make it even more difficult for her to cope when she returns home. The mother and baby unit provides an ideal opportunity for focusing treatment on a disordered relationship. The nature of the difficulties can be directly observed and accurately diagnosed. The mother can readily ventilate her emotions, and express her obsessional thoughts, preoccupations and misinterpretations almost as they occur. Perhaps most importantly she can observe other mothers interacting with their babies and other staff interacting with her baby. She can thus learn by direct observation how to care for and play with him, and thus receive the powerful reinforcement which a baby provides for those who please him. Not only is the milieu of the unit a great opportunity for providing this specific treatment, but it is hard to imagine any other way of providing it. The alternative would be to introduce a highly skilled professional person (nurse, social worker, doctor or psychologist) into the patient's home. Caring for mothers with difficulties in their relationship with their babies is the most obvious function of such a unit. It is also appropriate to admit mothers with psychiatric illness (usually depression) associated with other environmental difficulties such as an unhappy marriage or the lack of support from a husband or family, but no obvious problem in their feelings for the baby. Removal from the baby runs a high risk in these women of complicating their already considerable burden by adding the relationship problems which may develop during the period of separation.

In the Manchester unit, non-psychotic women comprised approximately half of the admissions; 47% of the mothers were in this group, of whom the majority (32% of all admissions) were suffering from major depressive illness, as defined by the Research Diagnostic Criteria. Thus an average of three beds per year apparently sufficed to meet this need in a population of 2 million. This figure is probably a considerable underestimate. Data presented elsewhere in Chapter 4 show that there is widespread depression among mothers of young children. The reason why they form so small a part of the work of the Manchester unit is probably because it is not adapted to their needs. It is an in-patient unit which cannot take babies over 12 months of age. Many of the depressed mothers have several young children, and their depression is not so severe (e.g. with delusions, severe biological symptoms or suicidal risk) that in-patient admission is judged necessary. What is required for the care of these women is a day hospital with day nursery where older children can be cared for, together with the provision of domiciliary visiting by appropriately trained nursing staff or social workers. The role of the in-patient unit would be to admit the most severe cases, and to train the staff in the diagnosis and care of mental illness or psychological disturbance in mothers.

Among the many unhappy and neurotic mothers there are a few who neglect or abuse their children. Unfortunately the mother and baby unit does not appear to be an appropriate place for the care of mothers who have actually "battered" their babies. At the present stage of uncertainty and unease about the safety of these units following the recent report of two non-accidental deaths, there must be a period when admission of potentially dangerous mothers is viewed conservatively. Ideally the unit should care for all types of mental disturbance within its field of interest, and it may eventually be able to do so, but not until further research has been carried out on the diagnosis and management of mothers at high risk.

The second large group of women treated on these units are those with puerperal psychosis. Although this is an uncommon illness, it accounts for about one third of the admissions (38% of the 245 studied by Margison). This disease, therefore, requires on the average only two beds to supply the needs of 2 million catchment population. In this group it is much less obvious that the unit serves a useful purpose. At Manchester certainly it has given the academic staff an opportunity to study puerperal psychosis, but this does not establish the service need. The risks to the baby appear to be less in these patients because the main risk comes from the mother rather than other patients and these mothers are not (as a rule) hostile to their babies. The babies are younger, however, and more vulnerable to infection. The pioneering work on admitting these women (Baker et al., 1961) was based on the idea that the poor prognosis was due to the practice of separating mother and baby, and their study provided some evidence that the mother–baby pairs fared better when jointly admitted. They were mistaken in believing that puerperal psychosis has a bad prognosis—all the evidence shows that it has an exceptionally good prognosis (see Chapter 3)—and their interesting findings have not yet been confirmed by other groups because no one else has researched the matter. Our own non-systematic observations seem to show that psychotic mothers often relate well to their babies during the illness, and have no difficulty in establishing a normal bond when they recover. The most obvious advantage of joint admission in these women is the convenience to the families. The birth of a new baby is always a difficult time for a family, and the difficulties are compounded by the absence of the mother. Often there is no one to take over and according to Bardon (1977) 116 children were taken into care in the North Western Metropolitan Region of London because of the admission of 75 mothers with puerperal illness during a 12-month period. The case for admitting babies with puerperal psychotic mothers, therefore, is less obvious than for mothers with late onset depressions, though later research may show that it has important benefits.

Another group of patients admitted to the Manchester unit is a small group of non-puerperal psychoses (15% of the admissions). A typical example would be a long-stay schizophrenic patient who became pregnant. The unit is an ideal solution to the management of such a patient who would otherwise have to be discharged from hospital, or deprived of her baby without even a trial of caring for him.

Finally, the unit has to some extent been used for the assessment of maternal competence and attitudes. Requests have been received from social services to admit mothers in whom there is uncertainty whether they can or should be given the custody of their babies. A well staffed unit with 24 hour observation is an ideal place to make this assessment and (as explained in Chapter 5) an observation routine was developed to enable an assessment to be made within 1–2 weeks. However, this is not work which the staff enjoy doing, because the orientation of nursing staff is towards treatment rather than assessment. We have taken a cautious approach and only been willing to undertake such an assessment if there was a definite possibility that the mother was mentally ill.

Conclusions

The introduction of the joint admission of mentally ill mothers and their normal babies or children had been an interesting development, mainly in Britain, since 1948. There have been two main streams of experience. One is the admission of babies and children up to the age of eight to general wards or day hospitals caring mainly but not exclusively for neurotic patients, these mothers and their babies comprising only a small proportion of the clientele. These units are appropriate wherever the population density is low. The problem has been to negotiate the policy of joint admission with the administration, with the nursing staff and with the other patients.

The other stream has been concerned with the specialized mother and baby unit. These units appear to work well, but are expensive. There is a case for developing them in any large city of, say, one million inhabitants. If they are restricted, however, to in-patient services and to babies under the age of one year (as at Manchester) they are bound to be very limited in scope; for example the Manchester unit provides treatment for only 50 patients a year at the most. There is a need for more research on the therapeutic effectiveness and the risks of both kinds of unit.

The present writers take the view that psychiatric mother and baby units are an innovation of considerable promise, but that their full potential has not yet been realized. An ideal unit would be located in a densely populated area, near its geographical centre. Because some of the psychotic mothers may, at least temporarily, be highly disturbed, it should be sited near to a general psychiatric unit. Because the mothers and babies are liable to medical illness, e.g. infections, it should form part of a general hospital. This ideal unit (which, to our knowledge, does not exist at the moment) should include day hospital and day nursery services as well as an in-patient unit, so that it can care for older children as well as babies, and for mothers with moderate levels of psychiatric disturbance not requiring admission. Such a unit could serve as a training centre enabling nurses and other professionals to obtain skills and experience which they could use in providing a domiciliary and community service as well as in-patient and day patient care. This is the kind of unit which would best serve the needs of the community, and such a unit would probably be more cost-effective, in that the same number of staff would treat or help a larger number of patients. There is a need to create a few units of this kind to explore their usefulness and cost effectiveness. As psychiatry becomes more differentiated and specialized, such units could serve a valuable function, but we need more empirical investigation and experience before we can recommend a general deployment of scarce resources in this way.

References

Baker, A.A., Morison, M. Game, J.A. and Thorpe. J.G. (1961). Admitting schizophrenic mothers with their babies. *Lancet* **ii**, 237-239.

Bardon, D. Glaser, Y.I.M., Prothero, D. and Weston D.H. (1968). Mother and baby unit: psychiatric survey of 115 cases. *Br Med. J.* **2**, 755-758.

Bardon, D. (1977). A mother and baby unit in a psychiatric hospital. *Nursing Mirror*

238   F. Margison and I.F. Brockington

(December 8th), 30-33.
Bowlby, J. (1953). *Child Care and the Growth of Love.*, Pelican Books, Harmondsworth.
Douglas, G. (1956). Psychotic mothers. *Lancet* **i**, 124-125.
Fowler, D.B. and Brandon, R.E. (1965). A psychiatric mother and baby unit. *Lancet* **i**, 160-161.
Glaser, Y.I.M. (1962). A unit for mothers and babies in a psychiatric hospital. *J. Child Psychol. Psychiat.* **3**, 53-60.
Grunebaum, H. Weiss, J.L., Cohler, B.J., Hartman, C.R. and Galland, D.H. (1975). *Mentally Ill Mothers and Their Children.* University of Chicago, Chicago.
Lindsay, J.S.B. (1975). Puerperal psychosis: a follow-up study of a joint mother and baby treatment programme. *Aust. N.Z.J. Psychiat.* **9**, 73-76.
Lindsay, J.S.B. and Pollard, D.E. (1978). Mothers and children in hospital. *Aust. N.Z.J. Psychiat.* **12**, 245-253.
Luepker, E.T. (1972). Joint admission and evaluation of postpartum psychiatric patients and their infants. *Hosp. Community Psychiat.* **23**, 284-286.
Main, T.F. (1958). Mothers with children in a psychiatric hospital. *Lancet* **ii**, 845-7.
Margison, F.R. (1981). Assessing the use of a psychiatric unit for mothers and their babies: risks to the babies. M.Sc. Thesis, University of Manchester.
Masson, D. Fivaz, E. and Ciola, A. (1977). Expérience d'hospitalisation conjointe mère-enfant dans un centre de traitement psychiatrique de jour (hôpital du jour) pour adultes. *Archives Suisses de Neurologie, Neurochirurgie et Psychiatrie* **120**, 83-100.
Mester, R. Klein, H. Lowental, U. (1975). *Israeli Annals of Psychiatry and Related Disciplines* **13**, 124-136.
Mitchell, N. and Turton, C. (1966). Children under five on an adult psychiatric ward. *Br. J. Psychiat.* **112**, 1117-1118.
Racamier, P.C., Sens, C. Carretier, L. (1961). La mère et l'enfant dans les psychoses du post-partum. *Evolution Psychiatrique* **26**, 525-570.
Robertson, J. (1958). Film: *A Two-Year Old Goes to Hospital.* Tavistock, London.
Schuurmans, M.J. (1966). The psychotic mother and the healthy infant on the psychiatric unit. *Persp. Psychiat. Care* **4**, 22-26.
Spitz, R.A. (1946). *Anaclitic Depression.* IUP, New York.
Van der Walde, P.H., Meeks, D. Grunebaum, H.U. and Weiss, J.L. (1968). Joint admission of mothers and children to a state hospital. *Arch. General Psychiat.* **18**, 706-711.

9

Drug Addiction and Psychotropic Drug Treatment during Pregnancy and Lactation

I.F. Brockington and R. Kumar

Introduction

Whenever drugs are prescribed to a pregnant or lactating woman, the foetus is put at risk in a number of different ways. Some drugs may cause mutations, affecting the ovum even before fertilization (mutagenicity), or they may cause toxic damage during the first few weeks of intra-uterine life, killing the foetus (miscarriage) or causing major malformations (teratogenicity). Drugs can sometimes have toxic effects during the later stages of pregnancy, resulting in foetal death *in utero*, or in impaired growth. Towards the end of pregnancy they may precipitate labour through toxic effects on the mother, for example, by increasing uterine irritability, resulting in the birth of a premature baby with increased risks of perinatal mortality, mental retardation and mother–baby bonding disturbances. If prescribed during labour they may intoxicate the newborn, causing breathing and sucking difficulties. If prescribed or abused for some time before delivery, they may induce drug dependence in the infant who can then develop withdrawal symptoms after delivery. If prescribed to a lactating mother, certain drugs may be excreted in the milk and exert toxic effects on the baby in this way. Finally, a drug's adverse effects may not declare themselves in the child for years, as in the case of diethylstilboestrol or dienoestrol given during pregnancy which carries an increased risk of vaginal malignancy in female offspring when they reach adolescence and, similarly, it has been suggested that prolonged behavioural and psychological consequences may be found in the children of women who have taken certain drugs during pregnancy.

In this chapter we will review various drugs of psychiatric interest, starting with drugs of addiction or abuse (alcohol, nicotine, barbiturates, opiates, lysergic acid diethylamide, cannabis), and then consider some psychotropic agents

239

(lithium, neuroleptics, tricyclic antidepressants and benzodiazepines) and electroconvulsive therapy. The authoritative reviews of Nishimura and Tanimura (1976) on teratogenicity, Ananth (1978) and Arena (1980) on breast feeding, Glass and Evans (1979) on drug abuse and the more general reviews by Goldberg and DiMascio (1978) and Hill and Stern (1979) are the main sources of information.

Drug Dependence and Abuse

Alcohol

The teratogenicity of alcohol was first suspected by Lemoine and his colleagues at Nantes in France; for several years before their report (1968) they had been impressed by the resemblance between children born to "alcoholic" mothers. Their report concerned 127 cases from 69 families in 29 of which both parents were alcoholic, in 25 only the mother and in 15 (less well documented) only the father was alcoholic. The four characteristics which they noticed in the children were: unusual facial appearance, short stature, frequent malformations and psychomotor disturbance. Seeing these children sometimes led them to diagnose previously unsuspected maternal alcoholism, and "social enquiries always confirmed the fact."

The same discovery was made independently at the University of Washington in Seattle. Ulleland (1972) observed a number of small infants, who were admitted with failure to thrive and failed to grow even when given special attention to their feeding and care. She then collected 47 undergrown infants from 1641 pregnancies and found that 10 of them were born to chronic alcoholic women; the frequency of low birth weight was 2.3% in the non-alcoholics and 83% (10 out of 12) in the alcoholics. A team at Seattle embarked on a systematic study of the children of alcoholics, and by 1974 had collected 11 cases, six of whom were American Indian. They were all small for dates and failed to catch up after birth. They had low IQs and most were tremulous and poorly coordinated. Among the congenital malformations the most common were short palpebral fissures (indicating deficiencies in eye growth) and maxillary hypoplasia (small nose, hypoplastic upper lip and thin vermilion border). In 1976 they reported 41 cases of the "Fetal Alcoholism Syndrome". All of the mothers were "chronic alcoholics" and most had secondary complications such as cirrhosis, gastritis, pancreatitis and delirium tremens. Microcephaly with head circumference more than two standard deviations below the mean was found in 90%, and 44% had mental retardation. Malformations in other organs were common, for example 20 (49%) had cardiac anomalies. By 1979 Smith had collected 618 cases from the world literature, including a large series from Tübingen in West Germany (Bierich *et al.*, 1976).

Post mortem studies in these infants have been reported by Smith (1979) and Peiffer *et al.* (1979). There were no constant pathological findings, but neuroglial heterotopias, cerebellar dysplasia and absent corpus callosum were all reported more than once in the 10 cases.

Clinical reports of this kind must be substantiated by prospective surveys demonstrating an association between maternal drinking and foetal damage. There have been at least two large surveys. Kaminski *et al.* (1978) followed through 9236 women of whom 5.5% were heavy drinkers. The heavy drinkers were older, of lower social class, more often unmarried, of higher parity and more often smokers. They had more bleeding in early pregnancy and more stillbirths. Birth weight was slightly lower, but there was no increase in neonatal mortality or congenital malformations. Sokol *et al.* (1980) followed through 12 127 pregnancies of which 204 were complicated by maternal alcoholism. The same associated risk factors were present as in the French study (older, separated, smoking etc.). Bleeding during the first or second trimester was increased (17.3% compared with 6.2%, $P < 0.0001$). The mean birth weight was only slightly reduced (2903 g compared with 3090 g) but the number born under 2500 g was increased (31.3% compared with 19.6%, $P < 0.0005$), in spite of the fact that the babies were not premature; 11.3% were small for their gestational age, compared with 4.2% in the controls ($P < 0.00001$). Neonatal infection was more common (7.1% compared with 0.6%, $P < 0.001$). There was an increase in oral and genito-urinary abnormalities and 38% had some form of congenital abnormality. Only five infants (2.5%) had the full foetal alcohol syndrome. These surveys suggest that maternal alcoholism has to be severe (or possibly severe at a particular time) to cause teratogenic effects.

The foetus is likely to be most "at risk" during the early stages of pregnancy when many women may not be aware that they have recently conceived. Women who reduce their consumption to "moderate" levels or those who continue to take moderate amounts of alcohol have smaller babies and this effect is independent of tobacco smoking (Hanson *et al.*, 1976; Little, 1977; Oullette *et al.*, 1977). Little *et al.* (1980) found evidence that babies born to former alcoholic women who abstained during pregnancy still showed evidence of intra-uterine growth retardation, with birth weights of 3137 g average, compared with 3391 g for normal women and 2898 g for current alcoholics. Rosett *et al.* (1980), however, compared the babies of 25 women who reduced their drinking during pregnancy with those of 44 who continued to drink heavily and found a much reduced frequency of low birth weight (8% compared with 45%, $P < 0.001$).

Breast-feeding may have ill effects on the infants when the mother is drinking. Abnormal sleep, liver damage and pseudo-Cushing syndrome (Binkiewicz *et al.*, 1978) have been reported. Kesäniemi (1974) has measured the concentrations of alcohol in breast milk after mothers were given various amounts to drink and concluded that the equivalent of two glasses of wine or cocktails a day is not likely to harm a breast-feeding infant.

There is, therefore, a great deal of evidence that maternal alcoholism damages the foetus. Some believe that alcohol is the most frequent and serious teratogen, and third after Down's syndrome and neural tube defects as a cause of mental retardation, and are recommending therapeutic abortion in addicted women. More evidence is required on this point, because it is not known what quantity, duration or timing of alcohol abuse is necessary to cause abnormalities. It is also not clear how other associated factors, such as nutritional deficiences or the habitual ingestion of other substances, interact with the toxic effects of alcohol. Criteria for heavy or moderate drinking are notoriously difficult to define and self-reports by patients are often unreliable. Nevertheless, there is substantial evidence in favour of a link between excessive intake of alcohol and harm to the foetus and every effort should be made to persuade alcoholic pregnant women to cut down their intake. Withdrawal from alcohol during the second trimester is not known to harm the infant, but disulfiram is contraindicated because of reports of limb reduction defects in the babies.

Barbiturates

Barbiturates may be taken by the mother throughout pregnancy either for the treatment of epilepsy, or as drugs of addiction. They pass freely into the foetal circulation.

The question of their teratogenicity is controversial. While some have described major malformations including anencephaly, cleft lip and palate, congenital heart disease, face and ear anomalies and congenital dislocation of the hip, these may be associated with the epilepsy itself (and its inherited causes) rather than anticonvulsant treatment (Shapiro et al., 1976). In this American study of 305 children born to epileptic mothers, the rate for major malformations was increased (6.6% compared with 2.7% in about 50 000 controls), but it was no higher in the epileptics taking barbiturates than it was in those taking other drugs or no drugs. A Japanese study, however, (Nakane, 1979) compared 657 children born to treated epileptics with 162 born to epileptic mothers who did not take anticonvulsants during pregnancy. The malformation rate was very much higher in the treated group (11.5% compared with 2.3%), as was the abortion rate too (13.5% compared with 4.3%). If mothers taking trimethadione were excluded, the malformation rate fell to 6.8% which was about the same as the mean for 13 other studies of barbiturates, involving a total of 3514 live births. It was hard to tease apart the effects of the many drugs prescribed (frequently in combination) but there did seem to be an association between phenobarbitone and malformations.

Barbiturates have been claimed to have other adverse effects at delivery and after. Lack of movement by the intoxicated foetus has been linked with abnormal foetal position in labour. After birth, intoxication may lead to hypotonia and diminished sucking. A barbiturate withdrawal syndrome with restlessness, tremors, hypertonia, hyperreflexia, crying and disturbed sleep has been described in the neonate (Bleyer and Marshall 1972; Desmond *et al.*, 1962).

Tobacco Smoking

There has been a steady increase in cigarette smoking by women in Britain in recent years and this trend has been more prominent in women belonging to the lower socio-economic groups (Royal College of Physicians, 1977). Special compaigns have been directed at pregnant women which have had a small impact (Health Education Council, 1976) and the pregnant cigarette smoker continues to place not only herself but also her baby "at risk". Maternal tobacco smoking can harm the foetus in several ways: both nicotine and carbon monoxide are potentially harmful substances which can adversely affect the baby directly by their presence or by affecting placental or uterine function (see reviews by Royal College of Physicians, 1977; Holsclaw and Topham, 1978).

Miscarriage

The rate of spontaneous abortion is raised in women who smoke and it may be related with the amount of smoking. It is, however, difficult to partition out the effects of social class, parity and age. It may be possible to explain the finding that women who smoke are less likely to develop pre-eclampsia than women who do not, in terms of a high rate of early spontaneous abortion amongst the smokers; such women might otherwise have gone on to develop pre-eclampsia (Palmgren *et al.*, 1973).

Congenital Malformations

Links between smoking and cardiac and facial abnormalities have been suggested but the evidence is not convincing and there have been several surveys which have not demonstrated any such associations.

Perinatal Mortality

The risk of stillbirth or neonatal death is clearly higher in smokers. Butler *et al.* (1972) found that there was a 30% increase in perinatal mortality in women who continued to smoke in the second half of pregnancy and that, up to a point, the amounts smoked determined the degree of risk. A reduced placental blood flow and antepartum haemorrhage are thought to be mainly responsible. There is less risk in women belonging to social classes 1 and 2 and Butler *et al.* (1972) found that women who gave up smoking by the 4th month of pregnancy avoided such risks altogether.

Reduced Birthweight

The effect of smoking on birth weight is also greatest in the second half of pregnancy. It hs been calculated that each daily cigarette reduces the baby's weight by about 8 g. The frequency distribution of birth weights is shifted to the left (Holsclaw and Topham, 1978) and the numbers of babies weighing less than 2.5 kg is almost doubled in smokers (Butler and Alberman, 1969). Neonatal mortality increases as birth weights fall. The action of smoking in producing "small for dates" babies is by causing a delay in growth rather than by shortening gestation (Royal College of Physicians, 1977) but it is not known how this effect is brought about. Placental blood flow may be reduced by nicotine through a vasoconstrictor action on blood vessels and placental size has also been reported as reduced in smokers. Nicotine releases oxytocin which increases uterine contractility; blood flow through the uterus and placenta may be reduced as a consequence. Smokers have raised concentrations of carbon monoxide in their blood and an increase in carboxyhaemoglobin in foetal blood results in a lowered oxygen carrying capacity. Other constituents of tobacco smoke may also affect the foetus directly if they can cross the placental barrier, or indirectly through actions on the mother or on the placenta.

Long Term Effects of Maternal Smoking

Butler and Alberman (1969) followed up the children of mothers who took part in a perinatal mortality study. Mothers who had regularly smoked 10 or more cigarettes in pregnancy had children who were about 1 cm shorter than their counterparts at seven and eleven years of age. At age seven years their ability to read was retarded by four months and at eleven years by three months. Such children also had difficulties with mathematics and they were noted as being clumsier and in having more problems at school.

In the face of such powerful evidence for undesirable effects of smoking in pregnancy it seems imperative to counsel mothers to stop smoking.

Opiates

The effects of opiate drugs on pregnancy and the newborn have been the subject of several excellent American studies including those of Cobrinik et al. (1959), Zelson et al. (1971) and Strauss et al. (1974). The matter has been reviewed recently by Blinik et al. (1976) and the management of the pregnant narcotic addict has been reviewed by Connaughton et al. (1977). As with alcoholics, these women have multiple social problems (poor education, poor housing and poverty) as well as emotional problems, and 75% do not seek antenatal care. They may suffer medical complications of addiction, such as hepatitis and endocarditis, and they often abuse other drugs such as barbiturates, amphetamines, cocaine and alcohol. Narcotics are apparently not mutagenic or teratogenic (for example Zelson et al. found only four major malformations in 384 infants), but they cause foetal death and growth impairment and very commonly lead to withdrawal syndromes in the newborn.

Heroin has considerable effects on foetal growth *in utero*. The stillbirth rate is three times the normal rate. A high proportion of the infants are of low birth weight, e.g. 49% of Zelson's series (compared with 15% of their controls) and 29% of Blinik's series (compared with 11% of their controls) were under 2500 g. This could not entirely be attributed to premature labour, because 41% of the underweight babies studied by Zelson *et al.* (1971) were full term, i.e. they were "small for dates". Heroin is therefore thought to bring about intra-uterine growth retardation. Its long term effects in these babies are unknown, but Fitzhardings and Steven (1972) have shown that small-for-dates babies in general have a 25% incidence of minimal cerebral dysfunction as shown by hyperactivity, poor fine motor coordination, speech defects and learning difficulties in spite of normal intelligence, and 65% had mild diffuse electroencephalographic abnormalities. Methadone maintenance on the other hand does not appear to lead to low birth weight (Strauss *et al.*, 1974).

After birth, the infants do not usually need resuscitation, nor do they develop hyaline membrane disease, but signs of withdrawal develop in 50–90%. In heroin addicts withdrawal may appear within 12 hours of delivery, and the mean is about three days after (some say earlier); rarely they appear as late as seven or ten days after. Withdrawal symptoms are less common if the mother has been addicted for less than a year, uses less than five bags daily or took the last dose more than 48 hours before delivery. Affected infants feed poorly with an unsustained sucking reflex. They are irritable, jittery, tremulous and have a high-pitched cry. There is a great increase in muscle tone, and the jaws clamp down on the examining finger. Sneezing and vomiting are common. Sweating, fever, yawning, respiratory distress, and diarrhoea may occur. In severe cases there may be convulsions and excoriation of the skin caused by constant movement. There is no increase in neonatal deaths, and a comparatively low incidence of jaundice, possibly due to the intra-uterine induction of glucuronyl transferase. The infants of addicted mothers are at additional risk because of the presence of impurities and adulterants in the "bags" of drugs that are purchased from dealers and pushers (Primm and Bath, 1973). They are also likely to be adversely affected by maternal malnutrition, concurrent infections and a failure to participate in antenatal health care.

With the introduction of methadone maintenance programmes, many infants are now born dependent on this drug. According to Kandall *et al.* (1977) these infants are of more normal birth weight (mean 2937 g compared with 2490 g for heroin addicts and 3170 g for normal women). Connaughton *et al.* (1977) quote other studies with low incidences of underweight infants and their own figure was 19%; they attribute this to the relatively constant blood level of the narcotic so that premature labour was less often induced by maternal withdrawal states. Withdrawal symptoms, however, may be more severe in methadone addicted infants. Some studies have shown that withdrawal occurs more frequently, lasts longer (ten days instead of five) and has a greater frequency of diarrhoea and seizures; for example Herzlinger *et al.* (1977) found that myoclonic jerks or generalized seizures occurred between days three and 34 (mean ten) in 18 babies out of a total of 302 born to addicted women, and ten of these were on methadone (10/127), only one on heroin (1/83). Kandall and Gartner (1974) say that about 10% of methadone babies have a very late onset of withdrawal 10–32 days after delivery; of the seven babies in their series, four had seizures and one died. However, Connaughton *et al.* (1977) with their moderate doses of methadone and comprehensive treatment programme did not encounter severe withdrawal syndromes.

Connaughton and his colleagues have set out the principles for the management of the pregnant narcotic addict. The patients should be admitted to hospital for thorough evaluation. If addicted to other drugs (e.g. barbiturates), these should be gradually withdrawn. Withdrawal from heroin is not recommended because the patients default, and because in the third trimester there is a risk of foetal distress and meconium aspiration if the mother is suffering from withdrawal symptoms. If it is decided to withdraw the drug, it should be done slowly, and in the second trimester. Heroin is replaced by moderate doses of methadone, beginning with 10 mg daily and increasing it as little as possible and only to prevent withdrawal symptoms. A social worker is assigned to each patient to help her attend the clinic and to cope with her social problems. After birth the infants are kept in hospital for 14 days.

Many clinicians favour planned induction of delivery so that the birth can take place in a hospital where the mother's drug history is known and there are good facilities for the care of sick babies. Glass (1975) has drawn attention to the high incidence of venereal disease amongst addicts and to the need for early recognition and treatment in the neonate of gonococcal ophthalmic infections or of congenital syphilis. Sometimes, diarrhoea during withdrawal may be due to an infection and the infants are also prone to suffer from pneumonia. Such infants are liable to become dehydrated and require careful monitoring of their electrolyte balance and appropriate replacement therapy together with the maintenance of calorie intake.

The treatment of withdrawal symptoms (only necessary in 50%) has been described in detail by Blinick *et al.* (1976). They recommend diazepam in a dose of 0.5–1 mg every 12 hours, and state that 1–2 days treatment is usually sufficient, though rarely it has been necessary to continue for nine days. The main indications are irritability and loss of weight, and treatment is gauged by a reduction in these symptoms. Infants exposed to methadone *in utero* are more likely to have seizures on withdrawal than are babies of heroin-dependent mothers. Paregoric (camphorated tincture of opium) is more effective than diazepam in controlling and preventing such seizures (Herzlinger *et al*, 1977) but giving an opiate to an infant when the diagnosis of opiate dependence is uncertain can create a problem where none existed before.

Opiate antagonists, such as naloxone, should only be given to a pregnant addict if there is clear evidence of risk to her life from an overdose; they will precipitate an abstinence syndrome in the foetus. Similar considerations apply to the neonate and a small dose of naloxone 0.01 mg/kg can be given parenterally if there is evidence of respiratory depression from opiate drugs (Gerhardt *et al.*, 1977).

Heroin and methadone readily appear in the milk but in very low doses (e.g. 50μg methadone daily). The dose to the infant can be minimized by giving the mother's treatment after the evening feed. No ill effects have been noted in breast-fed infants (Ananth, 1978). The long term outlook for these children is uncertain. There have been two reports of an increased rate of "sudden infant death syndrome" in these infants. Rajegowda *et al.* (1978) found that 8/383 such infants died in this way (21/1000 births which compared with the general rate of 3.8/1000). Chavez *et al.* (1979) found that 17/688 died suddenly between one and six months (25/1000 births compared with their control group's rate of 5/1000). However, it has been pointed out by Peterson (1980) that adolescent multiparous mothers have an exceptionally high rate of sudden infant death, 10–18 times the risk of older primiparous mothers, and the deaths may not be related to the delayed effects of narcotics.

Lysergic Acid Diethylamide (LSD)

The are individual case reports of unusual deformities of the extremities in babies born to women taking LSD during pregnancy; they include the absence of the radius and tibia, of the left arm, and of a hand, absence of the ends of the fingers, amputation deformities of the fingers and toes, fibular aplasia, short humerus and aplasia of the fingers, club foot, "lobster claw deformity" and syndactyly. Studies quoted by Nishimura and Tanimura (1976) found rates of 10% and 21% for major structural abnormalities if the drug was taken during pregnancy and 13% when it was taken before conception. Twenty studies in animals were inconclusive. No definite conclusion can be drawn, because the patients came from deviant subcultures who were also using other drugs including "street" drugs of uncertain composition. The fathers were often multiple drug abusers.

Cannabis

Although some of 16 animal studies reviewed by Nishimura and Tanimura showed CNS and limb abnormalities, marihuana has only once been claimed to be associated with congenital abnormalities in man and in this case other drugs were taken as well.

Therapeutic Drugs and ECT

Lithium

Lithium is used as a prophylactic agent in manic depressive psychosis and, since this condition starts before the age of 30 in about half the patients, there is every possibility that women will become pregnant while taking the drug. There has, therefore, been great concern about its possible teratogenic effects. There are reports that it is teratogenic in amphibians, but 13 studies in mammalian experimental animals (reviewed by Nishimura and Tanimura) have produced inconsistent results. To monitor the effects in man, an International Register of Lithium Babies was set up collaboratively by Schou in Denmark and Weinstein and Goldfield in San Francisco. By 1977 (the last time the group reported), a total of 217 babies had been registered, of whom 18 were malformed (11%), at least three times the rate in the general population (Schou and Weinstein, 1977). Eighteen of the malformations involved the cardiovascular system. A report on the first eleven was written by Weinstein & Goldfield (1975): they comprised four cases of Ebstein's anomaly (atrialization of the right ventricle), two of mitral atresia (one with rudimentary left ventricle and other defects), two of ventricular septal defect, and one each of tricuspid atresia, coarctation of the aorta and single umbilical artery. Thus seven of them involved the atrio-ventricular valves. By 1977 there were six babies with Ebstein's anomaly. As the authors point out, there is every reason that there would be preferential registration of abnormal babies, but no reason to expect that these particular unusual malformations would be so frequent. Ebstein's anomaly is present in about 1/20 000 births and 1/80 congenital heart lesions. Thus there is a definite possibility that lithium has teratogenic effects on the heart.

The next point of danger is the time of delivery. The clearance of lithium by the kidney alters during pregnancy, rising steadily up to the time of labour, when it reaches about 30 ml min^{-1}, then abruptly falling to the normal level which is half that figure. This means that a pregnant woman will tolerate a higher dose of lithium for the same blood level. After delivery the blood levels will rise without any change in dosage. There is a remarkable instance of lithium levels, which had been maintained at or below 1 mEq L^{-1} during pregnancy, rising to 3.4 mEq L^{-1} on the day of delivery; at this point the drug was stopped but the serum level continued to rise to 4.4 mEq L^{-1} and the mother became stuporose with clonic twitching. The baby was flaccid and cyanotic and had a poor sucking reflex; his lithium level was 2.4 mEq L^{-1} on the second day. He had recovered completely by the eighth day (Woody et al., 1971).

Lithium is one of the drugs which can exert its toxic effects on the infant through the breast milk. Schou and Amdisen (1973) state that the infant's blood level is one tenth to one half that of the mother. Infection, however, (e.g. an attack of diarrhoea, with sodium loss) may cause the serum level to rise sharply.

One might expect to find thyroid insufficiency in these children; in fact only two cases of goitre have been reported (Amdisen, 1969; Nars and Girard, 1977). Schou has searched for other side effects in the short and long term. Comparing five year outcome with their siblings, he found that a small proportion (6/60) had transitory abnormalities such as stuttering or delay in gaining weight, and four had permanent anomalies, but they were not statistically more common than in the siblings. Thus there is no evidence at present of long-term adverse effects.

In conclusion, women should use contraception when taking lithium. If they wish to become pregnant, they should stop the drug during the first trimester. If the drug must be prescribed during pregnancy—and the reasons should be pressing—it should be given in divided doses to avoid transient peaks, and the blood level checked frequently. Sodium depletion should be avoided. The drug should be stopped at the first signs of labour. After delivery, treatment with lithium should not be started until renal function has reverted to normal. A mother who is receiving lithium should not breast-feed.

Neuroleptic Drugs

The possible teratogenic effects of phenothiazines and other neuroleptics have been extensively investigated because there are many women of childbearing age taking these drugs for long term prophylaxis against schizophrenia. Nishimura and Tanimura reviewed 23 animal studies with the conclusion that there was no consistent trend for phenothiazines to induce teratogenicity. In man there have been a number of large surveys including those of Favre-Tissot *et al.* in 1964 (287 women taking various neuroleptics), Schrire in 1963 (410 patients on trifluoperazine), Moriarty and Nance in 1963 (480 women on trifluoperazine) and Rawlings *et al.* in 1963 (341 women on trifluoperazine). All failed to show any ill effects. Nishimura and Tanimura were able to find 13 isolated instances of major abnormalities, but these could all have been coincidental. Ananth concludes that "the almost total absence of teratogenicity of phenothiazines is conspicuous".

One might expect these drugs to cause extrapyramidal symptoms in the newborn babies. These have been described, but very rarely. Hill *et al.* (1966) reported the occurrence of prolonged hypertonia, tremors, posturing and other motor symptoms in two successive infants born to the same schizophrenic mother; they postulated a familial predisposition to drug-induced parkinsonism. Cleary (1977) published a similar case in a baby born to a mother who was receiving intramuscular fluphenazine.

Neuroleptics enter the breast milk but only in small quantities. Ananth concluded, after reviewing several studies, that a daily oral dose of 200 mg chlorpromazine would give a minute dose of the drug to the infant. Stewart *et al.*

(1980) reached a similar conclusion for haloperidol, calculating that an infant suckled by a mother taking 30 mg day^{-1} would receive only 0.005 mg day^{-1}. Whalley *et al.* (1981) found that a mother who had taken 10 mg haloperidol daily for three weeks secreted about 20 μg litre^{-1} of the drug in her milk. Treatment of this duration did not seem to have any harmful effects on the infant's development which was assessed up to a year after delivery.

Tricyclic Antidepressants

In 1972 there was concern about the possible teratogenic effects of tricyclic antidepressants started by McBride in Australia, who published three cases of amelia or reduction deformities of the limbs, all the cases being poorly documented (Morrow, 1972). In the same year Barson reported an anencephalic still-born child whose mother had taken imipramine. These isolated reports caused the matter to be thoroughly investigated all over the world. Surveys in England, Scotland, USA (Atlanta and Los Angeles) and Canada showed no evidence of teratogenicity. In a large Finnish study (quoted by Nishimura and Tanimura) five of 2784 children with birth defects were exposed to tricyclics compared with only one among a comparison series of normal babies, but in no instance was the tricyclic the only drug used. A review of 21 animal experiments showed that some teratogenic effects were found when very high doses were used. Tricyclic antidepressants are very commonly prescribed, and the evidence for their teratogenicity is very slim indeed. Neonates born to mothers receiving tricyclics in the last month of pregnancy may show withdrawal symptoms including restlessness, irritability, insomnia, abdominal cramps and fever.

Tricyclic drugs can be detected in breast milk, but in very small quantities and no adverse effects have been reported in infants of mothers who continued to breast-feed while continuing to take these drugs (Bader and Newman, 1980).

Benzodiazepines

Some reports have claimed that these drugs, which are among the most commonly prescribed, lead to an increased risk of cleft lip and palate, both in mice and men. Safra and Oakley (1975) found that diazepam was more frequently used by mothers of babies with this anomaly than those with other congenital malformations, though it was pointed out that the incidence was not above the rate in the general population (Goldberg and DiMascio, 1978). Safra and Oakley's finding was confirmed by Saxén & Saxén (1975) analysing the Finnish register of oral cleft defects, and by a Norwegian study (Aarskog, 1975). Milkovitch and van den Berg (1974) reporting on 19044 live births found that the overall rate of severe abnormalities was rather high among women taking chlordiazepoxide during early pregnancy (11.4% compared with 2.6% not on this drug). According to Goldberg and DiMascio the records of the Roche

Research Laboratories showed only three abnormal births among 671 women taking this drug during the first 84 days of pregnancy. The large surveys of Crombie *et al.* in 1975 (21 911 pregnancies) and Hartz *et al.* in 1975 (50 282 pregnancies) failed to show any ill effects of this drug. However, the American Food and Drugs Authority thought it wise to advise against the use of diazepam and chlordiazepoxide in pregnant women, especially in view of the fact that their use is rarely a matter of urgency.

Diazepam is often used late in pregnancy for the treatment of pre-eclamptic toxaemia. This has two hazards for the infant—"the floppy infant syndrome" due to diazepam intoxication, and withdrawal symptoms due to addiction. The effects of intoxication were demonstrated by Cree *et al.* (1973) who compared 14 infants whose mothers were given more than 30 mg parenterally in the 15 hours before delivery with 18 who were given less than this amount. Ten of the 14 on a high dose required endotracheal intubation to assist their breathing and two had secondary apnoeic spells. Twelve had marked hypotonia with depressed reflexes for 36–48 hours and ten required tube feeding for 36–72 hours because they failed to suck. The temperature fell to 35° or less in 8 infants (an effect also shown by Owen *et al.* in 1972). Clearly such large doses are dangerous to the infant, but adverse effects have been noted with smaller doses too. Gillberg (1977) reported a child who was "floppy" for 14 days after birth, born to a mother who took 6 mg daily for the last trimester and had 10 mg rectally at delivery; the infant's serum diazepam and desmethyldiazepam were high on the 12th day. This infant also developed hyperbilirubinaemia and there is a possible connection here because diazepam is eliminated by the same pathway as bilirubin. According to Patrick *et al.* (1972) diazepam may exert its ill-effects (lethargy and weight loss) via the breast milk.

A withdrawal syndrome has been described by Rementeria and Bhatt (1977) in three infants whose mothers were taking 20 mg daily for 4½ months, 10–15 mg daily for five months and 15 mg daily for three months. The main symptom was tremor, starting 2½ to 6 hours after birth and persisting for 10 days in two of the infants and at least 16 days in the third. The most severely affected infant also had loose stools, vomiting, irritability and hypertonicity.

Electroconvulsive Therapy

Severe depressive psychosis is rather uncommon during pregnancy, but it does occur and may even lead to suicide (Goodwin and Harris, 1979). Electroconvulsive therapy has often been given to such women, and the matter was well reviewed by Impastato *et al.* in 1964.

Electroconvulsive therapy (ECT) is a complex treatment involving anaesthesia with short-acting barbiturates, muscle relaxation with succinylcholine, a *grand mal* convulsion and the possibility of anoxia. As for the convulsion, there is no evidence that spontaneous epilepsy leads to abortion or damages the foetus

(Clemmesen, 1927). Attempts to cause abortion in pigs and rabbits with repeated convulsions have failed. The uterus does not contract during the convulsion. It is possible that strong contractions of the abdominal muscles could affect the pregnancy, but this possibility should be eliminated by muscle relaxation.

Succinyl choline does not cross the placental barrier, and, during Caesarian section (for example) does not affect the uterus or foetus. Anoxia which might be a danger in the first trimester can be avoided by fully oxygenating the patient before the convulsion. The effects of barbiturates have been discussed earlier in this chapter.

There is no reason, therefore, to expect any untoward effects of properly administered ECT. Impastato's review of 318 patients confirmed that there is no evidence of any ill effects. Foetal damage was found in 4% which was less than a control series. Seventy-one children were followed up, and all were found to be normal except for two who were mentally retarded and four neurotic. The mother of one of the retarded children had been exposed to 35 insulin coma treatments starting at the eighth week, and the other had not received ECT until the sixteenth week. Five patients treated in the eighth month went into labour or suffered abdominal pain or vaginal bleeding, but they delivered normal babies.

Remick and Maurice (1978) recently wrote to the American Journal of Psychiatry recommending that an obstetrician routinely be consulted before ECT is given in pregnancy, and that external foetal monitoring be used during this treatment.

References

Aarskog, D. (1975). Association between maternal intake of diazepam and oral clefts. *Lancet*, **ii**, 921.

Amdisen, A. (1969). In a discussion of a paper by Sedvall. *Acta Psychiat. Scand. Suppl.* **207**, 67.

Ananth, J. (1978). Side effects in the neonate from psychotropic agents excreted through breast-feeding. *Am. J. Psychiat.* **135**, 801-805.

Arena, J.M. (1980). Drugs and chemical excreted in breast milk. *Pediat. Annals* **9**, 452-457.

Bader, T.F. and Newman, K. (1980). Amitriptyline in human breast milk and the nursing infant's serum. *Am. J. Psychiat.* **137**, 855.

Bierich, J.R., Majewski, F., Michaelis, R. and Tillner, I. (1976). Das embryofetale Alkoholsyndrom. *Europ. J. Pediat.* **121**, 155.

Binkiewicz, A., Robinson, M.J. and Senior, B. (1978). Pseudo-Cushing syndrome caused by alcohol in breast milk. *J. Pediat.* **93**, 965-967.

Bleyer, W.A. and Marshall, R.E. (1972). Barbiturate withdrawal syndrome in a passively addicted infant. *J. Am. med. Ass.* **221**, 185-186.

Blinik, G., Wallach, R.C., Jerez, E. and Ackerman, B.D. (1976). Drug addiction in pregnancy and the neonate. *Am. J. Obs. Gyn.* **125**, 135-142.

Butler, N.R. and Alberman, E.D. (Eds.) (1969). *Perinatal Problems.* The second report of the 1958 British Perinatal Mortality Survey. Churchill Livingstone, London.

Butler, N.R., Goldstein, H. and Ross, E.M. (1972). Cigarette smoking in pregnancy: its influence on birth weight and perinatal mortality. *Br. med. J.* **2**, 127-130.

Chavez, C.J., Ostrea, E.M., Stryker, J.C. and Smialek, Z. (1979). Sudden infant death syndrome among infants of drug-dependent mothers. *J. Pediat.* **95**, 407-409.

Cleary, M.F. (1977). Fluphenazine decanoate during pregnancy. *Am. J. Psychiat.* **134**, 815-816.

Clemmesen, C. (1927). Epilepsy in pregnancy. *Ugeskrift fur Laeger*, **88**, 939-945.

Cobrinik, R.W., Hood, Jr, R.T. and Chusid, E. (1959). The effect of maternal narcotic addiction on the newborn infant; review of the literature and report of 22 cases. *Pediatrics* **24**, 288-304.

Connaughton, J.F., Reeser, D. Schut, J. and Finnegan, L.P. (1977). Perinatal addiction: outcome and management. *Am. J. Obs. Gyn.* **129**, 679-686.

Cree, J.E., Meyer, J. and Hailey, D.M. (1973). Diazepam in labour: its metabolism and effect on the clinical condition and thermogenesis of the newborn. *Br. med. J.* **4**, 251-255.

Crombie, D.L., Pinsent, R.J., Fleming, D.M., Rumeau-Rouquette, C., Goujard, J. and Huel, G. (1975). Fetal effects of tranqillizers in pregnancy. *New Eng. J. Med.* **293**, 198-199.

Desmond, M.M., Schwanecke, R.P., Wilson, G.S., Yasunaga, S. and Burgdorff, I. (1972). Maternal barbiturate utilization and neonatal withdrawal symptomatology. *J. Pediat.* **80**, 190-197.

Favre-Tissot, M., Broussolle, P., Robert, J.M. *et al.* (1964). Psychopharmacologie et teratogenèse, bilan d'une première enquête clinique. *Annls Méd-psychol.* **122**, 398-400.

Fitzhardinge, P.M. and Steven, E.M. (1972). The small-for-dates infant: II Neurological and intellectual sequelae. *Pediatrics* **50**, 50-57.

Gerhardt, T., Bancalari, E. and Cohen, H. (1977). Use of naloxone to reverse respiratory depression in the newborn infant. *J. Pediat.* **90**, 1009-1012.

Gillberg, C. (1977). 'Floppy infant syndrome' and maternal diazepam. *Lancet*, **ii**, 244.

Glass, L. (1975). The neonate in withdrawal—identification, diagnosis and treatment. *Pediat. Ann.* July, 384-390.

Glass, L. and Evans, H.E. (1979). Perinatal drug abuse. *Pediat. Ann.* **8**, 84-92.

Goldberg, J.L. and DiMascio, A. (1978). Psychotropic drugs in pregnancy. *In Psychopharmacology: A Generation of Progress*, pp. 1047-1055 (M.A. Lipton, A. DiMascio and K.F. Killam, eds). Raven, New York.

Goodwin, J. and Harris, D. (1979). Suicide in pregnancy: the Hedda Gabler syndrome. *Suicide and Life-threatening Behaviour*, **9**, 105-115.

Hanson, J.W., Jones, K.L. and Smith, D.W. (1976). Fetal alcohol syndrome: experience with 41 patients. *J. Am. med. Ass.* **235**, 1458-1460.

Hanson, J.W., Streissguth, A.P. and Smith, D.W. (1978). The effects of moderate alcohol consumption during pregnancy on fetal growth and morphogenesis. *J. Pediat.* **92**, 457-460.

Hartz, S.C., Heinonen, O.P., Shapiro, S., Siskind, V. and Slone, D. (1975). Antenatal exposure to meprobamate and chlordiazepoxide in relation to malformations, mental development and childhood mortality. *New Eng. J. Med.* **292**, 726-728.

Health Education Council (1976) *Anti Smoking in Pregnancy Campaigns. Pre- and post-campaign study*. Health Education Council, London.

Herzlinger, R.A., Kandall, S.R. and Vaughan, H.G. (1977). Neonatal seizures associated with narcotic withdrawal. *J. Pediat.* **91**, 638-641.

Hill, R.M. and Stern, L. (1979). Drugs in pregnancy: effects on the fetus and newborn. *Drugs* **17**, 182-197.

Hill, R.M., Desmond, M.M. and Kay, J.I. (1966). Extrapyramidal dysfunction in an infant of a schizophrenic mother. *J. Pediat.* **69**, 589-595.

Holsclaw, D.S. and Topham, A.L. (1978). The effects of smoking on fetal, neonatal, and childhood development. *Pediat. Ann.* **7**, 201-222.

Impastato, D.J., Gabriel, A.R. and Lardaro, H.H. (1964). Electric and insulin shock therapy during pregnancy. *Dis. Nerv. Sys.* **25**, 542-546.

Kaminski, M., Rumeau-Rouquette, C. and Schwartz, D. (1978). Alcohol consumption in pregnant women and the outcome of pregnancy. *Alcoholism* **2**, 155-163.

Kandall, S.R. and Gartner, L.M. (1974). Late presentation of drug withdrawal symptoms in newborns. *Am. J. Dis. Child.* **127**, 58-61.

Kandall, S.R., Albin, S., Gartner, L.M., Lee, K.S., Eidelman, A. and Lowinson, J. (1977). The narcotic-dependent mother: fetal and neonatal consequences. *Early Human Development* **1**, 159-169.

Kesäniemi, Y. (1974). Ethanol and acetaldehyde in the milk and blood of lactating women after ethanol administration. *J. Obst. Gynec. Br. Commonw.* **81**, 84-86.

Lemoine, P., Harousseau, H., Borteyru, J.P. and Menuet, J.C. (1968). Les enfants de parents alcooliques: anomalies observées. *Ouest-Médical* **25**, 476-481.

Little, R.E. (1977). Moderate alcohol use during pregnancy and decreased infant birth weight. *Am. J. publ. Hlth.* **67**, 1154-1156.

Little, R.E., Streissguth, A.P., Barr, H.M. and Herman, C.S. (1980). Decreased birth weight in infants of alcoholic women who abstained during pregnancy. *J. Pediat.* **96**, 974-977.

Milkovitch, L. and van den Berg, B.J. (1974). Fetal effects of tranquillizers in pregnancy. *New Eng. J. Med.* **291**, 1268-1271.

Moriarty, A.J. and Nance, M.R. (1963). Trifluoperazine and pregnancy. *Can. med. Ass. J.* **88**, 375-376.

Morrow, A.W. (1972). Limb deformities associated with iminodibenzyl hydrochloride. *Med. J. Aust.* **1**, 658-659.

Nakane, Y. (1979). Congenital malformation among infants of epileptic mothers treated during pregnancy—the report of a collaborative study group in Japan. *Folia Psychiat. Neurol. Japonica* **33**, 363-369.

Nars, P.W. and Girard, J. (1977). Lithium carbonate intake during pregnancy leading to a large goitre in a premature infant. *Am. J. Dis. Child.* **131**, 924-925.

Nishimura, H. and Tanimura, T. (1976). *Clinical Aspects of the Teratogenicity of Drugs.* Elsevier, New York.

Ouellette, E.M., Rosett, H.L., Rosman, N.P. and Weiner, L. (1977). Adverse effects on offspring of maternal alcohol abuse during pregnancy. *New Eng. J. Med.* **297**, 528-530.

Owen, J.R., Irani, S.F. and Blair, A.W. (1972). Effect of diazepam administered to mothers during labour on temperature regulation of neonate. *Arch. Dis. Child.* **47**, 107-110.

Palmgren, B., Wahlen, T. and Wallander, B. (1973). Toxaemia and cigarette smoking during pregnancy: prospective consecutive investigation of 3927 pregnancies. *Arch. Obstet. Gynec. Scand.* **52**, 183-185.

Patrick, M.J., Tilstone, W.J. and Reavey, P. (1972). Diazepam and breastfeeding. *Lancet*, **i**, 543.

Peiffer, J., Majewshi, F., Fischbach, H., Bierich, J.R. and Volk, B. (1979). Alcohol embryo- and fetopathy. *J. Neurol. Sci.* **41**, 125-137.

Peterson, D.R. (1980). SIDS in infants of drug-dependent mothers. *J. Pediat.* **96**, 784.

Primm, B.J. and Bath, P.E. (1973). Pseudoheroinism. *Int. J. Addict.* **8**, 231-242.

Rajegowda, B.K., Kandall, S.R. and Falciglia, H. (1978). Sudden unexpected death in infants of narcotic-dependent mothers. *Early Human Development* **2**, 219-225.

Rawlings, W.J., Ferguson, R. and Madison, T.G. (1963). Phenmetrazine and trifluoperazine. *Med. J. Aust.* **1**, 370.

Rementeria, J.L. and Bhatt, K. (1977). Withdrawal symptoms in neonates from intrauterine exposure to diazepam. *Pediat. Pharmac. Ther.* **90**, 123-126.

Remick, R.A. and Maurice, W.L. (1978). ECT in pregnancy. *Am. J. Psychiat.* **135**, 761-762.

Rosett, H.L., Weiner, L., Zuckerman, B., McKinlay, S. and Edelin, K.C. (1980). Reduction of alcohol consumption during pregnancy with benefits to the newborn. *Alcoholism: Clinical and Experimental Research* **4**, 178-184.

Royal College of Physicians of London (1977). *Smoking or Health.* Pitman Medical, Tunbridge Wells.

Safra, M.J. and Oakley, G.P. (1975). Association between cleft lip with or without cleft palate and prenatal exposure to diazepam. *Lancet* **ii**, 478-480.

Saxén, I. and Saxén, L. (1975). Association between maternal intake of diazepam and oral clefts. *Lancet* **ii**, 498.

Schou, M. and Amdisen, A. (1973) Lithium and pregnancy—III, lithium ingestion by children breast-fed by women on lithium treatment. *Br. Med. J.* **2**, 138.

Schou, M. and Weinstein, M.R. (1980). Problems of lithium maintenance treatment during pregnancy, delivery and lactation. *Agressologie* **21A**, 7-10.

Schire, I. (1963). Trifluoperazine and foetal abnormalities. *Lancet* **i**, 174.

Shapiro, S., Slone, D., Hartz, S.C., Rosenberg, L., Siskind, V., Monson, R.R., Mitchell, A.A., Heinonen, O.P., Idanpaan-Heikkila, J., Hero, S. and Saxen, L. (1976). Anticonvulsants and parental epilepsy in the development of birth defects. *Lancet* **i**, 272-275.

Shaywitz, S.E., Cohen, D.J. and Shaywitz, B.A. (1980). Behaviour and learning difficulties in children of normal intelligence born to alcoholic mothers. *J. Pediat.* **96**, 978-982.

Smith, D.W. (1979). The fetal alcohol syndrome. *Hosp. Pract.* **14**, 121-128.

Sokol, R.J., Miller, S.I. and Reed, G. (1980). Alcohol abuse during pregnancy: an epidemiologic study. *Alcoholism: Clinical and Experimental Research* **4**, 135-145.

Stewart, R.B., Karas, B. and Springer, P.K. (1980). Haloperidol excretion in human milk. *Am. J. Psychiat.* **137**, 849-850.

Strauss, M.E., Andresko, M., Stryker, J.C., Wardell, J.N. and Dunkel, L.D. (1974). Methadone maintenance during pregnancy: pregnancy, birth, and neonate characteristics. *Am. J. Obstet. Gynec.* **120**, 895-900.

Ulleland, C.N. (1972) The offspring of alcoholic mothers. *Ann. N.Y. Acad. Sci.* **197**, 167-169.

Weinstein, M.R. and Goldfield, M.D. (1975). Cardiovascular malformations with lithium use during pregnancy. *Am. J. Psychiat.* **132**, 529-531.

Whalley, L.J., Blain, P.G. and Prime, J.K. (1981). Haloperidol secreted in breast milk. *Br. med. J.* **282**, 1746-1747.

Woody, J.N., London, W.L. and Wilbanks, G.D. (1971) Lithium toxicity in a newborn. *Pediatrics* **47**, 94-96.

Zelson, C., Rubio, E. and Wasserman, E. (1971). Neonatal narcotic addiction: 10 year observation. *Pediatrics* **48**, 178-189.

Index